THE COMPLETE

Recipe Writing Guide

*Mastering Recipe Development, Writing,
Testing, Nutrition Analysis, and Food Styling*

RAEANNE SARAZEN, MA, RDN, FAND

eat right. Academy of Nutrition and Dietetics

ACADEMY OF NUTRITION AND DIETETICS
CHICAGO, IL

eat right. Academy of Nutrition and Dietetics

Academy of Nutrition and Dietetics
120 S. Riverside Plaza, Suite 2190
Chicago, IL 60606

The Complete Recipe Writing Guide
ISBN 978-0-88091-200-6 (print)
ISBN 978-0-88091-074-3 (eBook)
Catalog Number 200623 (print)
Catalog Number 200623e (eBook)

10 9 8 7 6 5 4 3 2

For more information on the Academy of Nutrition and Dietetics, visit eatright.org.

Names: Sarazen, Raeanne, author.
Title: The complete recipe writing guide : mastering recipe development,
  writing, testing, nutrition analysis, and food styling / Raeanne
  Sarazen, MA, RDN, FAND.
Description: Chicago, IL : Academy of Nutrition and Dietetics, [2023] |
  Includes bibliographical references and index.
Identifiers: LCCN 2023001058 (print) | LCCN 2023001059 (ebook) | ISBN
  9780880912006 (paperback) | ISBN 9780880910743 (ebook)
Subjects: LCSH: Food writing.
Classification: LCC TX644 .S27 2023 (print) | LCC TX644 (ebook) | DDC
  808.06/6641–dc23/eng/20230404
LC record available at lccn.loc.gov/2023001058
LC ebook record available at lccn.loc.gov/2023001059

Contents

Foreword

Thorough, engaging, and inspiring, Raeanne Sarazen's *The Complete Recipe Writing Guide* is a long-awaited addition to the library of culinary arts and communication. No doubt it is destined to become an essential resource for anyone wishing to develop, write, and publish compelling recipes.

Recipes are everywhere—not only in cookbooks but also in blogs and social media posts, in newspapers and magazines, and on television. Food and recipes can also be a key part of travel and cultural exploration. Many cooks, however, are unfamiliar with certain ingredients, techniques, and flavors. How can a recipe developer provide this information accurately to ensure a successful cooking and eating experience? And what about the cook with minimal cooking background and confidence: how much explanation is necessary (for example, what terms should be used to describe proper measuring techniques and equipment)?

As a dietitian, I became aware of my own recipe writing limitations when my first book, *The Art of Cooking for the Diabetic*, was published in 1978. I was guided by my coauthor Kay Middleton, a retired food editor. Since then, many food writers, editors, and culinary dietitians have relied on two classic books for guidance: *Recipes Into Type* (published in 1993) and *The Recipe Writer's Handbook* (published in 2001). Today, however, we need more. Enter *The Complete Recipe Writing Guide*, a state-of-the-art reference that provides comprehensive guidance on recipe development, writing, testing, nutrition analysis, food styling, photography, and video.

Author Raeanne Sarazen has a unique and diverse background in food communication that made her an ideal author for this book. Raeanne is a registered dietitian as well as a professional chef and food writer with expertise in creating consumer-friendly recipe content, a former public relations executive, a former test kitchen director at the *Chicago Tribune*, a cook at the renowned Chicago restaurant Charlie Trotter's, a television cooking personality, and a curriculum developer and educator at several charities that teach children to how to cook. She brings her extensive knowledge and experience plus the advice and techniques of other food experts to the table with remarkable clarity and creativity. Her ability to synthesize the vast amount of information found in this book into a cohesive and easy-to-follow text exemplifies her expert communication skills. Raeanne provides the guidance needed to take your recipe writing to a whole new level.

The Academy of Nutrition and Dietetics has long been a source of nutrition and food expertise, but historically has focused on clinical nutrition, as a majority of its members worked in health care. As time passed, many dietitians gained positions throughout food industry, including food service, product development, marketing, sustainability, and agriculture and related fields. Culinary nutrition has also become an important career path. In 1997, I was the founding chair of the Academy of Nutrition and Dietetics Food & Culinary Professionals dietetic practice group, with the goal of providing advanced food and culinary education to dietitians. Raeanne was one of the 175 founding members of this group, which now boasts over 1,900 members, including many food writers, chefs, food and nutrition educators, and food industry professionals.

With interest in and demand for personalized nutrition growing, along with increasing emphasis on culinary medicine, the importance of focusing on taste and flavor in recipe development has never been greater. Whether there are dietary restrictions or not, every recipe should be delicious. *The Complete Recipe Writing Guide* helps recipe developers meet this challenge, enabling them, like artists, to work with a limited palette to create palate-pleasing food.

Everyone who writes or publishes recipes can benefit from the words of wisdom found in this book. Raeanne walks you through the recipe production workflow—from recipe concept to development and testing to presentation in print, digital, or other formats. Many dietitians along with prominent chefs and food personalities have contributed their expertise, as you will see in the abundant tips highlighted throughout the book. Even experienced recipe developers will learn new tricks of the trade; I know I did!

I am honored to provide this foreword to a book that is a manual of best practices for developing, writing, and producing recipe content. And I salute its dedicated and brilliant author.

Mary Abbott Hess, LHD, MS, RDN, LDN, FAND
Founder, Food & Culinary Professionals Dietetic Practice Group
Former President, The American Dietetic Association
Former Chairman of the Board, American Institute of Food & Wine

Introduction

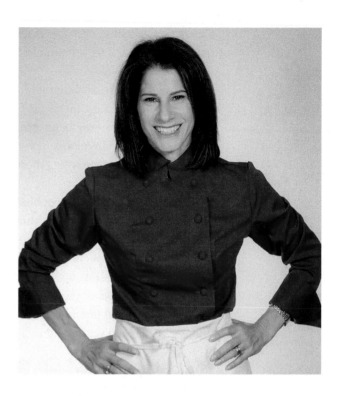

You are here because we share a connection: the desire to create and document recipes that work. Perhaps you're a food professional—a chef, nutritionist, editor, cookbook author, or marketing expert. Or maybe you want to turn your love of food into a career. No matter, you are in the right place.

Over the years I've come to appreciate different styles of recipe writing. Yet I'm a purist when it comes to the ultimate goal of the written recipe:

A written recipe must be accurate, readable, and reproducible—a set of instructions that translates the act of cooking into words.

My clarity-first approach reflects a career immersed in the science of nutrition and the culinary arts. I've worked as a clinical dietitian; recipe developer, writer, editor, and tester; professional chef; food stylist; and as a television and video host. I'm also an avid home cook and mother of three—two of whom have celiac disease.

I wrote *The Complete Recipe Writing Guide* because I wanted to pay it forward. I wished I'd had a book like this early in my career, a single source of truth for developing recipes—from kitchen to plate, and finally, to publication. Today, endless information on food, health, and nutrition is only a click away. Yet much of this information is overwhelming, contradictory, and confusing at best. Nowadays, it's easy to become an "expert" simply by creating a digital presence. No education or experience is needed thanks to easy-to-use platforms, nutrition analysis software, and smartphone cameras. Don't get me wrong, there are some great food and recipe sites out there. But there are many that contain misleading or just plain inaccurate food, nutrition, and recipe information.

Writing this book, I passionately approached every topic like an investigative journalist, interviewing top industry professionals, reading research studies and books, and attending professional conferences and webinars. I wanted to curate and share not only what I've learned over the years but also share the expertise of others. And I wanted those in the field of recipe writing to have professional standards of practice that incorporate the science of nutrition. Inside these pages, you'll learn how to develop recipes for plant-based diets, diabetes management, celiac disease, food allergies, and everything in between.

I hope you'll use *The Complete Recipe Writing Guide* to build a foundation of knowledge and expand your skill set. Once you master the principles, I encourage you to add your own personal style and creativity to the mix.

Food Is My Passion and My Profession

Food is medicine. The array of nutrients in food supports good health and can help prevent, manage, or even reverse disease. Yet, food is so much more. Food is memory. Food is cultural identity. Food is community. And, of course, food is joy. People don't eat nutrients; they eat food.

For me, food has always been the lens through which I view and understand life. I am curious about everything as it relates to food—from how it grows to its meaning and place in history. What I love about food is that there's always more to know and to experience, which no doubt explains why I've taken so many different career paths in the food industry and have sought out culinary adventures around the world. My husband and children have come to accept (and even embrace) that we'll return from our travels with stories sure to regale our friends—fried scorpions in Beijing, testicle meatballs in Arizona, or the culinary and cultural discoveries from cooking alongside local home cooks (the true experts).

Most toddlers outgrow the *why* phase of development. I never did. Even at age seven, I wanted to know why the popcorn stuck together in the popcorn balls my friend Susan's mother made. I looked through my mom's few cookbooks and found nothing. Later, I was at another friend's house flipping the pages of one of her mother's cookbooks. There I discovered the answer: Karo syrup. *WOW!* Liquid sugar. How cool. I remember reading that popcorn balls were originally made with molasses. Even as a young girl, when it came to questions about food, I could go down a rabbit hole like nobody's business.

Growing up, my grandmother Sonia's kitchen was an endless source of fascination. There I discovered pickling salt, kosher salt, and sour salt (citric acid). We only had table salt at our house. She used pickling salt to preserve the cucumbers from her garden, sour salt to balance the sweetness of her meatballs rolled in cabbage, and kosher salt for everything else—veal brisket, *kneidlach* (matzo balls), beet borscht, and chicken soup. She also loved to bake. Stashed in her kitchen drawers were bags of semisweet chocolate chips and chips I'd never seen before—butterscotch, peanut butter, white chocolate, mini chocolate. There was not only vanilla extract but also almond and mint. What could I make with these?

The truth was that my grandmother was far more interested in cooking and baking for her family than teaching me how to do it. Most of the time, her goodies just appeared. They arrived in sturdy boxes mailed from Ottumwa, Iowa, to our home in Chicago, Illinois,

filled with chocolate chip cookies, rocky road bars, *mandelbrot* (an Eastern Europe cousin of biscotti), and *hamantaschen* (three-cornered pastries filled with poppy seeds or prunes). Why did the rocky road bars remain moist and tasty long after they arrived, but the other cookies dry out so quickly?

When we visited her in Ottumwa, these same treats emerged from a coffin-sized freezer in the basement. How long could you freeze cookies and bars? Why did the spaghetti she cooked, frozen and then defrosted, change in texture? What was the liquid inside the jars of dill pickles, tomatoes, and peaches that lined the cool walls of the basement?

The magic she performed in her kitchen was hard to replicate. She didn't use measuring cups or spoons. And I never saw her use a recipe. Yet I watched intently as she sprinkled sugar in her spaghetti sauce (that's why I must have liked it!) and smeared butter on bread so the tuna sandwiches, wet with pickle juice, didn't get soggy. Years later, with the help of my brother, a documentary filmmaker, I translated her pinch-of-this and handful-of-that creations into recipes, some of which I shared with my readers when working as the test kitchen director for the *Chicago Tribune*.

It wasn't until many years later, after she'd passed away, that I found she actually did have recipes—magazine and newspaper clippings taped to 3" × 5" notecards or hand copied from the back of food packaging—stored in a recipe box. I discovered that her recipes were not *hers*, per se, but ones she'd adapted to make her own.

When I look back, the genesis of this book began when I was a girl enthralled with the mysteries inside Grandma Sonia's kitchen. It was there that I first had the urge to pull back the curtain, to discover the *whys* and *hows* behind the magical dishes and treats she lovingly prepared for us. I believe that recipes (like my grandmother's) are meant to be shared. For recipes to live on, they must be accurately recorded.

How to Use This Book

Inside these pages you'll learn how to create professional recipes from development to publication with accuracy and confidence. I use the term "publication" loosely to encompass the many ways we consume content these days, whether flipping the pages of a cookbook, reading an online publication, or watching a recipe video.

While each chapter of this book stands on its own, to get the most out of this book, read (or reference) Chapters 1 through 6 together. They contain the building blocks of recipe development with a special focus on health and wellness. If you're more experienced, simply open to the section of the book where you're looking for guidance. Be sure to take in the Quick Tips throughout the book for advice and insights from top industry professionals. Here's a quick overview of the contents:

Chapters 1 through 6: Recipe Development

With the growing interest in eating for better health, as well as rising rates of diet-related diseases, food allergies, and food intolerances, recipe developers need reliable resources. These chapters show you how to develop recipes for health and wellness, while keeping the focus on flavor, including plant-based diets; food allergies and food sensitivities; fat, sodium, and sugar modifications; celiac disease (gluten-free); and FODMAP intolerance.

Chapter 7: Recipe Writing

Learn how to translate the act of cooking food into words with clarity, consistency, and original voice. You'll find answers to questions on grammar, spelling, punctuation, and recipe writing styles.

Chapter 8: Recipe Testing

Learn the recipe testing process and how professional testers ensure a recipe can be replicated with consistent results every time. Access recipe testing forms and tips on how to use home cook recipe testers for your cookbook projects.

Chapter 9: Nutrition Analysis

There are many types of analysis options. This chapter teaches you how to evaluate and use them. You'll learn the guidelines professionals use to analyze recipes with complex ingredients and preparation methods.

Chapter 10: Food Styling, Photography, and Videos

Food photos and videos take center stage when it comes to recipes. While there are entire books written on these topics, this guide wouldn't be complete without professional secrets and tips for improving your skills in food styling, photography, and videos.

Appendixes

Turn to these helpful go-to resources when you're developing, writing, and testing recipes:
- Common ingredient equivalencies and conversions
- Recipe writing style guides
- Food safety instructions in recipes
- Understanding meat cuts for recipe development

PLEASE PROVIDE FEEDBACK

Nutrition science is constantly evolving. So, too, are consumer preferences based on current values, beliefs, and culinary trends. If there is anything you believe is missing or needs further explanation or detail, please email your suggestions and feedback to me at raeanne@raeannesarazen.com. There is always the next edition!

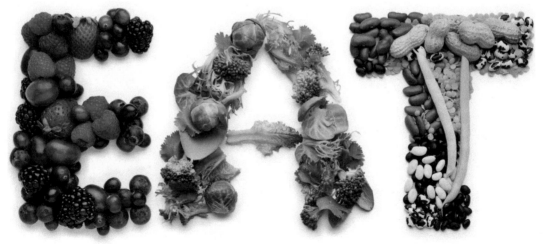

Photo credit: Renée Comet Photography

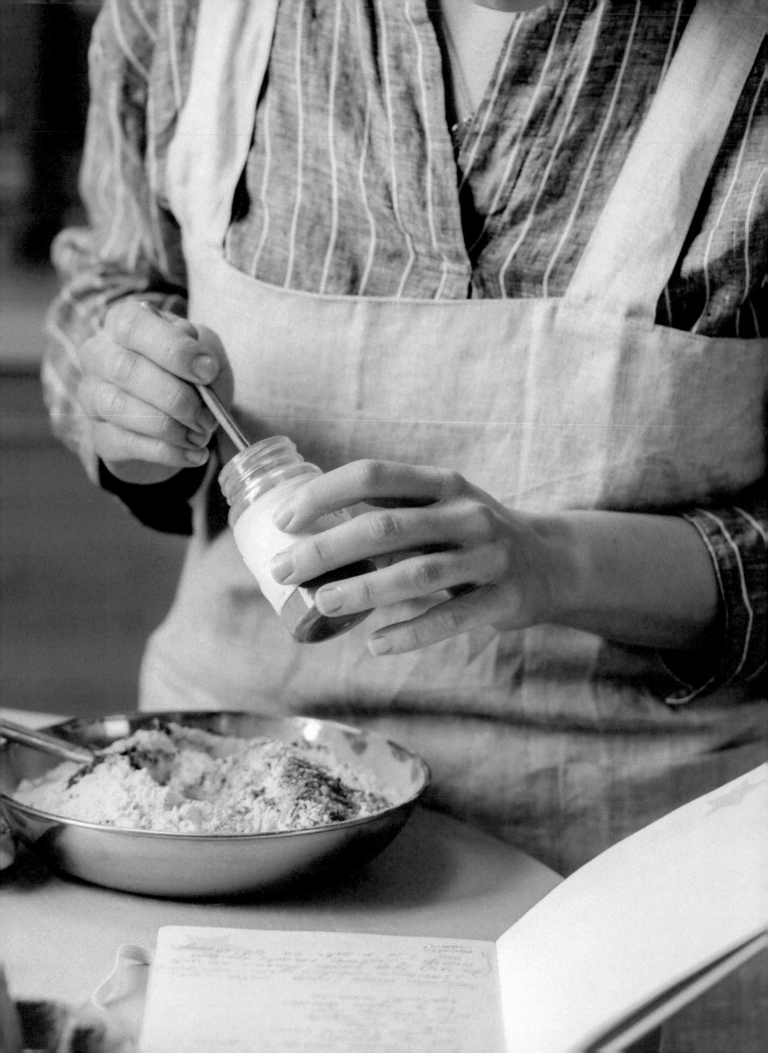

Chapter 1
Guidelines for Recipe Development

IN THIS CHAPTER, LEARN ABOUT:

- The key steps involved in the recipe development process

- The importance of celebrating and respecting global cuisines in recipe development

- How to develop an original recipe or adapt an existing one

- Recipe copyright and professional best practices for recipe attribution and recipe sharing

Recipe development is both an art and a science. Creativity, inspiration, and open-mindedness contribute to the art, a process that is unique to each recipe developer. The science is in the culinary techniques and strategies that are shown to be effective. While there is no one right way to develop a recipe, the objective is always the same—the final recipe should taste good and work consistently. To meet this goal, the ingredients, amounts, and instructions need to be communicated clearly. This process includes writing out the "bones" of the recipe, preparing it, making adjustments, preparing it again, and perhaps adjusting and preparing again as needed. This is true whether developing recipes for restaurants, hospitals, schools, senior living centers, cookbooks, websites, trade associations, food companies, or print or online newspapers or magazines.

Aspiring and seasoned recipe developers alike always have room to further develop their craft. Recipe developers should recognize, however, that it takes time to develop and hone recipe development skills. Through a process of constant experimenting and tasting in the kitchen combined with reading and researching about food and cooking, experienced food professionals and chefs continually improve their recipe development skills and increase the breadth and depth of their food and culinary knowledge.

The Recipe Development Process

The skill of recipe development is distinct from the ability to properly write and edit a recipe (see Chapter 7). This chapter is not intended to teach professional cooking principles and techniques; instead, it will show how to develop an original recipe or modify or adapt an existing one.

The recipe development process can be divided into three key steps, each of which will be discussed in more detail:

Step 1: Build Culinary Knowledge

Step 2: Create a Recipe Strategy

Step 3: Start the Creative Recipe Development
Process

Recipe Development Step 1: Build Culinary Knowledge

Cooking, tasting, and learning about food will strengthen your culinary knowledge and expertise in flavor and technique, which are essential skills for recipe development. Build your culinary skills by spending time cooking, refining your tasting skills, and exploring culinary resources.

Cook: Master the Culinary Basics

Extensive cooking experience allows a recipe developer to know instinctively which recipe steps or culinary techniques can be shortened and changed. Cooking is based on a foundation of objective techniques we refer to as culinary rules. Culinary rules, once mastered, can be tweaked/tailored to create new recipes.

Following are some basic and essential culinary rules that every recipe developer must understand and apply.

Kitchen equipment Know which knives, pieces of cookware, appliances, or tools are appropriate for which kitchen tasks.

Heat and foods Understand what happens to different foods when they are heated in various ways—the relationship and effects of heat and heat transfer. For example, the various forms of heat (roasting, baking, grilling, frying, searing, conduction, convection, radiation, microwaving, and steaming) cause proteins to coagulate, starches to gelatinize, sugars to caramelize, water to evaporate, or fat to melt.

Cooking methods Recognize why different cooking methods are chosen for different types of foods and choosing the technique that will best capture a food's flavors. Methods include moist heat (poaching, simmering, blanching, boiling, steaming, or braising), dry heat (roasting, baking, broiling, grilling, cooking on a griddle, or air frying), dry heat using fat (sautéing, panfrying, or deep-frying), and microwaving.

Principles of seasoning and flavoring Understand when to season and add flavor to heighten the natural flavors of the foods being cooked, and the common seasonings (salt, pepper, acids) and flavoring ingredients (fats, herbs and spices).

Sanitation and food safety Know the rules of proper food handling and storage as well as cleaning and sanitizing procedures.

Culinary knowledge for recipe development can be acquired in many ways: attending culinary school, working in professional kitchens or alongside other food professionals, or becoming self-taught with cookbooks and recipe trial and error. Various cookbooks or culinary textbooks can provide the why, the how, or the food science behind cooking, as well as information on fundamental techniques (see Recipe Development Resources on page 23). Major food publications invest in test kitchens, so their food information is quite reliable, and their recipes deliver consistent results. Reading and trying tested recipes allows a recipe developer to experience the expertise of other professionals, assess what works, and learn their own preferences for cooking styles.

A mix of curiosity, interest in experimentation, and a desire to perfect basic culinary techniques through repetition and refine skills over time will form the foundation needed for a career as a recipe developer. Keep in mind that recipes must align with the cooking skills of the target audience; this is discussed in more detail in Chapter 7 on recipe writing.

Taste: Develop Your Palate

You will become a better cook and recipe developer by experimenting with flavor combinations, learning how to season foods—especially with salt—and seizing every opportunity to taste foods. Over time, it will become clear when an ingredient can stand on its own and when to add some flavor to enhance the dish. Food that tastes "just okay" may be underseasoned or it may be the choice of ingredients or the cooking method.

Some recipe developers follow the rule of tasting at the start of cooking, again when halfway through, and then again at the end. Others taste and adjust each time an ingredient is added if it is appropriate

CULINARY KNOWLEDGE FOR RECIPE DEVELOPERS

Following are a few examples of the culinary knowledge recipe developers should acquire.

Stocks, sauces, and soups	Learn techniques for preparing their foundations (e.g., roux or gravy)
Meats*	Get familiar with the basic cuts, know which cooking methods to use for each, and how to determine doneness
Poultry	Understand how to cook light versus dark meat and determine doneness
Fish and shellfish	Recognize the common varieties and the few basic cuts for fish, select appropriate cooking methods, and determine doneness
Vegetables	Understand methods of preparation; how to control texture, flavor, and color
Beans, peas, lentils, and soy products	Identify the varieties and types and learn different techniques for preparation
Pasta, rice, and other grains**	Identify the types and characteristics of each when cooking
Salads and salad dressings	Identify the types of salad greens available (e.g., endive, butter, frisée) and the method and preparation of various types of salads and dressings (e.g., vinaigrette, emulsified, or mayonnaise based)
Breads, desserts, and other baked goods	Learn the principles of baking, including proper measurement or weighing of ingredients and the function of key ingredients, such as flour, fat, sugar, eggs, liquids, and leavening agents

* See the appendix Understanding Meat Cuts for Recipe Development on page 381 for more information.
** See Guide to Cooking Whole Grains on pages 78 and 79 for more information.

and safe. Determining seasoning, especially with salt, is a matter of personal taste. Seasoning can turn a dish that tastes bland and flat into something special.

Your palate will become more discerning and developed as you taste foods while cooking. By tasting, you learn when a dish needs more seasoning (e.g., salt to enhance the flavor, or herbs, spices, or pepper to add flavor) or how and when to balance flavors by adding an acidic ingredient (e.g., lemon juice, wine, vinegar, Parmesan cheese, tomato, or Dijon mustard) that contributes a sour flavor or puckery sharpness (the culinary description for which is brightness).

The creative process of recipe development should consider all factors that influence flavor: taste, aroma, mouthfeel, and the sensory stimulation of food. How food is experienced is a fusion of all these factors.

Aroma

Aroma is the odor perceived when inhaling through the nose. The senses of smell and taste work together to influence perception of flavor. Olfactory cells located at the ends of the nasal passages detect the aromas of foods, and the information gathered by these cells is also relayed to the mouth via a process called olfactory referral. The sense of smell is believed to be responsible for 75% to 95% or more of the sense of taste. You can test this by plugging your nose while eating: an inability to detect the aroma of foods will directly influence your ability to taste them. Chefs often add fresh herbs, spices, citrus zest, or other aromatic ingredients to enhance the aroma of a dish because doing so also enhances the dish's flavor.

Mouthfeel

The temperature and texture perceived while eating—the mouthfeel of food—stimulates sensory cells located alongside taste cells and activates the perceived qualities of enjoyment, such as heat, spiciness, creaminess, crunchiness, and crispness.

FIVE TASTE SENSATIONS

Taste buds, located on the tongue and roof of the mouth, respond to the five basic taste sensations of sweet, salty, sour, bitter, and umami. When we eat, our taste buds become activated, and we perceive the flavors of these types of foods and ingredients.

Taste		Common foods	Culinary uses
Sweet		sugar, honey, jams, jellies, syrups	mellows acidic or bitter tastes
Salty		salt, soy sauce, miso	enhances flavor, counteracts bitterness, accentuates sweetness
Sour		lemon, lime, and orange juices; tomatoes; yogurt; sour cream; vinegars	adds brightness, reduces saltiness, balances spiciness, counterbalances sweetness
Bitter		cocoa, coffee, beer, and various greens, including kale, endive, radicchio, spinach	provides color, complexity, depth
Umami		anchovies, Parmesan cheese, fish sauce, miso, seaweed, mushrooms, tomatoes, cured meats (bacon)	adds savory sensation

Experience

The experience of eating includes aspects of the visual ("eating with your eyes") and emotional (evoking memories of food) as well as the rituals of eating. These characteristics enhance a food's palatability and enjoyment.

Quick Tip

"When I develop recipes, I always look for ways to create what I call the Big Taste . . . food that is deeply satisfying, and that appeals to all the senses. I like dishes that leave their flavor with me, whose tastes and aromas I will never forget." —Paula Wolfert, *Paula Wolfert's World of Food*

Factors That Influence Flavor

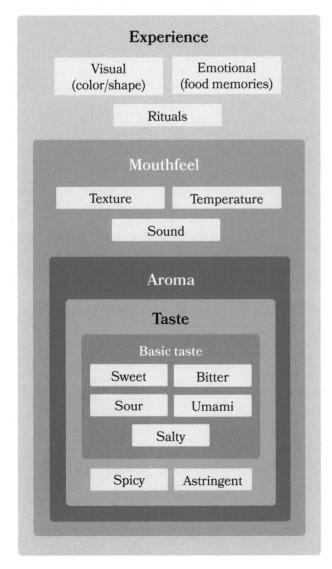

Experience

Visual (color/shape)

Emotional (food memories)

Rituals

Mouthfeel

Texture

Temperature

Sound

Aroma

Taste

Basic taste

Sweet

Bitter

Sour

Umami

Salty

Spicy

Astringent

Read: Expand Your Food Knowledge

Recipe developers can expand their culinary knowledge and improve their kitchen skills by reading books about food—cookbooks, food and ingredient reference books, food science books, cultural history books, and food memoirs—and by watching food media, including online cooking tutorials, cooking shows, and food-themed movies and documentaries. In addition to the obvious benefits of skill improvement, acquiring culinary knowledge through reading and visual media can inspire developers to push the traditional boundaries of their culinary knowledge base. These resources can teach you about food and cooking and can serve as a source of wisdom. Think of them as a starting point for gathering recipe ideas from other experts and gaining a better understanding of how successful recipe developers think. (See Recipe Development Resources on page 23 for examples of reference books.)

While reading about food and watching food media provides wonderful opportunities to learn, eating in restaurants and traveling to places with different culinary styles and traditions puts eating and food in the context of experiential learning about the flavors, ingredients, and techniques of a specific region. When traveling, try to learn about the local cuisine's traditional preparation methods not only by eating at restaurants but also by cooking alongside the people who live there. Food-themed travel or tours led by chefs or local food experts offer a blend of cultural and culinary knowledge that can yield taste memories and inspiration for future recipe development.

Recipe Development Notes

To help generate ideas for future recipe development projects, create your own system of organizing your food and recipe notes. Some professionals, many of whom say they are always thinking about food, find it helpful to store future ideas for recipe development projects on their smartphones or in notebooks. Consider keeping notes about interesting ingredient combinations, flavors, techniques, and food presentations so you can reference them when brainstorming new recipe ideas.

Recipe ideas or general thoughts about food may arise after enjoying a great meal, visiting a market while on a trip, eating at a friend's house or a new restaurant, seeing something new at a trade show or conference, or even dreaming about a new recipe. Any experience might inspire a food idea or a memory, so always be prepared to write them down. Take and attach pictures, if possible, to complement your notes and help jog your memory.

A recipe development notebook can be maintained in various ways: for example, using a note-taking, task management, or organizational smartphone app (e.g., the Notes app), or recording in a spreadsheet or paper notebook. Regardless of how you keep food notes, they can be useful to reference when you need recipe development inspiration at a later time.

ORGANIZE RECIPE DEVELOPMENT IDEAS

Following are examples of ways to organize and document your food and recipe ideas to more easily reference them for future recipe development projects.

By Season
(Seasonal ingredients and dish ideas)

Fall: molasses, maple syrup, pecans, pumpkin, figs, apples, brisket, pork
Dish idea: grilled pork chops with maple butter and pickled apples

Spring: asparagus, peas, spinach, eggs, lamb
Dish idea: asparagus and pea frittata

Summer: raspberries, blueberries, watermelon, corn, broccoli
Dish idea: watermelon salad (watermelon, cucumber, corn, and feta cheese)

Winter: beans, butternut squash, celeriac, pomegranates, barley
Dish idea: Bean stew with barley and winter squash

By Culture or Region
(Ideas for ingredient combinations and cooking methods)

Spain/Mediterranean:
Squid, paprika, and olive oil
Asparagus, orange, and Ibérico ham
Sautéed breadcrumbs, garlic, chorizo, roasted pepper, and poached egg

North African or Moroccan:
Chickpea, eggplant, couscous, lentils, and mint (cold salad)
Chicken, harissa, almonds, and dates (braised)
Roasted lamb, coriander, lime, and mayonnaise

Vietnamese:
Tofu, pickled carrots, rock sugar, fish sauce, lemongrass, chili, and mint
Chicken, shrimp paste, red Thai chili, fried shallots, cinnamon, and lime

By Recipe Category

Appetizers or starters
Soups
Eggs
Main dish: vegetarian, fish, seafood, beef, pork, and poultry
Salads
Vegetables
Pastas
Sweets
Breads
Beverages

By Meal, Recipe Type, or Occasion

Breakfast
Lunch
Dinner
Snacks
Desserts
Fast/easy
Healthy
Special occasion/holiday

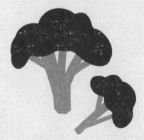

Recipe Development Step 2: Create a Recipe Strategy

Mastering the culinary basics, developing your palate, and committing to lifelong culinary learning through reading and experimenting with food will enhance your recipe development skills. With this foundational culinary knowledge, you can move on to step two—the recipe strategy. The recipe strategy involves thinking through the objectives of the recipe and the profile of its intended audience: essentially, the who, what, when, where, and why of the recipe. Getting these questions answered first will help guide your recipe's content.

First, understand the audience and their needs—including their problems and frustrations, particularly the ones that a recipe developer can solve. Recipe success is more than just a summary of clicks, shares, and page views. **Rather, the end goal of a recipe, whether it's for a print or digital publication, social media platform, or food company, is that it must work as written, taste good, look appealing, and provide replicable results.** After preparing the recipe, the end user should feel successful as a cook.

A professional recipe developer must strive to be a trusted resource whom cooks can count on.

A recipe strategy should answer the following questions:

- **Who** is the target audience?
- **What** recipe is needed?
- **When** will the recipe be used?
- **Where** will the recipe be published?
- **Why** develop this recipe?
- **How** will you know if the recipe is successful?

The Target Audience

Recipes are like formulas, with instructions that tell a story using the active voice. When creating a recipe strategy, it is best to start by identifying the people who will most likely prepare the recipe: its target audience. Clearly defining the target audience helps the recipe developer meet their interests and needs. Today, this step is more important than ever before, since consumers can access hundreds of recipes a day through a variety of platforms but may only choose to use one or two.

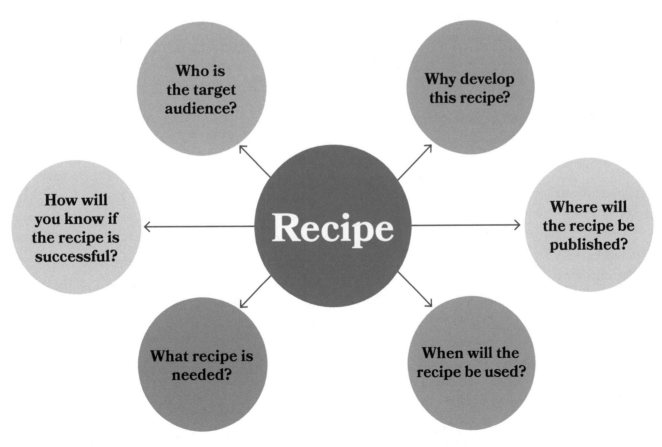

If a recipe is being developed for a food company or food association, it's likely that they will have their own research and data on the target audience. Brands are tightly bound to their understanding of their customers' needs, and any recipe developed for a brand must adhere to that understanding. A recipe developer should ask the client for as much audience data and product insights as they can provide. If audience data is unavailable, the recipe developer should personalize the ideal cook as much as possible by visualizing what the ideal cook will do with, think about, and want from the recipe.

Begin by identifying and exploring audience demographics and the various lifestyle and behavioral characteristics of the target group. Defining these demographics and behavioral traits is critical. Developing a recipe for a family with young children is very different from developing a recipe for a retired couple, just as developing a recipe for someone with good access to many quality ingredients is different from developing a recipe for someone on a strict budget or who lives in an area with limited food access. A clear understanding of the target audience is critical to the recipe strategy.

Demographics

Consider the following factors first when establishing the basic profile of the target audience:

- age
- gender
- cultural background
- where they live (country, region, whether they live in cities or rural areas)
- education level
- estimated income level
- household size
- age of household members

Lifestyle and Behavioral Characteristics

Next, answer the following questions to further narrow or segment the recipe's audience.

What is the ideal cook's culinary skill level? For example, do they understand more esoteric culinary terms (supreme an orange, julienne a vegetable)? How much detail should be included in the recipe's instructions?

What type of equipment will the ideal cook have on hand? For example, are they likely to own a blender to puree a soup or make a frozen smoothie? Do they own specialized pans, such as a popover pan or a roasting pan with a rack?

What measurement system is used by your audience? Does your audience understand and use metric (kilograms, grams, milliliters) or US customary measures (pounds, ounces, cups, tablespoons, teaspoons) or both?

What are the ideal cook's shopping habits? Does the ideal cook have easy access to a well-stocked grocery store? Do they shop daily or biweekly, or do they make weekly visits to the grocery store?

When will the recipe be prepared? Is the recipe intended to be made on an average weeknight or is it a prep-heavy recipe intended for a weekend or a special occasion when the cook would have more time?

What is the availability or accessibility of the ingredients of the recipe? Are there cost considerations when choosing ingredients?

Is the recipe trying to solve a consumer challenge? For example, is it making dinner at the end of a workday in 20 minutes or less? Or creating a lunch item that can be eaten using one hand?

Does the audience have dietary restrictions? Does the recipe need to meet different dietary requirements for each family member?

RECIPE CONSIDERATIONS FOR AN AUDIENCE WITH LIMITED COOKING EXPERIENCE

Consider the following factors:

- Use basic cooking equipment and appliances.
- Make sure recipes are easy to read and follow.
- Limit the number of ingredients—for example, five or fewer.
- Limit the total preparation time to 20 or fewer minutes, with the finished dish ready and on the table within 30 to 40 minutes.
- Whenever possible, try to use the entire amount of an ingredient in the package specified in order to prevent waste, such as 1 (14.5-ounce) can chicken broth instead of 1¼ cups.
- Ensure that the recipe is flexible: it should be able to accommodate fresh, frozen, or canned versions of the ingredients and provide practical suggestions, including easy substitutions (e.g., bouillon cubes for canned broth).
- Include tips and additional educational information when appropriate.
- Include information on handwashing and food safety.
- Offer suggestions on what parts of the recipe can be made ahead of time or how leftovers can be used in a second meal.
- Provide general nutrition information in the recipe's headnote.

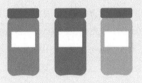

The Purpose of a Recipe

Just like other forms of communication, recipes convey a message by fulfilling a specific purpose for an audience, publisher, or company. A recipe's primary purpose might be to inspire action on the part of the audience—eating more vegetables, buying a specific product or appliance used in the recipe, or supporting marketing goals on social media. Secondary purposes or goals could include a desire on the part of a publisher or company to create a new audience or to encourage its existing audience to seek out other content on a website or on social media.

Before starting a recipe development project, consider the what, why, when, and where of the recipe. Finding the answers to these questions will help clarify the recipe's purpose. If the client is a food company or restaurant, many of these answers can be found on their media outlets or in their publications. Do your own research to ensure you are familiar with their goals.

What?

What features of the recipe may be most appealing to the target audience?

Should the number of ingredients in the recipe be limited?

Does the recipe need to meet certain nutrient criteria for a specific audience?

Should the cook use a specific piece of equipment (e.g., a handheld blender) or technique (e.g., a no-bake pie recipe)?

Should this recipe showcase a particular ingredient or product? If it's a brand recipe, what image, budget, and branding guidelines must be followed? How will the recipe showcase the brand's promise or message?

How visually appealing is the end product? Depending on how the recipe will be used, the accompanying photo of the dish may be just as important as the dish's flavor.

How will this recipe differentiate itself from others?

Why?

Should the recipe convey a feeling or emotion, such as love, comfort, warmth, fun, or joy?

Should the recipe solve a problem for its audience?

Will the recipe convey a message or educate its audience about a specific culture, ingredient, family tradition, cooking technique, or any other important factor?

Should the recipe tell a story?

Will the recipe highlight a new food trend, regional foodway, or seasonal ingredient?

When?

When will the audience use the recipe? Think through the consumer's entire experience with the recipe, from when and how the consumer finds the recipe on through to shopping, prepping, cooking, eating, and cleanup. Recipes can be brand ambassadors that help consumers experience, taste, and buy into a brand's message.

When will the finished recipe be served? Will it be served at a picnic, a potluck, an elegant or casual dinner party, or a holiday gathering? This may alter certain ingredient and cooking method choices.

Where?

Where will the recipe be available once it is complete? Will it exist digitally or in print to be used by employees in food service; on a food company's website; on a food product package; in a consumer brochure; in an online or print magazine or newspaper; or in a cookbook, an email newsletter, or on social media? The number of possible platforms for where a recipe can exist continues to grow, and different platforms have different space constraints and word count limits. If the platform includes food photography and video capabilities, the space devoted to the recipe may be affected as well.

MEASURING RECIPE SUCCESS

How will you know if a recipe is successful? A key "ingredient" often missing in recipe development is follow-up with the target audience to determine both whether the recipe ends up being used and if so, the audience's reactions to the recipe in terms of its taste, cost to prepare, and ease of preparation. Ask a publisher, food company, or foodservice establishment if they have data on their most popular and most-requested recipes. It may be nearly impossible to measure a recipe's impact on sales of a specific product featured, but recipe developers can assess a recipe's performance in a variety of ways, including consumer engagement with the recipe (including clicks, likes, and ratings), posts about the recipe, comments, or inquiries.

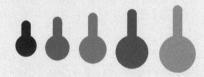

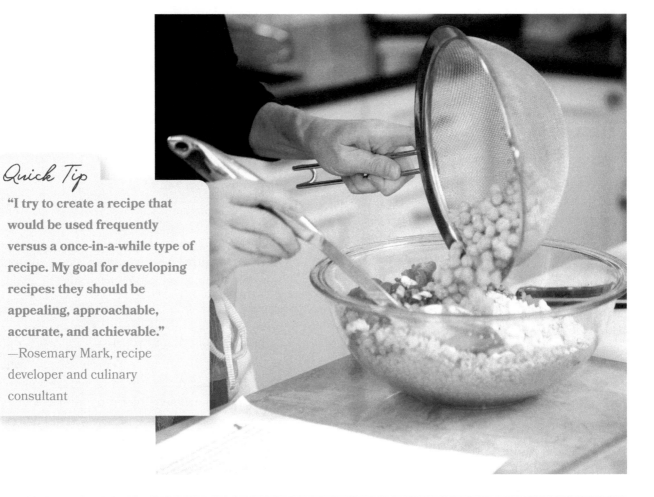

Quick Tip

"I try to create a recipe that would be used frequently versus a once-in-a-while type of recipe. My goal for developing recipes: they should be appealing, approachable, accurate, and achievable."
—Rosemary Mark, recipe developer and culinary consultant

STAYING ON TOP OF CONSUMER FOOD TRENDS

Following consumer food trends can help a recipe developer pitch ideas, gain a better understanding of a recipe's intended audience, or provide a rationale for a specific recipe.

- Monitor companies and associations that perform market research and gather industry insights, data analytics, and trend reports on food and beverage; restaurants and food service; food retail; and consumer eating and drinking behavior. (Examples include Circana, SPINS, Data Essentials, Hartman Group, Deloitte, McKinsey & Company, Food Genius, Mintel Food and Drink/Mintel Menu Insights, Food Navigator, Sterling Rice Group Culinary Trends, and the National Restaurant Association.)

- Read blogs and other online media outlets (e.g., Eater's Trends section, Food52, Kitchn, Allrecipes' Measuring Cup Consumer Trends Report).
- Scan online platforms, such as Instagram, TikTok, and Pinterest trends, Pinterest100.com (annual report), Substack (for food e-newsletters), Google Analytics, or Google Trends.
- Customize social media feeds so they display trending topics. (Search trend hashtags like #foodtrends or #trendyfoods.)
- Read trade journals, trade newsletters, cookbooks, and consumer magazines.
- Eat out at local and out-of-town restaurants.
- Become a keen observer of other people and their eating habits.

Recipe Development Step 3: The Creative Process

From Vision to Revision to Final Recipe

The creative process of recipe development involves taking your vision on through to revision and ultimately to the creation of the final recipe. It can begin once the recipe's target audience and purpose have been clearly defined and the platform where the recipe will appear has been identified. As the recipe developer, you are what makes the next step in the recipe development process unique—your culinary skills and kitchen experience, the books you like to reference, your food notes on ingredients and flavor combinations, and your personal taste memories.

No recipe developer follows the exact same creative process every time, so documenting the "art" of a successful recipe developer's process is impossible. However, certain approaches and strategies commonly used by a variety of food professionals—from home economists and chefs to test kitchen professionals—can serve as a good start.

Brainstorm and Research

The brainstorming and research process of recipe development can start in a variety of ways. Here are some examples:

- Jot down recipe ideas while referencing your food notes or taste memories of a recent amazing dish. Start with a group of written ideas and choose one or two to focus on, including tweaking ingredients and cooking methods. Of course, there are endless flavor combinations to experiment with in the kitchen, but consider changing up the technique, presentation, temperature, texture, or any combination of these elements when brainstorming a new recipe.

- Turn to books for reference while researching or when generating new recipe ideas. Begin by researching what has already been published on the subject, using books as a jumping-off point.

Just be sure that your own personal stamp goes into the final recipe. Read more about copyright law pertaining to recipes on page 20.

- Consider creating a chart of different existing versions of the same recipe so that you can compare them side by side. While this process is time-consuming, it can be especially helpful when learning about recipes from unfamiliar cultures. The process can help inform recipe development because it allows you to clearly see the different authentic ingredients and techniques used in each version. Taking the process a step further and testing and tasting each version is a good opportunity to note the strengths, weaknesses, similarities, and differences of each.

- Alternatively, make notes about the differences among recipes, including variations in ingredient amounts, techniques, and temperatures, in one version of the recipe, using different colors of text or ink to highlight the differences.

- Read about different cuisines and create a completely unique blend of your own. Consider merging different flavors, ingredients, and cooking techniques when creating a new recipe, and use its headnote to describe and acknowledge any cultural inspirations. Read more about avoiding cultural appropriation on page 15.

- Start with a main ingredient and pair it with three to four complementary flavor profiles. To avoid confusing the palate with too many competing flavors, think about flavor balance, color, and texture. Next, move on to the cooking technique and put your own spin on it.

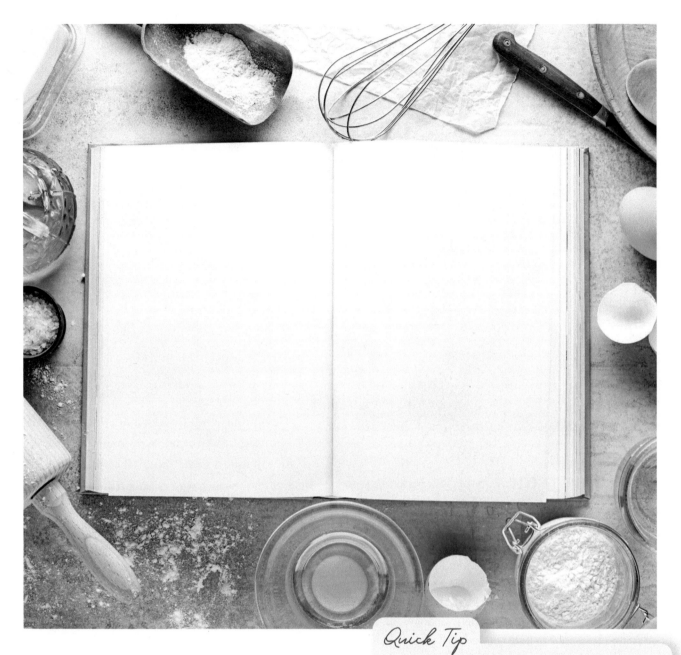

- When adapting an existing recipe, first understand how the recipe is traditionally prepared and where there may be opportunity to experiment and improvise. A methodical approach could involve using different ingredients, perhaps to avoid a food allergen, or an alternative cooking technique or serving method. Just be sure to rename the final recipe appropriately, since removing or substituting key or authentic ingredients in a traditional dish makes it no longer that dish.

- Finally, be sure to file away the recipe ideas that don't make the cut, as they may help inspire future recipes.

Quick Tip

"For help when developing a recipe, read dozens of recipes, take careful notes, spend time comparing ratios, techniques, and temperatures. Then, write out your own recipe, test it, and retest it. If one particular recipe influenced you—give proper credit. If not, there is no need to credit anyone specifically." —Kathryn Pauline, cardamomandtea.com recipe blogger and cookbook author

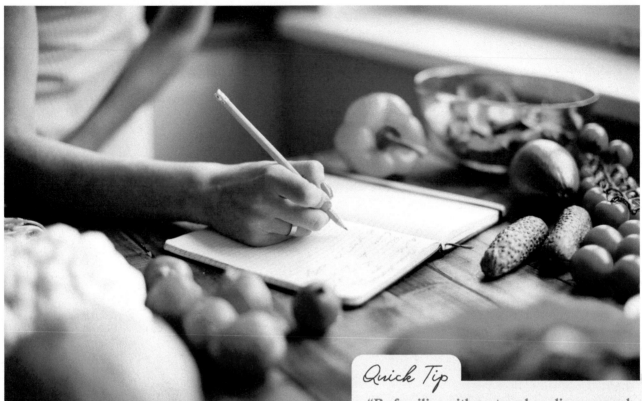

Write Down the Recipe

Regardless of which brainstorming and research approach you choose, all of your ideas, inspirations, and thoughts should be translated to a written form. Sit down in front of a blank computer screen or piece of paper and create a list of ingredients and general instructions. This step gives you a framework or out-line to begin testing in the kitchen. Changes to this draft are likely once testing begins (see Chapter 8). For example, it might become clear that the recipe needs more vegetables, more acid, or a contrasting textural ingredient, but writing it down provides a record where you can add notes and ideas. It's a starting place.

Experiment With the Recipe

Don't be afraid to mess up. A recipe developer does not always know whether new flavor combinations will work together without tasting them or whether a different cooking method will turn out without testing it. Sometimes a new recipe will work fairly well as planned, and many times the draft recipe leads the recipe developer down a whole new creative path.

Quick Tip

"Be familiar with on-trend appliances, such as standard and electric pressure cookers, slow cookers, grills (both electric and gas), and air fryers. Many clients will ask for recipes specific to certain appliances."
—Rick Rodgers, cookbook author and recipe developer

Quick Tip

"A food professional has a recipe base that can and should be repurposed because each use generates income. I try to use a recipe three times during the course of its life in various venues, changing the recipe up each time." —Rick Rodgers, cookbook author and recipe developer

Along the way, take time to taste for flavor, balance, and texture and document the steps during each stage of the recipe process. Be sure to write down your notes or take photos or record (on video or audio) observations at different stages of the cooking process. Always keep in mind the visual image of the recipe and how it will photograph.

Celebrate and Respect Global Cuisines

In recipe development, the lines between cultural appreciation and appropriation can become blurred. *Cultural appropriation* is the act of taking or using elements from another culture without showing an understanding of and respect for the culture, especially when it leads to personal gain or profit. Cultural appropriation may be evident anywhere that recipes and food are found.

Ken Albala, a food historian and professor of history at the University of the Pacific, advises that this does not imply that individuals should only cook or develop recipes from their own heritage, but it does mean that research, respect, and sensitivity should be evident along with providing cultural context and source attribution. See Authenticity in Cooking: Avoiding Cultural Appropriation for more on how to avoid cultural appropriation in recipe development.

AUTHENTICITY IN COOKING: AVOIDING CULTURAL APPROPRIATION

When developing a recipe that features or stems from a different culture, be as honest and transparent as possible. Provide the audience with the recipe's origin story, if possible, to authenticate your relationship to and understanding of its heritage. The more idiosyncratic the story is, the better. Descriptive language can quickly shift from archetypal to stereotypical, so be careful. There are bound to be many different versions of a recipe, so avoid making assertions about the one best way to do something. The best advice is to keep it professional and respectful. In most cases, recipes are in the public domain and do not belong to any one individual, but if you find a recipe or idea in a favorite cultural cookbook, tell the audience about it. Tell a story—was it fun, exciting, intimidating? If so, how and why? Invite an insider from the culture—what anthropologists refer to as a person with an emic view—to dialogue, offer advice, and consult with you on the recipe. The recipe headnote is the perfect place to share how a classic recipe for a dish may have inspired your own version. Explain the choices you made with the recipe's technique and ingredients and where your innovative recipe veers from traditional versions. This might include substitutions for ingredients that are not readily available in the US, thus making it different (but avoid language that suggests you "cleaned up," "improved," or "upscaled" the recipe). Recipe developers whose creations are inspired by lesser-known dishes should be straightforward about their origins and never claim that their versions are exact replicas.

—Krishnendu Ray, PhD, Associate Professor and Chair of the Department of Nutrition and Food Studies at New York University Steinhardt School of Culture, Education, and Human Development

RECIPE DEVELOPMENT: AN ILLUSTRATION OF THE CREATIVE PROCESS

My Inspiration

After enjoying an incredibly simple side dish at an Italian restaurant—bagna cauda served with crusty bread—I write down the ingredients in the dish, according to the server: olive oil, anchovies, and garlic. I read more about bagna cauda and decide to create a pasta dish using the flavors from this traditional Italian dipping sauce as the base.

The idea starts in my head, first by thinking about a dish called aglio e olio that I make often for my family. It's convenient because the ingredients—olive oil, garlic, salt, pasta, and Parmesan cheese—are always in my pantry or refrigerator.

I think of how I've used anchovies before—maybe one or two, just to add some depth to a dish—but as I reference my taste memory of the dipping sauce, I recall how prominent the anchovy and lemon flavors were.

My Brainstorming Process

I start brainstorming ingredients and making food notes about the potential ingredients for my new pasta dish. Some ingredients (and notes about them) that come to mind based on my own preferences and consideration of a complementary flavor profile include:

- Olive oil, garlic, anchovies (traditional ingredients in bagna cauda)
- Unsalted butter (for some additional richness and a different fat source)
- Crushed red pepper (for heat—also used in aglio e olio)
- Capers or olives (might provide too much saltiness?)
- Lemon juice (for acid)
- Sherry vinegar (for mellow acid)
- Pasta types: spaghetti, bucatini
- Roasted cauliflower and roasted fennel (for a caramelized flavor)
- Cheeses: Parmesan, feta, burrata, Manchego
- Toasted slivered almonds or toasted breadcrumbs (for texture)
- Chopped parsley, mint, basil, rosemary (for color and flavor)

After this step, I might peruse some Italian cookbooks to get more inspiration about ingredients and techniques. Finally, I may again reference my taste memories and reread my brainstorming notes.

Instead of using just olive oil, as is traditional for bagna cauda, I decide to use a combination of butter and olive oil and also add some fresh lemon juice and crushed red pepper. I want to make it my own and add elements that I like—roasted vegetables and Parmesan cheese. Many other additions could be made, but I decide to keep my recipe fairly simple and limit the number of ingredients.

Following is the first draft of the new recipe, with approximate ingredient amounts, short recipe instructions, and some notes I made along the way.

Pasta with Garlic, Anchovies, and Roasted Cauliflower

Draft version #1

2 to 5 tablespoons extra-virgin olive oil
2 to 4 tablespoons unsalted butter
2 to 4 cloves garlic, thinly sliced
3 to 6 anchovies
½ to 1 teaspoon crushed red pepper
Juice from 1 to 2 fresh lemons
1 head cauliflower, cut into bite-sized pieces (2 pounds?) (try other versions with fennel and/or escarole)
2 tablespoons extra-virgin olive oil
Salt
1 pound spaghetti
¼ to ⅓ cup chopped fresh herbs mint, basil, and parsley (or just use one?)
¼ to ¾ cup grated Parmesan cheese

1. Combine the anchovies, olive oil, butter, lemon juice, garlic, and red pepper flakes in saucepan; simmer mixture (or write recipe with bagna cauda left over to use for other dishes?).

2. Toss cauliflower with oil and salt. Roast at 425° F.

3. Cook pasta until al dente. Reserve some pasta cooking water.

4. Add cauliflower to the garlic and anchovy mixture. Add cooked pasta; pasta water as needed. Toss with fresh herbs and Parmesan cheese.

After testing this recipe several times, I make some small changes. I am precise and disciplined at this phase, making sure to translate changes to the written recipe. The recipe is finished once I know it's reproducible in anyone's kitchen. I finalize recipe edits using specific ingredient amounts, and I write the recipe headnote and instructions in my own style and voice. Read more about headnote writing in Chapter 7.

Here is the finished recipe:

Pasta with Garlic, Anchovies, and Roasted Cauliflower

By Raeanne Sarazen, MA, RDN

This pasta dish is inspired by bagna cauda, a hot dipping sauce made with anchovies and garlic and served with vegetables or crusty bread, often as part of a traditional appetizer in Italian American households who celebrate "The Feast of the Seven Fishes" on Christmas Eve. In my home, it inspires a quick weeknight meal tossed with pasta. This recipe won't take long to make, but if you want to get a future dinner on the table even faster, double or triple the sauce and store it in the refrigerator to use later. It's one less dish you'll need to wash on a busy weeknight!

Preparation time: 10 minutes
Cooking time: 30 minutes
Yield: 4 to 6 servings

1 head cauliflower (about 1½ pounds), trimmed and cut into bite-sized pieces (3 to 4 cups)
4 tablespoons extra-virgin olive oil, divided use
½ teaspoon kosher salt, plus more for pasta cooking water
2 tablespoons unsalted butter
Juice of 1 fresh lemon (about 2 tablespoons)
5 anchovy fillets
3 garlic cloves, thinly sliced
½ teaspoon crushed red pepper flakes
1 pound spaghetti
½ cup freshly grated Parmigiano-Reggiano cheese
⅓ cup chopped fresh basil
⅓ cup chopped fresh parsley

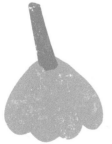

1. Heat the oven to 425° F. Line a baking sheet with nonstick aluminum foil (this prevents sticking, and also helps the cleanup).

2. On the baking sheet, toss the cauliflower with 2 tablespoons of the olive oil and the salt. Roast, turning the florets once, until tender and caramelized a bit on the edges, about 30 minutes. Remove from the oven and set the cauliflower aside.

3. While the cauliflower is roasting, heat the remaining 2 tablespoons olive oil, the butter, lemon juice, anchovies, garlic, and red pepper flakes in a small saucepan over low heat; cook, stirring with a wooden spoon, until the anchovies dissolve, about 2 minutes. Reduce the heat to the lowest setting and let the mixture simmer for about 10 minutes while flavors meld.

4. While the sauce is cooking, bring a large pot of water to a boil. Salt the water generously—about 1 tablespoon or more (it's not too much salt!). Add the pasta and cook according to package directions until al dente. Remove 1 cup of the starchy pasta cooking water and set aside. Drain the pasta and return to the pot.

5. Stir the cauliflower and garlic sauce into the pasta and mix to combine. Add the Parmigiano-Reggiano and enough of the reserved pasta water to moisten the pasta slightly and toss to coat the pasta with sauce. Add the basil and parsley and toss to combine. Serve immediately.

Notes: *It's an extra step, but well worth it to warm your bowls or plates in the turned-off oven that is still warm from roasting the cauliflower. Just set them in the warm oven for 10 to 15 minutes before serving the pasta.*

Use anchovies straight from the can or jar—any brand works equally well in this recipe. Store opened anchovies in a tightly sealed container in the refrigerator for up to 2 months. Alternatively, in a pinch, you can use 1 to 1½ teaspoons anchovy paste, but I prefer the fresher, less salty, and more complex flavor of the whole, canned anchovies.

Nutrition per serving (based on 4 servings): 680 calories, 26 grams fat, 8 grams saturated fat, 1,010 milligrams sodium (analysis includes salt in pasta cooking water), 92 grams carbohydrate, 7 grams fiber, 4 grams total sugar, 22 grams protein

RECIPE YIELD CONVERSION

Using a conversion factor is a common method for adjusting recipes to increase or decrease the yield (or number of servings) or change the serving size. The conversion factor is calculated by dividing the recipe's desired yield by the original yield. Once the factor has been determined, the recipe developer multiplies the quantity of each ingredient in the original recipe by that number.

desired yield (quantity of servings needed) ÷ original yield (original quantity of servings) = conversion factor

conversion factor × original ingredient quantity = new ingredient quantity

Example 1: Calculate conversion factor to change recipe yield from 25 servings to 60 servings

First, obtain the conversion factor:

60 servings ÷ 25 servings = a conversion factor of 2.4

Next, multiply the quantity of each ingredient in the original recipe by the conversion factor.

Example 2: Calculate conversion factor to change yield and serving size from 10 (4-ounce) servings to 20 (5-ounce servings)

First, calculate the total yield for the original and desired amounts:

Original: 10 × 4-ounce serving = 40 ounces

Desired: 20 × 5-ounce serving = 100 ounces

Next, divide the desired yield by the original yield.

100 ounces ÷ 40 ounces = a conversion factor of 2.5

Last, multiply the quantity of each ingredient in the original recipe by the conversion factor.

Recipe Conversion Tips

- For more accuracy, convert original ingredient quantities from volume to weight measurements whenever possible.
- After multiplying an ingredient's quantity in the original recipe by the conversion factor, the total quantity's unit of measure may need to be adjusted (e.g., teaspoons to tablespoons or ounces to pounds).
- When scaling recipes—especially upward—use your best cooking judgment to compensate for differences in measurement, equipment, cooking time, and seasoning.
- Always retest a recipe after it has been converted.
- The baker's percentage is the method used to scale a recipe for a baked good up or down. The baker's percentage calculates each ingredient amount based on its relative percentage of the recipe's flour weight, with the flour weight remaining constant at 100%.

For quantity recipes, some foodservice operations use spreadsheets or their own proprietary software to scale yield up or down. In these cases, the ingredient quantities are typically expressed in metric measurements, and the software or spreadsheet automatically recalculates the ingredient quantities based on the desired yield.

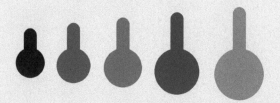

STANDARDIZED RECIPES

Quantity recipes developed to meet the nutritional requirements of hospitals, schools, senior living centers, or other foodservice operations are often "standardized" so they produce consistent, high-quality, and specific yields every time. A recipe is considered to be standardized when the written set of ingredients and instructions have been tested and verified to consistently prepare a known quantity and quality of food. See Chapter 8 for detailed information on recipe testing and Chapter 9 for information on nutrition analysis of recipes.

The benefits of standardizing recipes include:

- **consistent food quality** to help ensure the best possible dish is produced every time
- **predictable yield** in an effort to avoid food waste and shortages
- **accurate nutrient content** to ensure the recipe's nutritional requirements are met
- **food cost control** to keep the cost per serving consistent when the same ingredients and quantities are used each time
- **efficient purchasing** to calculate the quantity of ingredients needed for production based on the information provided in the recipe (this is useful for estimating food inventory as well)
- **labor cost control,** as having written procedures allows staff to make good use of their time, work more efficiently, and require less oversight
- **employee confidence,** as staff feel more independent and confident because a written set of ingredient amounts and instructions eliminates guesswork and decreases the likelihood of mistakes and poor food quality

Quick Tip

"We have a weekly creative meeting that includes recipe development. Sometimes an idea might be shaped by necessity: 'what we need on our menu, what is going to sell to our clients.' We brainstorm and talk about what we'd like to try—sometimes building off of existing recipes—and then experiment in the kitchen. Other times, we create recipes from our culinary travels. These trips are followed by extensive research on the region we visited. And sometimes, we start a creative meeting with a need to create a dish that evokes a specific emotion, such as nostalgia or comfort. We create and build from there." —Zach Steen, Culinary Director of Topolobampo, Frontera Grill, XOCO, and Bar Sotano

Quick Tip

"In my bakery, we start with an idea, which may come from simply tasting something we like. We'll gather several recipes—from books and online search[es]—and decide what we like best in each after making and comparing them side by side. We look at the ratios; get the base figured out; and then play with sugar, salt, spice, and fat, asking [ourselves], 'do we want more whole grain, less sugar, more add-ins,' and thinking about how this will affect our pricing. We always make notes on the recipe hard copy and then put in updates to recipes we store electronically." —Sandra Holl, chef and owner, Floriole Bakery, Chicago

Understanding the Legal Attributes of Recipes

Copyright law protects original works and gives their owner the exclusive right to reproduce and profit from the works. It's important to understand the nuances of copyright law and how it can apply to original recipes.

According to the US Copyright Office:

*A mere listing of ingredients is not protected under copyright law. However, where a recipe or formula is accompanied by **substantial literary expression** in the form of an explanation or directions, or when there is a collection of recipes as in a cookbook, there may be a basis for copyright protection.*

The first sentence of this message is very clear: an ingredient list in a recipe cannot be copyrighted. For instance, the ingredient list on the back of any commercial food product can be used by anyone to create a similar version.

The second part indicates that the headnote and method of preparation or directions *can* be copyrighted, especially if they include original and expressive elements, such as suggestions on presentation, advice on accompaniments, and information about the origin of the dish. This means you should obtain permission from a copyright owner if you print a recipe that is identical or substantially similar to a copyright-protected recipe in your own cookbook or website.

While an individual recipe may not be protected by copyright, collections of recipes (e.g., an entire cookbook or the entire content of a food blog) are always copyright protected, as is any kind of food photography that is not otherwise labeled as being in the public domain. Cookbooks fall into the category of literary works.

According to the US Copyright Office:

A literary work is a work that explains, describes, or narrates a particular subject, theme, or idea through the use of narrative, descriptive, or explanatory text, rather than dialog or dramatic action. Generally, literary works are intended to be read; they are not intended to be performed before an audience.

Quick Tip

"Due to changes in copyright law over the years, different copyright durations apply depending on the date of publication or creation of the particular work. As a general rule, any work published more than 95 years ago is in the public domain for United States purposes. For works created on or after January 1, 1978, copyright duration is tied to the life of the author—lasting for the lifetime of the author plus 70 years." —Joy R. Butler, attorney and author of *The Permission Seeker's Guide Through the Legal Jungle*

A self-published cookbook or other collection of recipes can be registered for protection under copyright law online via the Electronic Copyright Office (copyright.gov/registration).

Best Practices for Developing and Sharing Recipes

Regardless of copyright law protections, all food professionals—chefs, cookbook authors, food writers, food bloggers, and recipe developers alike—should adhere to ethical standards with respect to developing and sharing recipes.

Requesting Permission

Reprinting a recipe verbatim without citing the source and obtaining permission for use is considered plagiarism. If you are making reference to or including excerpts of someone else's recipe on a website, blog, or social media platform, provide a link to the original source giving appropriate attribution. Requesting special permission to link to another website is not required, but it is a professional courtesy.

Permission is necessary, however, if a complete recipe is to be posted verbatim on a social media platform, website, or email newsletter, magazine, or newspaper. Contact either the publisher or the author of the recipe and request permission to republish it, as well as the preferred method of citation. Many authors have a permissions section on their website.

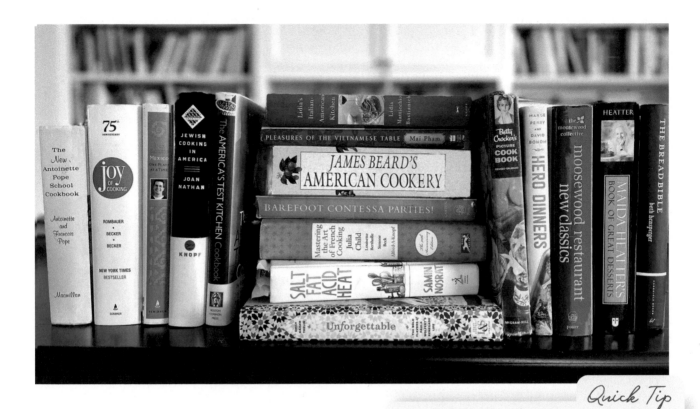

Following is a typical example of citation instructions for a website:

© 2019–2023 [Site Name]. All rights reserved. All words & images by [Full Name]. Unauthorized use and/or duplication of this material without express and written permission from this site's author and/or owner is strictly prohibited. Excerpts and links may be used, provided that full and clear credit is given to [Full Name] and [Site Name] with appropriate and specific direction to the original content.

Be aware that obtaining permission for older recipes might be difficult. For example, publishing rights generally belong to the original publisher unless otherwise stated, but some publishing houses no longer exist or have been consolidated. Most publishers have a permissions department; be aware that a fee is often required to secure permission. Permission is also required to reproduce or republish a photo or illustration that accompanies a recipe. Obtain permission from the original creator or copyright owner. See Chapter 10 for more information.

Creating Original Recipes

A persistent urban myth claims that only three ingredients must be changed in an existing recipe to make it your own. However, changing three ingredients in the recipe *does not* make it original.

A recipe is original when it's written in *your* own words, sharing details that reflect your personal experience, expertise on using specific ingredients, and recommendations for combining those ingredients. Simply adding a tablespoon of chopped fresh basil or changing pork to tofu is not enough to claim a recipe as your own. To make a recipe your own, you must start fresh, using your own language and voice, interpretations, measurements, and trial-and-error experimentation.

Attributing Reworked Recipes

"Adapted *from*" is to be used in the recipe headnote or in a note at the end of the recipe when modifying the structure of someone else's recipe. Note that it can be a fine line between someone else's original recipe and an acceptable "adapted from" recipe. There are different ways to adapt a recipe, including changing the title, headnote, ingredients, and method of preparation. If an adapted recipe is shared digitally, give proper attribution and link to the author's original recipe or link to where to purchase their book. This, too, is a professional courtesy. Following are two examples of proper adaptation:

- Modify the ingredient list: Start by changing one ingredient. Test the recipe and then see if you can change others. An easy place to start is the dish's main protein or vegetables. Can the ground beef be swapped for soft tofu? Could you use an entirely new type of vegetable, such as butternut squash instead of kale?

- Change the cooking method: For example, consider turning an oven-baked recipe into a slow-cooker dish, or make a recipe healthier by grilling the main protein instead of frying it.

"Inspired *by*" can be used when ideas originate from elsewhere. It's important to give credit to others where it's due, especially when taking ideas directly from a specific recipe. In the recipe headnote, mention that the idea was inspired by someone else's creation; for example, a headnote could read, "I started with the Nestlé Toll House cookie recipe . . . ," or "The wonderful Chicago-based Goddess and Grocer delicatessen inspired this seasonal version of chicken salad featuring dried fall fruits." Giving credit can also help the reader connect with the recipe and gives context.

Quick Tip

"Legally, there is no difference between adapted and inspired by—it's the level of tinkering. 'Adapted from' follows the structure of the (original) recipe ingredient list with small tweaks—maybe simplifying the ingredient list or changing the language in the directions. 'Inspired by' recipes have much bigger changes, such as significant ingredient changes and/or different cooking techniques and/ or equipment. Either way, readers like to know where the 'original' recipe or ideas came from; it's part of the recipe's story."
—Bonnie Benwick, former deputy food editor, *The Washington Post*

Quick Tip

"Keep a folder that includes documentation on your original recipe. This includes your recipe development process—recipes you were influenced by, books you used for research, your kitchen testing notes, and more. You are documenting the originality of your recipe and showing how it is unique."
—Rosemary Mark, recipe developer and culinary consultant

Quick Tip

"It's the way in which someone explains a technique—the way they construct and write their recipes—that is original. That is what people own and what distinguishes one recipe from another. A recipe becomes your own when you write the recipe as you would cook it, and it reflects your voice and experience. It's about telling a story through ingredients and instructions."
—Amanda Hesser, cofounder of Food52, interviewed by Dianne Jacob for her blog (diannej.com)

Recipe Development Resources

Following are just a few of the many resources that can help inspire recipe ideas; provide authenticity on history, ingredients, and techniques; and serve as reference guides for different types of foods, cuisines, and food writing.

General Cooking

The Food Substitutions Bible, 3rd Edition, by David Joachim. 2022. Robert Rose.

How to Cook Everything by Mark Bittman. 2013. Wiley.

The Joy of Cooking by Irma Rombauer. 2019. Scribner.

Kitchen Creativity: Unlocking Culinary Genius with Wisdom, Inspiration, and Ideas from the World's Most Creative Chefs by Karen Page. 2017. Little, Brown & Company.

Professional Cooking, 8th Edition, by Wayne Gisslen. 2014. Wiley.

Ratio: The Simple Codes Behind the Craft of Everyday Cooking, by Michael Ruhlman. 2010. Scribner.

The Smitten Kitchen Cookbook: Recipes and Wisdom from an Obsessive Home Cook by Deb Perelman. 2012. Knopf.

Flavor

The Complete Book of Herbs & Spices by Sarah Garland. 1986. Viking Press.

The Flavor Bible: The Essential Guide to Culinary Creativity, Based on the Wisdom of Americas Most Imaginative Chefs by Karen Page and Andrew Dornenburg. 2008. Little, Brown & Co.

The Flavor Matrix: The Art and Science of Pairing Common Ingredients to Create Extraordinary Dishes by James Briscione and Brooke Parkhurst. 2018. Houghton Mifflin Harcourt.

Salt, Fat, Acid, Heat: Mastering the Elements of Good Cooking by Samin Nosrat. 2017. Simon & Schuster.

Salted: A Manifesto on the World's Most Essential Mineral, with Recipes by Mark Bitterman. 2010. Ten Speed Press.

Food Science

CookWise: The Hows & Whys of Successful Cooking, The Secrets of Cooking Revealed by Shirley O. Corriher. 1997. William Morrow Cookbooks.

The Food Lab: Better Home Cooking Through Science by J. Kenji López-Alt. 2015. W. W. Norton & Company.

How Baking Works: Exploring the Fundamentals of Baking Science, 3rd Edition, by Paula Figoni. 2010. Wiley.

KitchenWise: Essential Food Science for Home Cooks by Shirley O. Corriher. 2020. Scribner.

On Food and Cooking: The Science and Lore of the Kitchen by Harold McGee. 2007. Scribner.

What Einstein Told His Cook: Kitchen Science Explained by Robert Wolke. 2008. W. W. Norton & Company.

Baking

Advanced Bread and Pastry by Michael Tuas. 2008. Cengage Learning.

The Baker's Appendix by Jessica Reed. 2017. Clarkson Potter.

The Baking Bible by Rose Levy Beranbaum. 2014. Houghton Mifflin Harcourt.

The Bread Baker's Apprentice: Mastering the Art of Extraordinary Bread, 15th Edition, by Peter Reinhart. 2016. Ten Speed Press.

Bread Revolution: World-Class Baking with Sprouted and Whole Grains, Heirloom Flours, and Fresh Techniques by Peter Reinhart. 2014. Ten Speed Press.

The Cake Bible by Rose Levy Beranbaum. 1988. William Morrow Cookbooks.

Maider Heatter's Book of Great Chocolate Desserts by Maider Heatter. 2006. Andrews McMeel Publishing.

Tartine All Day by Elisabeth Prueitt. 2017. Lorena Jones Books.

Tartine Bread by Chad Robertson and Eric Wolfinger. 2010. Chronicle Books.

Vegetarian/Vegan

The First Mess Cookbook: Vibrant Plant-Based Recipes to Eat Well Through the Seasons by Laura Wright. 2017. Avery.

How to Cook Everything Vegetarian, 2nd Edition by Mark Bittman. 2017. Harvest.

The New Vegetarian Cooking for Everyone by Debra Madison. 2014. Ten Speed Press.

Plenty: Vibrant Vegetable Recipes from London's Ottolenghi by Yotam Ottolenghi. 2011. Chronicle Books.

Veganomicon, 10th Anniversary Edition: The Ultimate Vegan Cookbook by Isa Chandra Moskowitz and Terry Romero. 2017. Da Capo Lifelong Books.

Seasonal Cooking

The Farm Cooking School: Techniques and Recipes that Celebrate the Seasons by Ian Knauer and Shelley Wiseman. 2017. Burgess Lea Press.

The Farmers Market Cookbook: The Ultimate Guide to Enjoying Fresh, Local, Seasonal Produce by Julia Shanks and Brett Grohsgal. 2016. New Society Publishers.

True Food: Seasonal, Sustainable, Simple, Pure by Andrew Weil, Sam Fox, and Michael Stebner. 2017. Little, Brown Spark.

Meat

How to Cook Meat by Chris Schlesinger and John Willoughby. 2000. William Morrow Cookbooks.

Meat: A Kitchen Education by James Peterson. 2010. Ten Speed Press.

Meat Illustrated: A Foolproof Guide to Understanding and Cooking with Cuts of All Kinds by America's Test Kitchen. 2020. Cook's Illustrated.

Regional/Cultural Cooking

Chinese
All Under Heaven: Recipes from the 35 Cuisines of China by Carolyn Phillips. 2016. Ten Speed Press.

Every Grain of Rice: Simple Chinese Home Cooking by Fuchsia Dunlop. 2013. W. W. Norton & Company.

Mastering the Art of Chinese Cooking by Eileen Yin-Fei Lo. 2009. Chronicle Books.

Filipino
Filipino Homestyle Dishes: Delicious Meals in Minutes by Norma Olizon-Chikiamco. 2003. Periplus Editions.

The Philippine Cookbook by Reynaldo Alejandro. 1985. Perigee Books.

French
La Varenne Pratique by Anne Wilan. 1989. Clarkson Potter.

Mastering the Art of French Cooking by Julia Child, Louisette Bertholle, and Simone Beck. 1970. Alfred A. Knopf.

Indian
50 Great Curries of India by Camellia Panjabi. 1994. Kyle Books.

Classic Indian Vegetarian and Grain Cooking by Julie Sahni. 1985. William Morrow and Company.

Tasting India: Heirloom Family Recipes by Christine Manfield. 2019. Simon & Schuster Australia.

Vegetarian India: A Journey Through the Best of Indian Home Cooking by Madhur Jaffrey. 2015. Alfred A. Knopf.

Italian
Essentials of Classic Italian Cooking by Marcella Hazan. 2012. Alfred A. Knopf.

La Cucina: The Regional Cooking of Italy by the Italian Academy of Cuisine. 2009. Rizzoli.

The Silver Spoon by the Silver Spoon Kitchen. 2011. Phaidon Press.

Japanese
Everyday Harumi: Simple Japanese Food for Family and Friends by Harumi Kurihara. 2019. Conran.

Japanese Cooking: A Simple Art by Shizuo Tsjui and Yoshiki Tsuji. 2012. Kodansha International.

Takashi's Noodle by Takashi Yagihashi. 2009. Ten Speed Press.

Jewish
Arthur Schwartz's Jewish Home Cooking: Yiddish Recipes Revisited by Arthur Schwartz. 2008. Ten Speed Press.

The Book of Jewish Food: An Odyssey from Samarkand to New York by Claudia Roden. 1996. Alfred A. Knopf.

Jewish Cooking in America by Joan Nathan. 1998. Alfred A. Knopf.

A Treasury of Jewish Holiday Baking by Marcy Goldman. 1998. Doubleday.

Korean
Dok Suni: Recipes From My Mother's Korean Kitchen by Jenny Kwak and Liz Fried. 1998. St. Martin's Press.

Growing Up in a Korean Kitchen: A Cookbook by Hi Soo Shin Hepinstall. 2001. Ten Speed Press.

A Korean Mother's Cooking Notes by Sun-Young Chang. 1997. Ewha Womans University Press.

Mexican
The Art of Mexican Cooking: Traditional Mexican Cooking for Aficionados: A Cookbook by Diana Kennedy. 2008. Clarkson Potter.

Authentic Mexican: Regional Cooking from the Heart of Mexico by Rick Bayless. 2007. William Morrow Cookbooks.

The Cuisines of Mexico by Diana Kennedy. 1972. Harper & Row.

Mexico: One Plate at a Time by Rick Bayless. 2000. Scribner.

Middle Eastern/Moroccan
Couscous and Other Good Food from Morocco by Paula Wolfert. 1973. Harper & Row.

The New Book of Middle Eastern Food by Claudia Roden. 2000. Knopf.

Palestinian
Falastin: A Cookbook by Sami Tamimi and Tara Wigley. 2020. Ten Speed Press.

Palestine on a Plate: Memories from My Mother's Kitchen by Joudie Kalla. 2016. Interlink Publishing Group, Inc.

Southeast Asian
Hot Sour Salty Sweet: A Culinary Journey Through Southeast Asia by Jeffrey Alford and Naomi Duguid. 2000. Artisan.

Southern United States
Heritage by Sean Brock. 2014. Artisan.

Mastering the Art of Southern Cooking by Nathalie Dupree and Cynthia Graubart. 2019. Gibbs Smith.

The Taste of Country Cooking: The 30th Anniversary Edition of a Great Southern Classic Cookbook by Edna Lewis. 2006. Knopf.

Spanish
Charcutería: The Soul of Spain by Jeffrey Weiss. 2021. Agate Surrey.

The Food of Spain by Claudia Roden. 2011. Ecco.

The Foods and Wines of Spain: A Cookbook by Penelope Casas. 1982. Knopf.

Taiwanese
The Food of Taiwan: Recipes from the Beautiful Island by Cathy Erway. 2015. Mariner Books.

Home-Style Taiwanese Cooking by Liv Wan. 2022. Marshall Cavendish Cuisine.

Thai
Real Thai: The Best of Thailand's Regional Cooking by Nancie McDermott. 1992. Chronicle Books.

Thai Food by David Thompson. 2002. Ten Speed Press.

Vietnamese
Into the Vietnamese Kitchen: Treasured Foodways Modern Flavors by Andrea Nguyen. 2010. Ten Speed Press.

Vietnamese Home Cooking: A Cookbook by Charles Phan. 2012. Ten Speed Press.

Food History and Memoirs

Food History

Consider the Fork: A History of How We Cook and Eat by Bee Wilson. 2013. Basic Books.

High on the Hog: A Culinary Journey from Africa to America by Jessica B. Harris. 2012. Bloomsbury.

Modern Food, Moral Food: Self-Control, Science, and the Rise of Modern American Eating in the Early Twentieth Century by Helen Zoe Veit. 2015. University of North Carolina Press.

The Omnivore's Dilemma: A Natural History of Four Meals by Michael Pollan. 2007. Penguin Books.

Perfection Salad: Women and Cooking at the Turn of the Century by Laura Shapiro. 2008. University of California Press.

The Rise: Black Cooks and the Soul of American Food by Marcus Samuelsson. 2020. Voracious.

Salt: A World History by Mark Kurlansky. 2003. Penguin Books.

Soul Food: The Surprising Story of an American Cuisine, One Plate at a Time by Adrian Miller. 2013. The University of North Carolina Press.

A Square Meal: A Culinary History of the Great Depression by Jane Ziegelman and Andrew Coe. 2016. Harper.

Sugar: A Global History by Andrew Smith. 2015. Reaktion Books.

Food Memoirs

The Cooking Gene: A Journey Through African American Culinary History in the Old South by Michael W. Twitty. 2017. Amistad.

Eating My Words: An Appetite for Life by Mimi Sheraton. 2004. William Morrow.

My Kitchen Wars: A Memoir by Betty Fussell. 2009. Bison Books.

My Life in France by Julia Child and Alex Prud'homme. 2007. Knopf Doubleday Publishing Group.

Tender at the Bone: Growing Up at the Table by Ruth Reichl. 2010. Random House Trade Paperback.

Bibliography

Butler J. Protecting your recipes: What culinary professionals want to know. Guide through the Legal Jungle website. January 2018. Accessed May 3, 2021. guidethroughthelegaljungleblog.com/2018/01/protecting-your-recipes.html

Chen E, Huang E, Dorsey J. Understanding cultural appropriation. Studio Atao website. February 15, 2021. Accessed June 2, 2021. studioatao.org/post/understanding-cultural-appropriation

Godbole N. How to avoid cultural appropriation in food writing. Dianne Jacob Will Write for Food website. April 27, 2021. Accessed June 2, 2021. diannej.com/2021/how-to-avoid-cultural-appropriation-in-food-writing

Jacob D. *Will Write for Food: Pursue Your Passion and Bring Home the Dough Writing Recipes, Cookbooks, Blogs, and More.* Hachette Go; 2021.

Lebovitz D. Recipe attribution. David Lebovitz website. April 10, 2014. Accessed May 3, 2021. davidlebovitz.com/recipe-attribution

Literary Works. US Copyright Office website. Accessed May 3, 2021. copyright.gov/registration/literary-works/index.html

Nosrat S. *Salt, Fat, Acid, Heat: Mastering the Elements of Good Cooking.* Simon & Schuster; 2017.

Ostmann BG, Baker JL. *The Recipe Writers Handbook.* Wiley; 2001.

Salt Types and Measurements. Cook's Illustrated website. Accessed May 3, 2021. cooksillustrated.com/how_tos/5799-salt-types-and-measurements

Small D. How does the way food looks or its smell influence taste? *Scientific American* website. April 2008. Accessed July 29, 2020. scientificamerican.com/article/experts-how-does-sight-smell-affect-taste

Spence, C. Just how much of what we taste derives from the sense of smell? *Flavour.* 2015;4:30.

What does copyright protect? US Copyright Office website. Accessed May 3, 2021. copyright.gov/help/faq/faq-protect.html

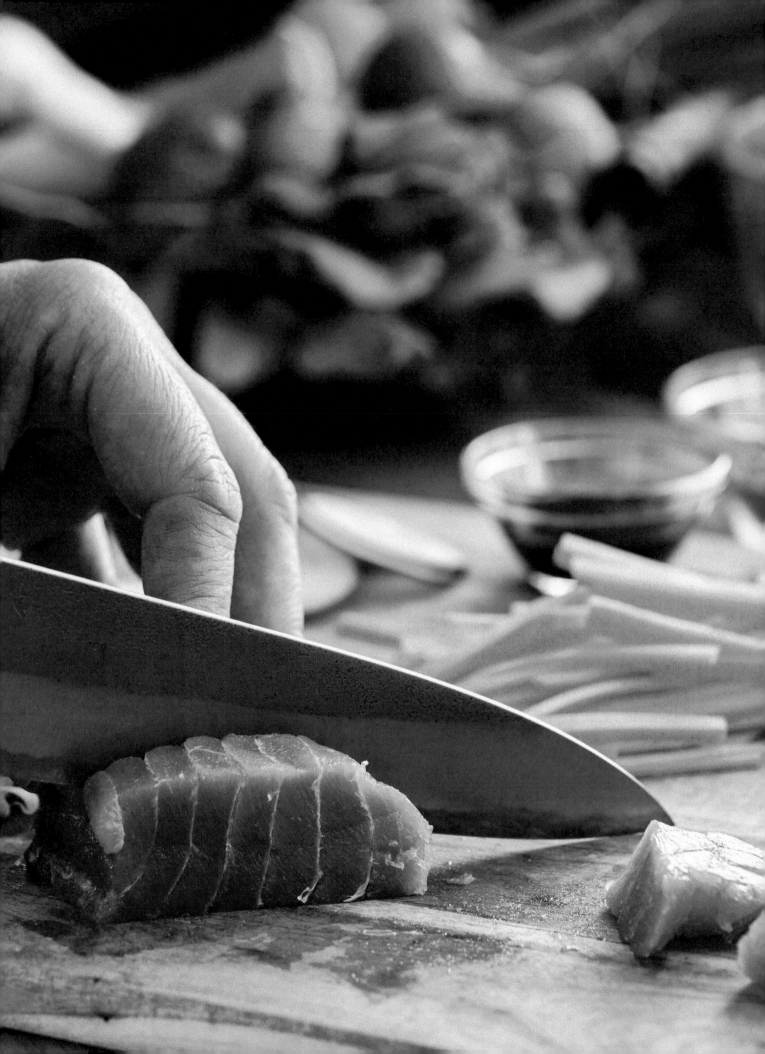

Chapter 2
Developing Recipes for Health and Wellness

IN THIS CHAPTER, LEARN ABOUT:

- How to use food-based guidelines, including the food label, for health- and wellness-focused recipe development

- Using nutrient criteria when developing health-focused recipes

- Techniques and tips for developing health-focused recipes

- Religious dietary considerations in recipe development

Consumers seeking health benefits from their food—whether their focus is on weight loss, heart health, digestive health, improved energy, or more—are driving increased demand for food products and recipes that appeal to a healthy lifestyle. Most food dishes can fit into a healthy diet, so every recipe you create does not have to be low in calories, saturated fat, added sugars, or sodium. It's the overall eating pattern that matters, whether foods are eaten in a balanced way throughout the day, over several days, or even over a week. So, why alter a dish that tastes delicious just as it is? For some, modified recipes are needed to treat a diet-related health condition or to reduce the risk of developing a chronic health problem linked to diet, such as obesity, high blood pressure, cardiovascular disease, or diabetes.

It's important to note that developing health-focused recipes for people with chronic illness or health conditions is an area of specialty within recipe development. It requires bridging knowledge in nutrition and food science with knowledge in the culinary arts as well as with cultural food traditions and preferences. Nutrition and culinary expertise are needed to translate the latest scientific evidence into recipes that people can enjoy preparing and eating. For this reason, it is necessary to have a thorough understanding of ingredients, cooking techniques and how to modify them, and how to read and use Nutrition Facts labels when developing recipes. Refer to Chapters 3 to 6 for information on recipe development for plant-based and therapeutic diets.

Quick Tip

"The science around guidelines for healthy eating will continue to evolve as new nutrition research on diet and health becomes available. For example, although there are conflicting studies on the effects of saturated fat on cardiovascular health, the totality of the evidence still points to the net benefit of reducing saturated fat intake." — *Scientific Report of the 2020 Dietary Guidelines Advisory Committee* (dietaryguidelines.gov/2020-advisory-committee-report)

Guidance for Developing Health- and Wellness-Focused Recipes

When developing health-focused recipes—whether they are intended for foodservice establishments, food companies, print or digital publications, or social media posts—using established guidelines or criteria can back up any references you make to health or nutrition. Food-based guidelines like the Dietary Guidelines for Americans; the American Heart Association (AHA) Dietary Guidance; the National Heart, Lung, and Blood Institute Dietary Approaches to Stop Hypertension (DASH) eating plan; and the Oldways' Mediterranean Diet Pyramid provide context-specific recommendations with a goal of promoting overall health and preventing chronic disease. All guidelines are based on sound evidence and can be referenced when developing recipes.

The specific guidelines used for recipe development will depend on the intended use and goals of the recipe. Most nutrition guidelines for healthy individuals consistently recommend consuming a variety of plant-based foods, with limits placed on added sugars, sodium, and saturated fats.

Dietary Guidelines for Americans

The *Dietary Guidelines for Americans*, first published in 1980 and updated every 5 years, provides food-based recommendations to promote health, helps prevent diet-related chronic diseases, and helps consumers meet their nutrient needs. The Dietary Guidelines are designed for use by health professionals and policymakers for outreach to the general public. They provide a foundation for federal food, nutrition, and health policies and programs, but they are not intended for the treatment of disease. While the Dietary Guidelines focus on overall healthy eating patterns, they can also serve as a general guide for developing health-focused recipes.

See the four Key Recommendations from the *Dietary Guidelines for Americans, 2020–2025* on the next page for more information.

KEY RECOMMENDATIONS FROM THE
DIETARY GUIDELINES FOR AMERICANS, 2020–2025

1. Follow a healthy eating pattern at every life stage.
2. Customize and enjoy nutrient-dense food and beverage choices to reflect personal preferences, cultural traditions, and budgetary considerations.
3. Focus on meeting food-group needs with nutrient-dense foods and beverages and stay within calorie limits. The core elements that make up a healthy dietary pattern include:

   - **Vegetables** of all types, including dark green, red, and orange vegetables; beans, peas, and lentils; starchy vegetables; and other types
   - **Fruits**, especially whole
   - **Grains**, at least half of which are whole grains
   - **Dairy**, including nonfat or low-fat milk, yogurts, and cheeses; alternatives include lactose-free versions and fortified soy beverages and yogurts
   - **Protein foods**, including lean meats, poultry, and eggs; seafood; beans, peas, and lentils; and nuts, seeds, and soy products. Include a variety of plant- and animal-based sources. (Limit intake of higher-fat and processed meats.)
   - **Oils**, including vegetable oils and oils found in foods, such as seafood and nuts

4. Limit intake of alcoholic beverages as well as foods and beverages that are higher in added sugars, saturated fat, and sodium.

   - **Added sugars:** Starting at age 2, fewer than 10% of the total calories consumed per day should come from added sugars. Limit intake of sugar-sweetened foods and beverages. Those younger than age 2 should avoid foods and beverages with added sugars altogether. Added sugars are of particular concern for adults because exceeding limits contributes to excess calorie intake.
   - **Saturated fat:** Starting at age 2, fewer than 10% of the total calories consumed per day should come from saturated fat to support heart-healthy eating. Substitute healthier choices, such as polyunsaturated and monounsaturated fats, for less healthy options such as saturated fats.
   - **Sodium:** For people age 14 and older, the limit for sodium consumption per day is 2,300 milligrams; it is even less for people younger than 14. A reduced dietary intake of sodium is a modifiable risk factor that can help improve blood pressure control and reduce risk of hypertension.
   - **Alcoholic beverages:** Adults of legal age can choose not to drink at all or to drink in moderation by limiting their intake to two or fewer drinks per day for men and no more than one drink per day for women. Some adults, such as people who are pregnant, should not drink alcohol.

US Department of Agriculture's MyPlate

This visual representation of the recommendations of the *Dietary Guidelines for Americans* indicates the variety and approximate proportions of the food groups that make up a healthy meal.

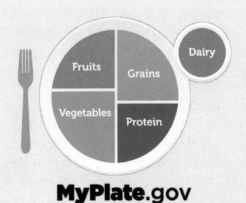

MyPlate.gov

Adapted from dietaryguidelines.gov

ARE PLANT-BASED MILKS INCLUDED IN THE DAIRY GROUP?

Plant-based "milks" are nondairy, alternative milk beverages made from plant ingredients, such as rice, soy, nuts or seeds (e.g., almond, hemp, flax), coconut, oats, peas, or blends of these ingredients. Many plant-based milks come in both sweetened and unsweetened varieties. Fortified soy milk and soy yogurt are included as part of MyPlate's Dairy Group because their nutrient content is similar to dairy milk and yogurt when they include added calcium and vitamins A and D. Other plant-based products sold as "milk" may contain added calcium and other nutrients, but they typically lack some of the nutrients found in dairy milk and yogurt and therefore are not included as part of the MyPlate Dairy Group. See page 74 for more on plant-based milks.

WHAT DOES NUTRIENT-DENSE MEAN?

The basic concept of nutrient density refers to the relative amounts of nutrients compared to the number of calories provided in foods. According to the Dietary Guidelines, nutrient-dense foods provide nutrients and other healthful substances, such as vitamins, minerals, dietary fiber, protein, and unsaturated fats. They also have little or no sugars, saturated fat, and sodium. Examples include beans, peas, nuts, seeds, eggs, fruits, vegetables, whole grains, lean meats, poultry without skin, seafood, fish, and nonfat and low-fat dairy products. Recipes that use more nutrient-dense foods and that are prepared without excessive saturated fats, added sugars, and sodium can provide beneficial nutrients without excess calories.

The DASH Eating Plan

The National Heart, Lung, and Blood Institute's DASH eating plan is a flexible, balanced, and heart-healthy eating plan that emphasizes vegetables, fruits, and whole grains, along with moderate amounts of low-fat dairy foods, fish, poultry, and nuts. The standard DASH eating plan is consistent with the Dietary Guidelines sodium recommendation of no more than 2,300 milligrams per day; a lower sodium version of the DASH diet sets the maximum at 1,500 milligrams per day. Daily and weekly menus for the DASH eating plan provide recommended servings from the food groups at various calorie levels.

Overall, the DASH eating plan emphasizes the following:

- vegetables, fruits, and whole grains
- nonfat or low-fat dairy products, fish, poultry, beans, nuts, and vegetable oils
- limiting foods that are high in saturated fat, such as fatty meats, full-fat dairy products, and tropical oils, such as coconut, palm kernel, and palm oils
- limiting sugar-sweetened beverages and sweets

American Heart Association
Eating Patterns to Promote Cardiovascular Health

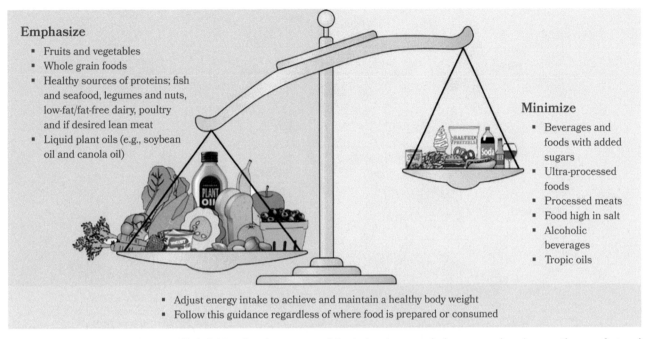

Emphasize

- Fruits and vegetables
- Whole grain foods
- Healthy sources of proteins; fish and seafood, legumes and nuts, low-fat/fat-free dairy, poultry and if desired lean meat
- Liquid plant oils (e.g., soybean oil and canola oil)

Minimize

- Beverages and foods with added sugars
- Ultra-processed foods
- Processed meats
- Food high in salt
- Alcoholic beverages
- Tropic oils

- Adjust energy intake to achieve and maintain a healthy body weight
- Follow this guidance regardless of where food is prepared or consumed

Note: There is no commonly accepted definition for ultra-processed foods but, in general, they are made using mostly manufactured ingredients and tend to be low in nutrients and higher in calories.

Adapted with permission from Lichtenstein AH, Appel LJ, Vadiveloo M, et al. Dietary guidance to improve cardiovascular health: a scientific statement from the American Heart Association. *Circulation.* 2021;144(23):e472-e487.

The American Heart Association Dietary Guidance

The AHA dietary guidance to improve cardiovascular health emphasizes the importance of dietary patterns beyond individual foods or nutrients. These guidelines reinforce the Dietary Guidelines for Americans, with added emphasis on consuming most protein from plants and minimizing ultra-processed foods. The AHA guidance also touches on the challenges in society that often make following their recommendations so difficult and ends with the statement that, "Creating an environment that facilitates, rather than impedes, adherence to heart-healthy dietary patterns among all individuals is a public health imperative."

The Mediterranean Diet

The principles of the Mediterranean diet reflect a style of eating based on the cuisines of Greece, Italy, and other countries that surround the Mediterranean Sea.

These principles include the following:

- plant-based foods as the foundation of the daily diet: whole grains, fruits, vegetables, beans, herbs, spices, and nuts
- olive oil as the main source of fat
- fish and seafood at least twice per week
- moderate portions of nonfat or low-fat dairy foods, eggs, and occasional poultry
- infrequent servings of red meats and sweets

The Mediterranean Diet Pyramid was first developed in 1993 by Oldways, a food and nutrition nonprofit organization, as an alternative to the original US Department of Agriculture (USDA) food guide pyramid. Oldways promotes "old ways" of eating that celebrate traditional diets rooted in wholesome and seasonal ingredients. Over the years, Oldways has added more food pyramids, including the African Heritage Diet, the Latin American Diet, the Asian Diet, and the Vegetarian/Vegan Diet. All of these heritage-based diet pyramids focus on vegetables, fruits, whole grains, dry beans and peas, nuts, seeds, herbs, spices, and other plant-based foods, and they respect culturally diverse recipes, flavor pairings, and ingredients.

The Mediterranean Diet Pyramid

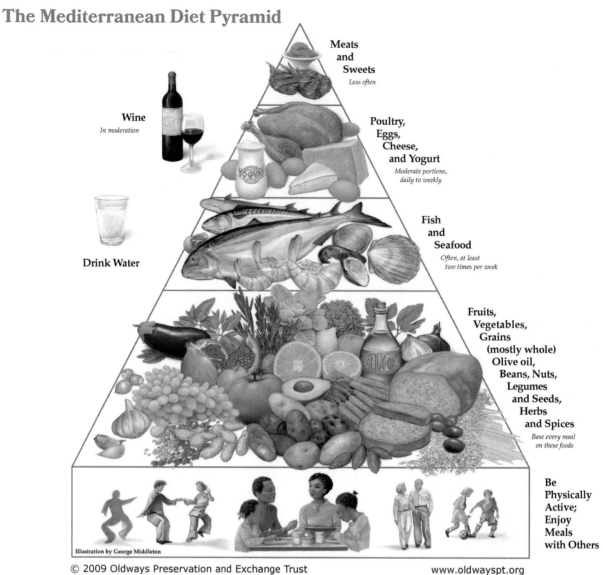

Meats and Sweets
Less often

Poultry, Eggs, Cheese, and Yogurt
Moderate portions, daily to weekly

Fish and Seafood
Often, at least two times per week

Wine
In moderation

Drink Water

Fruits, Vegetables, Grains (mostly whole) Olive oil, Beans, Nuts, Legumes and Seeds, Herbs and Spices
Base every meal on these foods

Be Physically Active; Enjoy Meals with Others

Illustration by George Middleton

WHAT IS A FLEXITARIAN DIET?

A flexitarian diet is a style of eating that is mostly vegetarian but allows for the flexibility of including meats occasionally. Sometimes referred to as semivegetarian, the flexitarian diet is similar to other dietary guidelines that recommend a mostly plant-based diet for overall health and focuses on adding more plants to the diet instead of eliminating animal sources. See Chapter 3 for more on plant-based recipe development.

Using Nutrient Parameters to Develop Health-Focused Recipes

No universal nutrient criteria exist for classifying a recipe as "healthy." Some magazines, websites, and other health organizations create their own recipe nutrient criteria using nutrition and health guidelines to classify recipes as healthy. Of these, some share their criteria and others consider their criteria to be proprietary. Depending on the recipes you are developing, consider developing your own specific nutrition parameters to meet recipe goals and document them clearly. Alternatively, consult other published criteria.

EATINGWELL NUTRIENT CRITERIA FOR A "HEALTHY" RECIPE

Category	Calories	Sodium (mg)
Entree	≤500	≤480
Combination meals	≤750	≤750
Side dishes	≤250	≤360
Muffins and breads	≤250	≤360
Desserts	≤300	≤360
Dips and salsas	≤100	≤140
Sauces	≤100	≤240
Salad dressings	≤100	≤140
Drinks	≤250	≤140
Appetizers	≤250	≤360

Source: Nutrition parameters and health considerations by *EatingWell:* eatingwell.com/our-food-and-nutrition
-philosophy-6746110

For example, *EatingWell* outlines its own criteria that the recipes it publishes must meet to be considered "healthy." *EatingWell* recipes start with mainly nutrient-rich, unprocessed, and seasonal whole food ingredients and are developed factoring in specific target goals for calories and sodium. Consider using these nutrient targets when developing health- and wellness-focused recipes. *EatingWell*'s team of registered dietitians also has created specific nutrient targets for special diets including heart-healthy, diabetes appropriate, and more.

Another example is the AHA Heart-Check Recipe Certification Program, which provides category-specific qualitative and nutrient requirements a recipe must meet to be certified as healthy. A nutrient analysis of each recipe must be submitted for review, including calories, sodium, saturated fat, added sugars, *trans* fats, and omega-3 fatty acids (for fish entrées). The American Heart Association Heart-Check Criteria for a Health Recipe can be a useful reference when developing recipes that promote heart health. Check the AHA's website for qualitative food dish descriptions for recipe categories.

AMERICAN HEART ASSOCIATION HEART-CHECK CRITERIA FOR A HEALTHY RECIPE

Category	Per serving amounts*			
	Calories	Saturated fat (grams)	Sodium (milligrams)	Added sugars (teaspoons)
Appetizers, soups, salads (with salad dressing), side dishes, muffins/quick breads, yeast breads	≤250	≤2 if they do not contain meats/fish/seafood ≤3 if they contain meats/fish/seafood	≤240	≤2
Entrées: One-dish entrées (e.g., stir-fry, casserole), entrée salads, entrée soups	≤500	≤3.5	≤600	≤2
Entrées: Meats, poultry, and seafood	≤350	≤3 for beef, poultry, pork, etc. ≤4 for fish or seafood ≤5 for fish entrées containing 500 milligrams omega-3 fatty acids	≤360	≤2
Desserts	≤200	≤2	≤240	≤2

* Criteria for *trans* fat for each category: <0.5 grams *trans* fatty acid and no partially hydrogenated oils (PHOs) or ingredient products that contain PHOs

Source: Heart-check recipe certification program nutrition requirements by American Heart Association website: heart.org/en/healthy-living/company
-collaboration/heart-check-certification/heart-check-certified-recipes/heart-check-recipe-certification-program-nutrition-requirements

Using the Food Label in Recipe Development

Another framework to consider when developing health- and wellness-focused recipes is the food label and the Food and Drug Administration (FDA) food-labeling guidelines for nutrient and health claims.

The Ingredient List

The ingredient list and Nutrition Facts label provided on a product food label are useful tools to help you choose ingredients for health-focused recipe development and modification. The ingredient list provides information about what is included in a product as well as an overall sense of an ingredient's contribution by amount, as the ingredients are listed in descending order by weight. So, scanning the first several ingredients of an ingredient list on a product's package gives you an idea of how much of each ingredient is contained in the product (generally, the first three ingredients in the list account for the largest portion).

It can be helpful to examine ingredient lists closely when developing specific types of recipes, such as one that requires "no added sugars." Be aware that different terms may be used to describe similar ingredients. For example, added sugars can be listed by many names—from barley malt syrup to cane juice—so it's important to know other names for key ingredients. See page 111 for more information on added sugars.

The ingredient list is also useful for identifying potential allergens quickly, easily, and accurately—critical for allergy-free recipe development. See Chapter 6 for information on recipe development for food allergies and intolerances.

The Nutrition Facts Label

The Nutrition Facts label is an equally useful tool for health-focused recipe development. A closer look at the label is helpful when developing recipes where amounts of calories, sodium, added sugars, fat, carbohydrate, protein, dietary fiber, and select vitamins and minerals matter in the final recipe. Once you know the estimated amount of a product or ingredient needed in a recipe, you can quickly calculate how much a specific nutrient will contribute, which can serve as a guide to ensure the nutrition parameters are met.

For example, consider a recipe that contains 3 tablespoons of soy sauce, which alone contributes 2,760 milligrams of sodium to the dish's sodium content. If the recipe serves four, then that single ingredient contributes 690 milligrams of sodium per serving. If the recipe must meet sodium requirements, extra attention to the recipe's remaining ingredients is critical. The recipe's final nutrition analysis will provide this information as well (see Chapter 9) but consulting the Nutrition Facts label first when evaluating ingredients can help even before recipe development begins.

How to Read a Nutrition Facts Label

The Daily Values (DVs) are the recommended amounts of nutrients to consume or not to exceed each day. The amounts of carbohydrates (including sugars), fats, and protein are based on a daily intake of 2,000 calories. See Daily Values: FDA Recommended Daily Amounts or Limits on the next page.

Nutrition Facts

(1) 8 servings per container
Serving size 2/3 cup (55g)

Amount Per Serving
Calories 230

% Daily Value*

(2)
Total Fat 8g		10%
Saturated Fat 1g		5%
Trans Fat 0g		
Cholesterol 0mg		0%
Sodium 160mg		7%
Total Carbohydrate 37g		13%
Dietary Fiber 4g		14%
Total Sugars 12g		
Includes 10g Added Sugars		20%
Protein 3g		

(3)

Vitamin D 2mcg	10%
Calcium 260mg	20%
Iron 8mg	45%
Potassium 235mg	6%

(4)

*The % Daily Value (DV) tells you how much a nutrient in a serving of food contributes to a daily diet. 2,000 calories a day is used for general nutrition advice.

(1) Start here.

(2) Watch or limit these nutrients when developing health-focused recipes.

"Total Sugars" includes naturally occurring and added sugars.

(3) Get enough of these nutrients.

(4) Take note of Daily Values:
 • Nutrient is low: DV is 5% or less
 • Nutrient is high: DV is 20%

DAILY VALUES: FDA RECOMMENDED DAILY AMOUNTS OR LIMITS

Daily Values for fats, carbohydrates, sugars, and protein are based on a 2,000-calorie diet. Other Daily Values are the amounts of a nutrient considered to be sufficient to meet the requirements of most healthy individuals (adults and children 4 years and older).

Nutrient

Mandatory nutrients on label	Daily Value (DV)
Total fat*	78 grams
Saturated fat*	20 grams
Cholesterol*	300 milligrams
Sodium*	2,300 milligrams
Total carbohydrate*	275 grams
Dietary fiber	28 grams
Total sugars	N/A (amount included in total carbohydrate; total sugars is naturally occurring and added sugars)
Added sugars*	50 grams
Protein	50 grams
Calcium	1,300 milligrams
Iron	18 milligrams
Vitamin D	20 micrograms
Potassium	4,700 milligrams

*These Daily Values are recommended limits.

Nutrient

Voluntary nutrients on label	Daily Value (DV)
Vitamin A	900 micrograms retinol activity equivalents (RAE)
Vitamin E	15 milligrams alpha-tocopherol
Vitamin K	120 micrograms
Thiamin	1.2 milligrams
Riboflavin	1.3 milligrams
Niacin	16 milligrams NE (niacin equivalents)
Vitamin B6	1.7 milligrams
Folate	400 micrograms DFE (Dietary Folate Equivalents)
Vitamin B12	2.4 micrograms
Biotin	30 micrograms
Pantothenic acid	5 milligrams
Magnesium	420 milligrams
Phosphorus	1,250 milligrams
Iodine	150 micrograms
Manganese	2.3 milligrams
Zinc	11 milligrams
Selenium	55 micrograms
Copper	0.9 milligrams
Chromium	35 micrograms
Molybdenum	45 micrograms
Chloride	2,300 milligrams
Choline	550 milligrams

Labeling Guidelines for Nutrient and Health Claims

The FDA's food labeling guidelines for nutrient and health claims are a helpful reference when developing recipes with specific nutrient claims or requirements. Published recipes are not required to follow labeling guidelines, but using the labeling requirements as a guideline provides credibility when making any kind of claim about a recipe you develop. FDA rules and laws define the use of these types of label claims.

Nutrient content claims either describe the level of a nutrient in a food using terms such as *low* or *high* or compare the level of a nutrient in a food to that of another food using such terms as *reduced* or *light*. See Food and Drug Administration Labeling Requirements for Nutrient Content Claims.

Health claims characterize a relationship between a substance (a specific food component or a specific food) and a disease or health-related condition—for example, sodium and high blood pressure. These claims are supported by scientific evidence, and each

FOOD AND DRUG ADMINISTRATION LABELING REQUIREMENTS FOR NUTRIENT CONTENT CLAIMS

Nutrient content claim	Requirement
Calories	
Low calorie	40 or fewer calories per serving
Reduced calorie	At least 25% less than reference amount per serving
Fat	
Nonfat	Less than 0.5 grams per serving
Low fat	3 grams or less per serving
Reduced fat	At least 25% less fat than reference amount per serving
Low saturated fat	1 gram or less saturated fat and no more than 15% of calories from saturated fat per serving
Reduced saturated fat	At least 25% or less saturated fat per serving
Light	At least 50% or less total fat per serving
Lean (seafood/poultry/ meats)	Less than 10 grams total fat, 4.5 grams or less saturated fat, and less than 95 milligrams cholesterol per 100 milligrams (about 3.5 ounces)
Extra lean (seafood/poultry/ meats)	Less than 5 grams total fat, 2 grams saturated fat, and 95 milligrams cholesterol per 100 milligrams (about 3.5 ounces)
Sugars	
Sugar free	Less than 0.5 grams per serving
Low sugar	Not defined by US Food and Drug Administration (FDA)
Lightly sweetened	Not defined by FDA
Reduced sugar	At least 25% less sugar than reference amount per serving
No sugar added	The terms "no added sugars" and "without added sugars" are allowed if no sugar or sugar-containing ingredients are added during processing. Products without added sugar can contain naturally occurring sugar.

BOX CONTINUES >

claim has specific requirements for foods or nutrient amounts depending on the claim. See Authorized Health Claims for Food Labels on page 38 for a list of approved health claims.

Structure or function claims describe the role of a nutrient or functional component in affecting or maintaining normal body structure or function or general well-being—for example, "calcium builds strong bones." These types of statements may be used only on the labels of dietary supplements or conventional foods when they meet specific requirements.

Quick Tip

"The terms 'superfoods' or 'functional foods' are unregulated and are mostly used as marketing terms. If these claims are used to promote ingredients or foods that offer benefits beyond their nutritional value, be aware that these have no defined meaning."
—Roberta L. Duyff, MS, RDN, food and nutrition consultant and author, *Academy of Nutrition and Dietetics Complete Food & Nutrition Guide*

FOOD AND DRUG ADMINISTRATION LABELING REQUIREMENTS FOR NUTRIENT CONTENT CLAIMS (CONTINUED)

Sodium

Sodium free	Less than 5 milligrams per serving
Low sodium	140 milligrams or less per serving
Reduced sodium	At least 25% less sodium than reference amount per serving
Light in sodium/lightly salted	At least 50% or less sodium per serving
Unsalted/no-salt-added	No salt is added during processing—but these products may not be salt/sodium-free unless stated

Other

"Good" source of a nutrient, or "contains" or "provides"	10% to 19% Daily Value per serving
"High," "rich," or "excellent" source of a nutrient	20% or more Daily Value per serving
Healthy	Under the *proposed rule* (as of September 2022), raw whole fruits and vegetables automatically qualify for the healthy claim. Other foods eligible for this claim must meet the following requirements: • Healthy foods must contain a minimum amount of food from at least one food group (e.g., fruit, vegetables, grains, dairy, protein foods, and oils); referred to as a "food group equivalent." • Healthy foods must adhere to upper limits for added sugars, sodium, and saturated fat. The limits vary depending on the food and are based on a percentage of the Daily Value (DV). Examples of requirements: • **Grain-based products:** ¾-ounce whole grain equivalent and limits of 2.5 grams added sugar (5% DV), 230 milligrams sodium (10% DV), 1 gram saturated fat (5% DV) • **Dairy food products:** ¾-cup equivalent and limits of 2.5 grams added sugar (5% DV), 230 milligrams sodium (10% DV), 2 grams saturated fat (10% DV) • **Fruit and vegetable products:** ½-cup equivalent and limits of 0 grams added sugar (0% DV), 230 milligrams sodium (10% DV), 1 gram saturated fat (5% DV) • **Meat and seafood products:** 1½-ounce and 1-ounce equivalents, respectively, and limits of 0 grams added sugar (0% DV), 230 milligrams sodium (10% DV), 2 grams saturated fat (10% DV) • **Mixed products, main dish products, and meal products:** require varying food group equivalents, and upper limits for added sugars, sodium, and saturated fat are based on the food groups included

To date, 12 health claims have been authorized by the US Food and Drug Administration to describe a relationship between a food or food component and a reduced risk of a disease or health-related condition.

- Fruits and vegetables *and* cancer
- Fiber-containing grain products, fruits, and vegetables *and* cancer
- Dietary lipids (fat) *and* cancer
- Saturated fat and cholesterol *and* coronary heart disease
- Soy protein *and* coronary heart disease

- Plant stanols/sterols *and* coronary heart disease
- Soluble fiber from certain foods *and* coronary heart disease
- Fruits, vegetables, and grain products that contain fiber and particularly soluble fiber *and* coronary heart disease
- Calcium and vitamin D *and* osteoporosis
- Sodium *and* hypertension
- Noncariogenic carbohydrate sweeteners (e.g., sugar alcohols) *and* dental caries
- Folic acid *and* neural tube defects

Developing Recipes with the Environment in Mind

The term *sustainability* is frequently used in discussions regarding food, health, and the environment, but its intended meaning can vary widely. For some, the term refers exclusively to environmental objectives or to particular aspects of environmental concerns, such as climate change (greenhouse gas emissions), land use, water use, energy use, or biodiversity loss. For others, it encompasses social and economic dimensions, including fair working conditions for farm laborers and food system workers, humane conditions for animals involved in food production, and the economic viability of small food production businesses.

For many consumers, following a sustainable diet requires more transparency throughout the supply chain so that they can understand where food comes from and decide whether its origins meet their own ethical and environmental demands. **Recipe developers should acknowledge the 3 R's of sustainability (reduce, reuse, and recycle) in their recipe development and writing.** Sustainable cooking allows home cooks to reduce the negative impact of their efforts on animals, other people, and the environment. Examples may include repurposing vegetable parts that might typically be thrown away (such as broccoli and cauliflower stems), reusing a roasted chicken carcass and vegetable trimmings to make a stock, or reducing the amount of meat in a recipe. See Resources Related to Sustainability and the Environment for more information when developing recipes that are healthy for both people and planet.

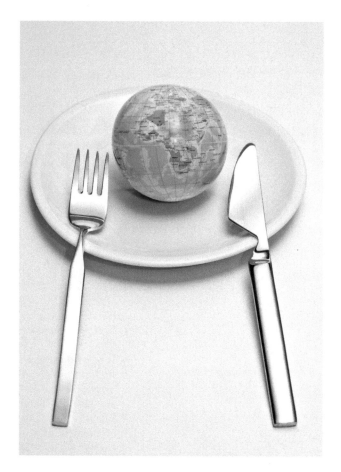

RESOURCES RELATED TO SUSTAINABILITY AND THE ENVIRONMENT

The State of America's Wasted Food & Opportunities to Make a Difference (2016): This report from the Academy of Nutrition and Dietetics Foundation Future of Food initiative highlights where food waste can potentially occur throughout the food supply chain, the environmental and economic impact of food waste, and opportunity areas for food and nutrition professionals to help reduce food waste.
eatrightfoundation.org/wp-content/uploads/2016/09/The-State-of-Americas-Food-Waste-Report.pdf

Healthy Diets From Sustainable Food Systems: Food, Planet, Health (2019): This report from the EAT Lancet Commission calls for a global shift toward healthy dietary patterns, large reductions in food loss and waste, and significant improvements in food production practices. With some similarities to other guidelines, the Planetary Health Diet recommends an optimal caloric intake and a diet that consists largely of a diversity of plant-based foods, low amounts of animal source foods, unsaturated rather than saturated fats, and limited amounts of refined grains, highly processed foods, and added sugars.
eatforum.org/content/uploads/2019/01/EAT-Lancet_Commission_Summary_Report.pdf

Plates, Pyramids, Planet: Developments in National Healthy and Sustainable Dietary Guidelines: A State of Play Assessment (2016): This joint publication of the Food and Agriculture Organization (FAO) and the Food Climate Research Network (FCRN) provides an in-depth review of how countries can incorporate sustainability into their food-based dietary guidelines, including a focus on seasonal and local foods, reduction of food waste, crop rotation, consumption of fish from sustainable stocks, and more.
fao.org/3/I5640E/i5640e.pdf

Food and Climate Change Infoguide (2021): This guide published by Columbia University's Center on Global Energy Policy provides background on the impact of the food system on climate change and vice versa. It includes strategies for reducing emissions from the food system and improving the resilience of the food system against climate change.
energypolicy.columbia.edu/sites/default/files/pictures/FoodandClimate-Infoguide-CGEP_v2G.pdf

Feed the Future: This US government-funded global hunger and food security initiative addresses the root causes of poverty, hunger, and malnutrition and helps people learn how to feed themselves while creating opportunities within agriculture sectors. The website includes a food security innovation center, annual progress reports, and AgriLinks, an online hub where professionals can share knowledge about food security and agriculture.
feedthefuture.gov

FoodPrint: This nonprofit organization is dedicated to research and education on food production practices. Its website includes resources on food labeling and the environment, as well as guidelines for sustainable shopping, dining, and cooking.
foodprint.org

Menus of Change: This website, a combined effort by the Culinary Institute of America and the Harvard T.H. Chan School of Public Health, includes principles and guidelines for creating menus that are tasty, healthy, and sustainable. Its resources, which are free to use, encourage foodservice operations to become more transparent and to use more plant-based foods.
menusofchange.org

Marketing Terms Related to Farming Practices, Animal Care, and Food Processing

Marketing claims related to how a food is grown or raised, produced, and processed can be confusing. More food companies are adding information about health and production methods to their packaging, a move that has been driven by consumer concerns for personal health, animal welfare, and environmental impact. Many of these terms are not regulated and have no standard definition. As a food professional, you must be cautious about using health associated buzzwords or unclear terms to define recipe qualities. If you use these terms with a recipe, you should provide education or further explanation, if possible.

When developing customized recipe development standards, document a proposed definition of a term you will use and use it consistently. See Glossary of Selected Food-Related Marketing Terms for examples of the complexity of certain terms and certifications that often appear on food products. Some are regulated by government agencies or third-party verification, but many others lack clear standards, verification processes, or independent oversight, allowing conditions and practices to vary widely.

GLOSSARY OF SELECTED FOOD-RELATED MARKETING TERMS

Artisanal	This unregulated term implies that products are made by hand in small batches, but the term is sometimes used by large manufacturers.
Cage free	Eggs labeled as cage free that also carry a US Department of Agriculture (USDA) grade must be produced by hens housed in a way that allows them unlimited access to food and water and freedom to roam indoors during the laying cycle. However, not all cage-free eggs are graded by USDA, so living conditions for these eggs are not verified by USDA through onsite farm visits.
Clean label/clean food	This unregulated term has no single definition. In general, the term *clean* implies that foods are close to their natural state, have few additional ingredients, and are made without artificial color or flavors and chemical-sounding ingredients. The use of *clean* might also refer to issues regarding animal welfare, organic status (not genetically modified [GMO]/bioengineered and no hormones or antibiotics), sustainability, and a food company's social and business ethics.
Conventionally grown	Conventionally grown foods have few restrictions. Foods with this designation may be grown using technological innovations to improve crop quality and decrease loss due to pests, weeds, and disease. Conventional farms may use GMO seeds, synthetic pesticides or herbicides, synthetic fertilizers, and monocropping. This term is often used as a contrast to organic growing methods. If a food is not labeled organic, assume conventional farming methods were used.
Fair trade	The definition of fair trade has been established by independent certifiers. It indicates that a product has been made according to certain social, environmental, and economic standards, including just compensation and fair treatment for farmers and workers, as well as investment in community development and environmental sustainability. It is typically referenced on products originating from less-developed countries, such as coffee, tea, chocolate, sugar, and bananas. Producers that sell products bearing the Fair Trade Certified seal may be certified according to Fair Trade USA or Fairtrade International standards (fairtradeamerica.org).
Free range	The term *free range* can be used on any meat or poultry food product by producers that can demonstrate that their animals have had continuous and free access to the outdoors for a significant portion of their lives. For poultry, access to the outdoors must be available, but no amount of outdoor time or space is specified. Eggs labeled as free range that carry a USDA grade must be produced by hens that are able to roam freely in indoor houses and that have access to fresh food and water and continuous access to the outdoors during their laying cycle.

BOX CONTINUES >

Functional	Functional foods are generally considered to provide additional health benefits beyond those covered by basic nutrition. The term itself is unregulated, but the Food and Drug Administration (FDA) regulates the claims that food manufacturers can make about functional foods' nutrient content and effects on disease, health, or body function.
Grass fed	The USDA provides criteria for certification on grass-fed only animals for small and very small livestock producers. In general, the term *grass fed* refers to weaned cattle, sheep, goats, or bison who subsist on a diet of grass and other forage (when fresh grass is unavailable), like clover, hay, or silage. Sometimes the term *pasture raised* is used interchangeably with grass fed, but this term may not indicate whether the animal was exclusively grass fed (e.g., cattle that were grass finished or grain finished).
Grass finished	Some grass-fed animals are grain finished, meaning that they are fed grains for a period of time before slaughter. If grass-fed animals are also grass finished, they were fed exclusively on grasses and forage for their entire lives.
Heirloom	Heirloom crop varieties have been developed by farmers through years of cultivation, selection, and seed saving; they are passed down through generations. Unlike hybrid crops and GMOs, heirloom varieties always produce seed with the same characteristics of the parent plant.
Heritage	Heritage labels are not officially recognized by USDA, but in general, the umbrella term is applied to pure breeds of livestock and poultry with a long history. Modern breeds have been selected for qualities that make them ideal for industrial meat production. Similar to heirloom fruits and vegetables, heritage meats typically have unique characteristics and flavors that make them highly desirable.
Humane	Producers and certifiers may use the unregulated term *humane* to imply that their animals were raised with compassion in a way that minimizes stress and allows them to engage in their natural behaviors. Humane certifications (e.g., Certified Humane and Animal Welfare Approved) have varying standards. These requirements may include nutritious feed, ample fresh water without added antibiotics or hormones, and sufficient space and shelter. The Humane Methods of Slaughter Act is enforced by the USDA's Food Safety and Inspection Service.
Hydroponics	The term *hydroponic* refers to vegetables and fruits (e.g., lettuce, tomatoes, or cucumbers) grown in water, rather than soil, with nutrients washing over the plants' roots.
Keto (e.g., keto certified, keto approved, certified keto)	This designation is undefined and generally describes foods that are low-carb and high in fat, consistent with a ketogenic (keto) diet. There is no universal or evidence-based definition for the term *keto*, so there are no criteria for testing and labeling. Food manufacturers may pay to have a keto certification applied to their product by an organization that establishes its own criteria to certify qualifying foods.
Local	Although no formal definition exists for *local* in food production, the term implies that the food has been grown and sold in a limited geographic area. The distance for local is not defined, but the concept connects farms and consumers through a broader philosophy of environmental sustainability and support for a local economy. While "eat local" is a common recommendation to reduce the carbon footprint of the diet, transportation of food tends to account for only a small amount of the greenhouse gas emissions from food.
Natural*	This USDA-regulated term for meats and poultry indicates that the product has no artificial ingredients or added colors and was not "fundamentally altered" during processing. If this term is used, the label must also explain why the term is used—for example: "no added coloring, minimally processed." The FDA does not have a formal definition for "natural" food products, but its longstanding policy considers the term *natural* to mean "nothing artificial or synthetic (including all color additives regardless of source) has been included in, or has been added to, a food that would not normally be expected to be in that food." However, this policy was not intended to address food production methods or whether the term *natural* should describe any nutritional or other health benefit.

* USDA-regulated term.

BOX CONTINUES >

No hormones* This USDA-regulated term verifies that no hormones were added during the cultivation of the product. Like humans, animals produce naturally occurring hormones. Look for "no added hormones" on labels.

Beef and lamb products: The label "no hormones administered" requires documentation on the part of the producer to show that no hormones were used in raising the animals. Hormone-free labels do not disclose what the animals were fed or if they had access to pasture.

Hogs and poultry: Food producers who raise hogs or poultry are not allowed to administer hormones to their animals. Therefore, the claim "no hormones added" cannot be used on pork or poultry products unless it is followed by a statement that reads, "federal regulations prohibit the use of hormones."

Milk products: The FDA-regulated terms *rBGH-free* or *rBST-free* (referring to recombinant bovine growth hormone and recombinant bovine somatotropin, respectively) may be voluntarily used; however, the guidance specifies inclusion of a disclaimer to clarify that the hormones may be naturally present in the milk product but that the animals were not treated with hormones to increase milk production.

No antibiotics added* This USDA-regulated term requires documentation on the part of the producer to demonstrate that its meats and poultry were raised without antibiotics. "Raised without antibiotics" does not describe the animals' living conditions or any other aspects of their lives. In conventional operations, antibiotics are sometimes given to treat and prevent diseases and to promote growth.

Organic* USDA oversees the National Organic Program, which governs organically produced crops and livestock. Organic meats, poultry, eggs, and dairy products come from animals that are given no antibiotics or growth-promoting hormones and are fed an organically grown diet (e.g., grass, grain, forage).

Organic plant foods are produced without using most conventional pesticides and without fertilizers made with synthetic ingredients or sewage sludge, bioengineering, or ionizing radiation. A US government–approved certifier must inspect the farm to ensure these standards are met. Farmers must practice organic methods for 3 years on a given piece of land before the products grown there can be certified as organic. The term transitional means that the farmland is in the midst of a transition period toward organic certification.

In addition to organic farming, there are USDA standards for organic handling and processing. All organic products must be certified by organizations accredited by the USDA. There are three types of organic claims, each with specific requirements:

- **100% Organic:** 100% organic ingredients and processing, no GMOs, all ingredients comply with National List of Allowed and Prohibited Substances
- **Organic:** 95% certified organic ingredients, no GMOs, non-organic ingredients comply with National List
- **Made with Organic:** must specify which ingredients are organic, at least 70% certified organic ingredients, no GMOs, and non-organic ingredients comply with National List

The USDA Organic seal is only allowed on products that meet the requirements for 100% Organic or Organic.

Paleo (e.g., "paleo certified," "paleo approved," "paleo friendly") There are no national standards for paleolithic (paleo) foods. This higher-protein, grain-free diet emphasizes foods such as lean meats, fish, shellfish, vegetables, eggs, nuts, and berries and eliminates all grains, legumes, dairy, salt, refined fats, sugars, and additives. The designation for paleo may be based on a food company's definition or certification relying on criteria set by a certifying body.

* USDA-regulated term.

BOX CONTINUES >

Pasture raised	This term is unregulated, and no standard definition exists for how much of an animal's life spent on pasture would qualify for the term. In general, a pasture-raised animal spent at least some time outdoors on pasture, feeding on grass or forage. This term is sometimes used by ranchers to differentiate their products from "free-range" products coming from animals raised primarily in a feed yard.
Pesticide free	The unregulated term *pesticide free* (or sometimes *no sprays*) implies that no toxic sprays have been applied to a produce item, at least not directly. Unlike the certified organic label, these claims are not verified by a third party.
Processed/ ultraprocessed	According to the USDA, a *processed* food item refers to a specific food that has undergone a change from its natural state. Some of the processing procedures may include washing, milling, cutting, chopping, heating, pasteurizing, blanching, cooking, canning, freezing, drying, dehydrating, mixing, and packaging. Minimally processed (or unprocessed) foods are only slightly altered primarily for preserving and do not have substantial changes in the nutritional content. Foods that undergo more significant processing, including the addition of sugar, fat, sodium, artificial colors and flavors, and preservatives (e.g., sugary drinks and chips), may be referred to as ultraprocessed.
Regenerative	The term *regenerative* refers to agriculture practices that lead to healthier soil and the production of high-quality, nutrient-dense food. It uses technologies that regenerate and revitalize the soil and the environment, helping to reverse the effects of climate change through carbon drawdown and improvement of the water cycle.
Sustainable	As it relates to food marketing, *sustainable* is an unregulated term. It may be used to describe the production of food or other plant or animal products using farming techniques and practices that help to conserve natural resources and have minimal impact on the environment. Sustainable eating refers to choosing foods that are healthful to the environment, to a healthy life for present and future generations, and to the human body in general.
Vertical farm	Vertical farming is the practice of growing crops indoors in vertically stacked layers without the aid of soil or sunlight. Farming techniques include hydroponics (plants grown without soil by submerging the roots in a liquid solution of water and nutrients), aquaponics (nutrient-rich wastewater from fish tanks is filtered and fed to plants and then recycled back to the fish tanks), and aeroponics (roots of plants are misted with water, nutrients, and oxygen without immersion in soil or water).
Vine- or tree-ripened	These terms refer to fruit that has been allowed to ripen on a vine or tree. Many fruits that are shipped long distances are picked while still unripe and firm and later treated with ethylene gas at the point of distribution to "ripen" and soften them.
Whole food	There is no regulatory definition of a whole food. *Whole foods* generally refer to foods that are not processed or refined and do not have any added ingredients. By most definitions, whole foods include fresh produce, dairy, whole grains, meats, and fish—any food that appears close to its original form with minimal processing.

* USDA-regulated term.

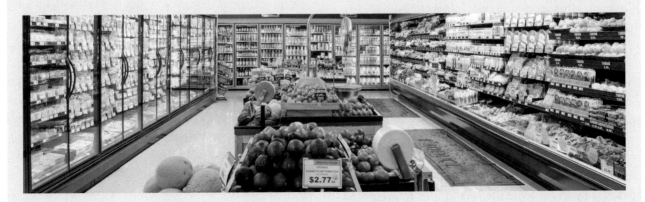

Methods for Developing Health- and Wellness- Focused Recipes

Once the type of recipe and the target audience is determined, consider using one of these ways to approach the recipe's health-focused modification or development:

- Adjust the serving size or ingredient proportions.
- Modify the ingredients.
- Alter the cooking technique.
- Modify the ingredients and the cooking technique.

These techniques can also be applied to recipe development for specific diets as addressed in Chapters 3 to 6.

Adjust the Serving Size or Ingredient Proportions

Many recipes can meet nutrition guidelines without requiring an ingredient modification or substitution. As an example, a simply prepared meal of grilled fish, vegetables, and rice can meet general guidelines for "healthy" and other therapeutic diets, such as low sodium or low in saturated fat. If a recipe doesn't meet the nutrition parameters being used, however, the first step is to look at the recipe's serving size. A nutrition analysis can confirm which nutrients do not meet the parameters.

Adjusting the recipe serving size is one method to modify a recipe. This alone may solve the issue. However, it's important to be realistic about serving size. Consumers may find a very small portion size to be impractical and unsatisfying—not an indicator of a successful recipe. It's also important to ensure that the serving size is very specific (e.g., listing the number of ounces or cups per serving), as people who are following a special diet often need this information. This detail is necessary for an accurate nutrition analysis and will also help teach consumers about appropriate portion sizes.

An alternate method to adjusting the serving size is to shift the ingredient proportions in a recipe when possible. For example, an apple crisp recipe could be modified by using a smaller amount of topping (see Recipe Example: Adjusting ingredient proportions or form) or by increasing the amount of fruit topping spooned over a smaller slice of cake.

Keep in mind that adjusting the serving size to make a recipe healthier isn't always about reducing the size. Sometimes simply adding more non-starchy vegetables, increasing water content, or incorporating more air in a recipe can improve the nutrient profile while keeping the serving size the same or possibly increasing it.

Modify the Ingredients

If adjusting the serving size will not make a recipe meet nutrition parameters, look closely at the ingredients to determine what can be modified or substituted. Understand what function and flavor those ingredients perform, as modifications and substitutions can affect the texture, mouthfeel, or flavor of a final dish. See Functional Role of Ingredients in Recipes on page 46 and Chapter 4 for additional details on ingredient functions and modifications.

If a recipe must meet specific nutrition requirements, start by moderately adjusting the amount of a specific ingredient. For other recipes, a substitution might be necessary. The latter is especially true with nutrient- or ingredient-specific restrictions in a recipe development project, such as sugar-free, gluten-free, dairy-free, or vegan recipes. If ingredient substitution is necessary, consider the role and function of the ingredient you need to eliminate or substitute. Does the recipe contain a liquid, flour, eggs, fat, sugar, or salt? These ingredients perform very specific functions in a final dish, so modifying or deleting any of them can significantly affect the final product.

Altering a baking recipe can also affect the liquid-to-dry ratio of ingredients. Having the right balance and proportions makes a difference—especially with baking recipes—so it's critical to understand the function of an ingredient you are modifying or eliminating to better predict the consequences of making a change.

Where should you begin? Start with a research approach by modifying one ingredient or variable at a time, and carefully record what happens to the dish when one specific variable is changed (e.g., using vegetable oil instead of butter). Changing two variables at once makes it difficult to determine the cause of the problem if a recipe does not turn out as desired—especially with baked goods.

Recipe Example: Adjusting ingredient proportions or form

Modifying ingredient proportions of classic recipes can be a straightforward health-focused recipe development technique. In this apple crisp, reducing the amount of the oat topping in relation to the apple filling was an easy way to reduce the calories, fat, and saturated fat per serving. Another health-focused recipe modification approach is changing the type or form of an ingredient typically used—in this case, using melted butter instead of the softened or chilled butter traditionally used in crisp toppings. Testing with melted butter resulted in a crisp with a crunchier topping, so using less topping was less noticeable. When modifying health-focused recipes, testing is very important to ensure modifications that make sense on paper produce the desired results in the kitchen.

Apple Walnut Crisp (Original)
By Raeanne Sarazen, MA, RDN

Preparation time: 25 minutes
Cooking time: 45 minutes
Yield: 6 servings

6 Granny Smith or Honeycrisp
   apples (about 3 pounds), peeled,
   cored, and sliced ⅓ inch thick
¼ cup granulated sugar
1 tablespoon fresh lemon juice

TOPPING
¾ cup old-fashioned rolled oats
¾ cup all-purpose flour
¾ cup packed brown sugar
¾ teaspoon ground cinnamon
¼ teaspoon kosher salt
6 tablespoons unsalted butter, cut
   into pieces, softened
¾ cup walnuts or pecans halves,
   chopped

1. Heat the oven to 375° F. Spray an 8-inch square baking dish with nonstick cooking spray.

2. Combine the apples, sugar, and lemon juice in medium bowl; scrape into the baking dish.

3. For the topping, stir together the oats, flour, brown sugar, cinnamon, and salt in the same bowl you used for the apples. Add the butter and blend the mixture together using one hand (always good to keep one clean to pick up the phone or whatever else!), a fork, or a pastry blender until well combined and forming clumps. Stir in the walnuts.

4. Spoon the topping over the fruit. Bake until the fruit juices are bubbling, the apples are tender, and the topping is crisp, 45 to 50 minutes. Let the crisp cool for about 10 minutes before serving.

Nutrition per serving: 550 calories, 21 grams fat, 8 grams saturated fat, 90 milligrams sodium, 87 grams carbohydrate, 9 grams fiber, 58 grams total sugar (35 grams added sugar), 6 grams protein

Modification of the Original Apple Walnut Crisp Recipe

Topping of original recipe	Topping cut by one-fourth (for a reduction of 130 calories, 7 grams fat, 3 grams saturated fat)	Topping cut by one-fourth and using melted butter for a crispier topping
¾ cup rolled oats	½ cup rolled oats	½ cup rolled oats
¾ cup all-purpose flour	½ cup all-purpose flour	¼ cup all-purpose flour
¾ cup packed brown sugar	½ cup packed brown sugar	½ cup packed brown sugar
¾ teaspoon ground cinnamon	½ teaspoon ground cinnamon	½ teaspoon ground cinnamon
¼ teaspoon kosher salt	⅛ teaspoon kosher salt	⅛ teaspoon kosher salt
6 tablespoons unsalted butter, cut into pieces, softened	4 tablespoons unsalted butter, cut into pieces, softened	4 tablespoons unsalted butter, melted
¾ cup walnut halves, chopped	½ cup walnuts halves, chopped	½ cup walnuts halves, chopped
Nutrition per serving: 550 calories, 21 grams fat, 8 grams saturated fat, 90 milligrams sodium,87 grams carbohydrate, 9 grams fiber, 58 grams total sugar (35 grams added sugar), 6 grams protein	**Nutrition per serving:** 420 calories, 14 grams fat, 5 grams saturated fat, 50 milligrams sodium, 71 grams carbohydrate, 8 grams fiber, 48 grams total sugar (26 grams added sugar), 4 grams protein	**Nutrition per serving:** 420 calories, 14 grams fat, 5 grams saturated fat, 50 milligrams sodium, 71 grams carbohydrate, 8 grams fiber, 48 grams total sugar (26 grams added sugar), 4 grams protein

FUNCTIONAL ROLE OF INGREDIENTS IN RECIPES

Being familiar with the role of key ingredients in cooking and baking allows recipe developers to make modifications that will meet health and nutrition goals and taste delicious.

Salt

Adds flavor: enhances the flavors and sweetness of other ingredients (increases the perception of sweetness by diminishing bitterness)

Strengthens gluten structure in baked goods: improves volume and crumb texture

Slows yeast fermentation in baked goods: increases browning

Sugar

Taste sensations: adds sweetness and balances acidity; contributes to brown color and caramelized flavors

In baking:
Tenderizer: interferes with and delays gluten formation, making a more tender product

Moistness: adds moisture due to the hydroscopic nature of sugar (it attracts and retains moisture), helping to improve shelf life

Assists in leavening: when butter and sugar are creamed together, the sugar granules cut through the butter and force air into the mix

Bulk: adds bulk to confections (e.g., sugary treats, such as cakes and candies) and icings

Stabilizer: stabilizes egg whites in meringues and adds volume and stability to cakes

Provides food: for yeast fermentation

Eggs

Adds nutritional value: contains protein; vitamins A, D, E, and B12; selenium; choline; and lutein and zeaxanthin (antioxidants)

Adds flavor and color: provides richness from the fat in the yolk as well as yellow color; the protein content contributes to the Maillard reaction (see Cooking Techniques to Boost Flavor on page 50) and produces browning

Leavening: when beaten with other ingredients, traps and holds air that expands during heating, such as in baked goods; air whipped into egg whites creates a foam that acts as a leavening agent in batters

Provides structure: binds with other ingredients (primarily flour) to create the supporting structure of cakes, quick breads, muffins, certain yeast breads, and cookies; coagulated (cooked) eggs provide thickness

Moisture and tenderness: adds moisture due to water content; the fat in the yolk acts as a shortener and improves the tenderness of the crumb

Binding and adhesive: conversion of a liquid egg into a solid form (coagulation) helps bind ingredients together (e.g., in a meat loaf or crab cakes); egg brushed onto a surface holds topically applied ingredients (e.g., breading, nuts, seeds)

Emulsification (yolk): provides stabilization and cohesiveness of liquid and fat, such as in mayonnaise and hollandaise sauce; also helps to properly blend ingredients in ice cream and baked goods

Wheat flour

Thickener: starch granules in flour absorb liquids and swell when heated

Builds structure: when the protein in flour is hydrated, gluten is formed; the gluten framework stretches to contain expanding leavening gases during rising, allowing baked goods to hold new and larger shapes and sizes

For more on types and uses for wheat flour, see page 81 in Chapter 3. For more on wheat flour substitutions, see Chapter 6.

Fat

Taste sensations: adds a creamy, rich, and smooth taste to savory dishes and baked goods; also adds crispness

Adds flavor: blends and distributes flavor (if using oil) or enhances flavor (if using butter)

In baking:
Tender crumb: oil and solid fat tenderize and provide moistness; butter can also provide flakiness by interfering with gluten formation by coating the proteins in flour responsible for forming gluten (butter for pies and crusts)

Assists in leavening: help baked goods rise (When butter and sugar are creamed together, the sugar granules cut through the butter and force air into the mix, creating air pockets that provide lightness and a natural leavening agent. However, oil does not act as a leavening agent and results in a moist and dense baked good.)

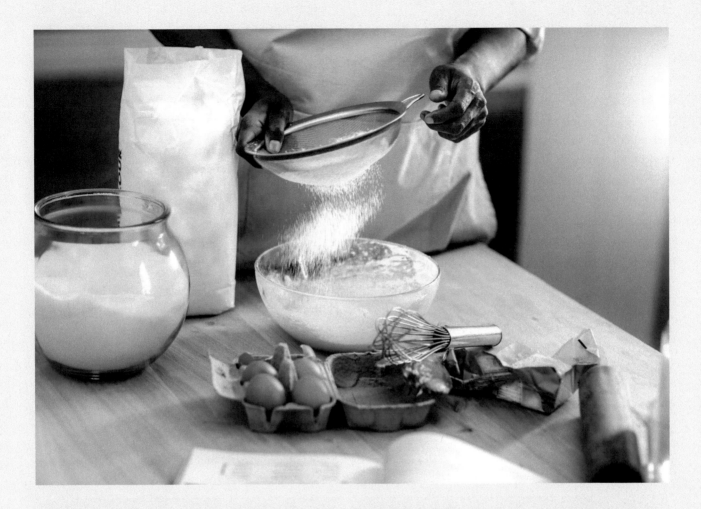

Liquids

Water or any liquid: hydrates protein and starch (providing structure and texture development); adds moistness to the texture and improves the mouthfeel of baked products; adds volume to a batter or dough by vaporizing into steam and expanding the air cells

Milk: aids in browning due to the protein content; the sugar and fat content helps tenderize and moisten baked goods

Juice: adds an acidic element

Acidic ingredients

For example, vinegar, lemon, honey, wine, buttermilk, yogurt, sour cream, molasses

Flavor: adds tanginess and brightens other flavors

Balance: competes with bitter flavors in foods and reduces the taste perception of them

Baking soda

Chemical leavening agent: produces a gas that creates leavening when combined with an acidic ingredient (e.g., vinegar, lemon juice, or molasses)

Baking powder

Chemical leavening agent: made of a mixture of baking soda and a dry acid; assists with leavening (Double-acting baking powder has two separate leavening reactions. The first reaction is when the baking powder gets wet at room temperature and the second reaction happens when it is heated.)

Adding Flavor

Taste should remain front and center when developing health-focused recipes. Instead of focusing on what to remove from a recipe, instead think about what could be added—for example, more whole grains, fruits, vegetables, beans, split peas, lentils, nuts, or seeds. Whenever possible, focus on using fresh, seasonal ingredients to maximize the dish's natural flavors, and choose ingredients that add layers to the flavor and turn something plain into something delicious. To enhance taste, try some of the following.

Brighten the dish. Instead of salt, perk up the flavor of a dish by adding a bit of acid, such as vinegar or citrus (lime or lemon) juice, to balance out bitter flavors.

Season with salt. Use kosher salt to season meats before cooking, as its larger granules add a burst of saltiness and cling well to the meat. For a quick hit of flavor, use a finishing salt like Maldon salt flakes, fleur de sel, or Himalayan pink salt. These salts, characterized by their large, flat flakes, can add a final touch of flavor and crunch to sweet or savory dishes.

Be generous with fresh herbs. Add heartier fresh herbs like rosemary, thyme, sage, marjoram, and oregano to a dish earlier in the cooking process to ensure the flavor has plenty of time to release, and reserve more delicate herbs like basil, cilantro, parsley, chives, and tarragon for the end to maintain their fresh flavor, color, and aroma. Dried herbs also add flavor, but they are more potent than fresh. Use a 1:3 ratio for dried to fresh herbs (1 teaspoon dried is equivalent to 1 tablespoon fresh).

Kick up the spices. To add flavor to rubs, marinades, and savory dishes, choose hot pepper flakes, ginger, cardamom, coriander, cinnamon, or garam masala. To change and enhance a dish's color and also add flavor, consider turmeric, smoked paprika, or dried chili peppers.

Use flavor-packed ingredients. Include ingredients that impart extra flavor, such as Dijon mustard, wasabi, chutneys, olives, salsas, flavored oils, or citrus zest.

Add heat. Use various concentrated and flavorful chili pepper sauces like harissa or gochujang or add chipotle peppers to give food another layer of flavor.

Use fresh and visually appealing ingredients. Add visual appeal and more full, fresh flavor to a dish with colorful vegetables, such as Chioggia beets, and a variety of colored greens that are bitter, sharp, or peppery.

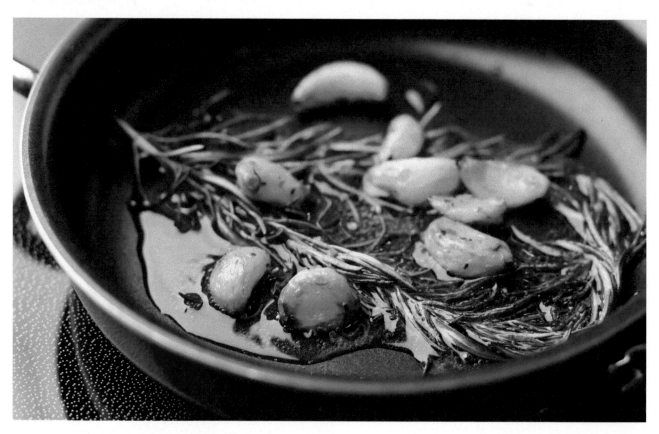

Finish with flavor. Be creative in jazzing up the flavor by using condiments and sauces. Examples include gremolata (made of fresh herbs, garlic, and citrus zest), pesto, sun-dried tomato relish (which provides a complex, concentrated flavor and light sweetness). Pickled vegetables like pepperoncini on salads, sandwiches, or grain dishes add a spicy, tangy crunch.

Add umami. Add some deliciousness and a savory umami boost to a dish by adding a small amount of anchovy, aged cheese (such as Parmesan), oyster sauce, fish sauce, soy sauce, miso, seaweed, dried bonito flakes, Marmite, Worcestershire sauce, mushrooms, tomato paste, or dried or cured meats (e.g., prosciutto or pancetta from Italy, jamón Serrano from Spain, or Jinhua ham from China). See page 4 for more on umami.

Consider Seasonality

Always consider the seasonality of ingredients when modifying or developing sweet or savory recipes. It's possible that you will be researching and writing months ahead of a recipe's publication date and testing the recipe out of season, but ultimately it's best to use ingredients close to the time they are harvested whenever possible. To help determine what is in season, focus on what's grown in your region of the country, especially if your recipes will be published locally. If the seasonal availability of certain ingredients—fruits and vegetables, for example—is limited, you can recommend them in their canned or frozen form, which can often serve as great substitutes. Just make sure the recipe is tested using the canned or frozen ingredient as well.

Minimizing Food Waste

Always give thought to food waste when choosing ingredients for recipe development. Whenever possible, provide strategies for reducing waste in the recipe headnote or directions. This could include simple tips to keep the dish or ingredients fresh and safe for as long as possible or recommendations for freezing leftovers or repurposing them in other recipes. For example, suggest some of the following:

- roasting leftover cuttings from broccoli or cauliflower instead of throwing them away
- using leftover pork in burritos or quesadillas
- repurposing unused fresh herbs in pesto, herbed butters, or smoothies or freezing them in ice cube trays

Encouraging and educating readers about food waste in recipes can make an impact.

Alter the Cooking Technique

Another health-focused approach to modifying a recipe is to see if an alternative cooking technique can help meet the nutrition parameters for the recipe. For example, can a deep-fried dish be baked instead? Could a panfried fish be steamed? Modifying a technique requires an understanding of an original recipe and why that technique was chosen in the first place.

Healthy Cooking Techniques

Microwaving, poaching, steaming, baking, roasting, broiling, grilling, pan grilling, a la plancha (high-temperature searing in a flat pan set over a grill grate), air frying, and pressure cooking are all healthy cooking techniques. Sautéing, panfrying, and stir-frying using a healthy fat in a stainless or aluminum pan can also be healthy options. A cast-iron pan is a good stick-resistant choice for high-heat searing or cooking, and nonstick skillets are preferred for delicate foods like crepes, eggs, and fish.

Flavor-Boosting Cooking Techniques

A healthy dish can be made more satisfying, with enhanced and deepened flavor, via two flavor-producing techniques known as the Maillard reaction and caramelization. While the browning adds visual appeal, the main focus is on the delicious flavors and aromas these techniques produce. The end result may be similar, but the science behind them is different. Maillard browning is a complex series of chemical reactions that occurs when sugars and proteins are heated together, and caramelization occurs when sugars are heated alone. See Cooking Techniques to Boost Flavor on page 50 for more details.

Modify the Ingredients *and* the Cooking Technique

If altering the cooking technique alone does not provide the desired healthier result, try changing one or more of the ingredients as well. Sometimes, both the ingredients and cooking techniques must be tweaked to meet nutrition requirements.

Expect multiple iterations when you're developing health-focused recipes, especially with baked goods. As with any recipe, continue to keep the dish's visual appeal, aroma, flavor, texture, and color in mind while modifying or developing a health-focused recipe.

Remember, a recipe may not need to be completely revised to become healthier. Tweaking parts of the recipe—the portion size, ingredients, cooking technique, or any combination of these—may make it fit the desired nutrition parameters. Sometimes small changes to a classic approach can produce big results. And if a recipe is too difficult to modify, consider developing a completely new recipe.

Oven-Baking Fried Foods

Consumers love the crispness and moistness of fried foods, so if an oven-baked version of a dish with the same ingredients doesn't provide the desired results, try changing one of the ingredients. For example, if you are creating an oven-baked "fried chicken" recipe, try replacing the flour coating with panko breadcrumbs, crushed cornflakes, or dried chickpea crumbs, all of which are naturally crunchy. Another option might be to mix a small amount of a healthy oil into the breadcrumbs or to experiment with a mixture of flour and cornstarch (usually replace about one-quarter of the flour with cornstarch). These small changes can help add a crispness to the coating and make up for all the oil that gets soaked into the food when it is deep-fried. You could also make changes to the baking temperature or adjust another ingredient to help the coating stick to the chicken, such as coating it with mustard, egg, or milk. Any of these changes could help lower fat and calories. For recipe examples that modify both the ingredients and cooking technique, see the recipes in Chapter 4 for Pecan-Crusted Chicken Tenders with Yogurt Dill Dip on page 97 and Corn Sorghum "Risotto" on page 100.

Quick Tip

"Aroma is sometimes a forgotten part of developing healthier recipes. Since the sense of smell is a key part of taste, I always consider what I can add to a recipe to make it more aromatic, such as finishing a dish with fresh herbs, a generous squirt of citrus juice, or perhaps freshly sautéed garlic 'chips.'"

—Jackie Newgent, RDN, chef and cookbook author

COOKING TECHNIQUES TO BOOST FLAVOR

Maillard Reaction

The Maillard reaction, also known as the browning reaction, takes place when proteins and sugars in foods are transformed by heat. The hotter the temperature is, the faster the Maillard reaction will take place, but take care to ensure that the food does not burn. Some foods that benefit from the Maillard reaction include meats, seafood, and other high-protein foods.

The browning that occurs when bread is baked is also caused by the Maillard reaction; while it is the same chemical reaction, it creates different aromas. This type of browning can be produced on a grill, on a stove, or in the oven.

BOX CONTINUES >

Searing provides the browning and flavor benefits of the Maillard reaction. There are important factors to consider when searing, such as the following:

- Make sure the food is dry. Blot meat, chicken, fish, or firm tofu with a paper towel to remove excess moisture before heating. Excess moisture will interfere with the Maillard reaction (the food will steam, not brown).

- Place the dry pan over high heat. Once it is hot, add a small amount of oil before adding the food. Make sure the oil approaches its smoke point before adding the food; if it is not hot enough, the food will soak it up.

- Once the food is placed in the pan, do not move it until it's finished searing on that side. Waiting until it is fully seared also allows it to release easily from the pan. If necessary, transfer the pan to the oven to finish cooking.

Sautéing or panfrying browns and seals in the flavor. Some important factors to consider when sautéing or panfrying include the following:

- Choose a pan large enough for all of the food to fit in a single layer. If the pan is too small, the food will not brown; instead, it will release water and steam.

- Place the dry pan over the heat first before adding the oil. Then, if sautéing, add enough oil to just cover the bottom of the pan; if panfrying, add about ¼ inch of oil to the pan. Warm the oil until a little water sprinkled into it makes a crackling sound. Once this happens, the pan is ready. (Another method is to shake the pan to see if the oil shimmers and moves as quickly as water.) The exception to heating the pan and oil before adding ingredients is if you are using butter or garlic. Both will burn if the pan is too hot.

- Choose the right oil. If you are using very high heat, consider oils with a higher smoke point, such as avocado, peanut, grapeseed, or canola. Extra-virgin olive oil has the potential to overheat since it has a lower smoke point but generally is fine when sautéing or panfrying.

- Cook at the right temperature. Chicken can be sautéed over medium-high heat, but foods that need less cooking time and that release more water, such as mushrooms, should be cooked over higher heat so they brown well without overcooking. Never cover the pan when you are sautéing or panfrying.

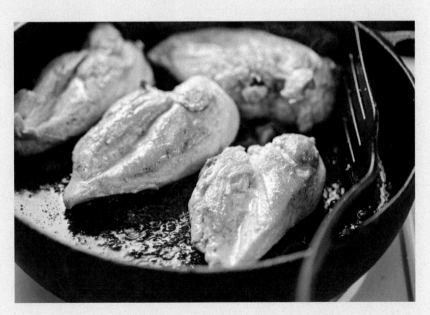

BOX CONTINUES >

Caramelization

Caramelization takes place at the point when most of the water content in the food evaporates and the natural sugars break down, ultimately producing a deep brown color and complex flavor. Foods that have been caramelized are sweeter than they are when raw. Onions caramelize beautifully; other high-sugar fruits or vegetables like apples and carrots also work well. Following are ways to obtain the complex and rich flavor of caramelization:

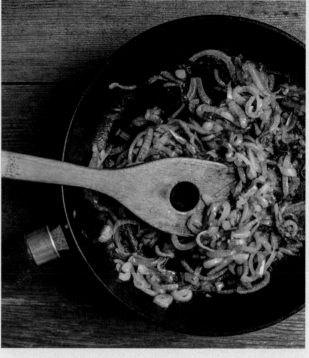

- **Roasting or grilling:** Toss the fruit or vegetable with a small amount of oil and then roast or grill over high heat until done. The time will depend on whether roasting and caramelizing root vegetables in the oven at 400° F or quickly cooking and caramelizing fresh peaches or pineapple on the grill.

- **Glazing:** Slowly cook the fruit or vegetable over low to medium-low heat in a small amount of liquid, fat (usually butter), and sugar so it caramelizes evenly. The natural sugars and water content of the food break down and release into the pan. As the liquid cooks down and becomes concentrated, it transforms into a light natural syrup that captures the food's natural sugars and glazes the food as it cooks. Any nutrients that leach into the syrup are reabsorbed into the food. Glazing works best with heartier vegetables like carrots, parsnips, turnips, beets, fennel, onions, and cauliflower. The classic white glaze technique uses a small amount of butter and sugar; for a slightly healthier version, use a small amount of olive oil instead of the butter and skip the sugar. The technique is as follows:

    1. Cut the vegetables into evenly sized pieces. Add 1 to 2 tablespoons butter and ½ to 1 teaspoon sugar per pound of vegetables, or simply drizzle the vegetables with 1 to 2 tablespoons of olive oil. Season the vegetables with a small amount of salt and black pepper.
    2. Place the vegetables in a pan large enough to fit all the food in a single layer and add enough liquid to come halfway up the sides of the vegetables. Place the pan over medium heat, partially cover, and simmer, checking the vegetables often to ensure the liquid does not evaporate before they are cooked. If it does, add more water. If you find that the vegetables are tender and too much water remains, uncover and cook until the liquid boils away.
    3. When the vegetables are done, remove from the heat and add 1 tablespoon water to the pan to help coat the vegetables with a shiny glaze. Add even more flavor by sprinkling chopped fresh herbs over the finished dish.

HOW TO USE DIFFERENT TYPES OF SALT

The two basic types of salt are:

- **Rock salt** (table, kosher, and specialty salts, like Himalayan pink), which is typically mined from underground salt deposits.
- **Sea salt** (flake, fine, or coarse), which is extracted from evaporated sea water.

All salts are about 40% sodium and 60% chloride by weight, but salts with larger crystal sizes contain less sodium by volume than finer-grained salts. For example, Morton table salt is denser than Morton kosher salt. The table salt's smaller grain size packs more tightly into a measuring spoon. According to USDA's FoodData Central 1 teaspoon of table salt contains 2,360 milligrams sodium, while 1 teaspoon of the Morton kosher variety contains 1,920 milligrams of sodium. Diamond Crystal kosher salt has a larger and more open crystal structure than Morton kosher salt, so 1 teaspoon of it contains even less at 1,120 milligrams of sodium.

Choosing the Type of Salt

Why choose one type of salt over the other when developing recipes? Depending on their training, chefs may use table salt for baking, kosher salt for cooking, and sea salt for finishing a cooked dish. Because of its smaller grain size, table salt dissolves easily into doughs and batters. The larger grain size of kosher salt makes it easier to pick up and sprinkle evenly over the food, which provides more control. The various grain sizes and colors of sea salt make it a good choice for sprinkling on food just before serving. Sea salt has a soft, flaky texture and provides a different crunch than kosher or table salt. When writing recipes, it is ideal to include the type and brand of salt recommended for use, but keep in mind that some publishers prefer not to include brand names.

Another difference to be aware of is whether a salt is iodized. Iodized salts are fortified with the nutrient potassium iodate to help prevent iodine deficiency. Iodized and non-iodized salts behave the same when used in recipes.

Salt Amount Guidelines

To keep track of how much salt is used in a recipe during development, measure a specific amount into a ramekin and then measure what's left after the recipe has been seasoned. Including specific amounts of salt is helpful for the home cook and is necessary to calculate an accurate nutrition analysis. Start with the suggestions in the chart below to enhance the natural flavor of foods with salt and adjust them according to personal taste and the type of recipe being developed.

Suggestions for using Morton kosher salt*

Per 1 pound of meat or vegetables	¾ to 1 teaspoon
Per 1 cup dry grains (e.g., rice, quinoa, barley)	½ teaspoon
Per 1 quart water for blanching vegetables or cooking pasta	1 to 1½ tablespoons
Per 1 quart soup or sauce	¾ to 1 teaspoon
Per 1 cup salad dressing	¾ to 1 teaspoon
Per 1 cup flour for doughs and batters	½ to ¾ teaspoon

* Use slightly less if using table salt (tiny grains mean more saltiness per 1 teaspoon) and slightly more if using Diamond Crystal kosher salt (larger grains mean less saltiness per 1 teaspoon). Use this reference guide to adjust the amounts based on type of salt being used:

1 teaspoon table salt =
1½ teaspoons Morton kosher salt =
2 teaspoons Diamond Crystal kosher salt

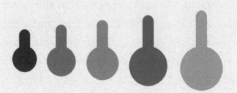

Developing Recipes to Address Religious Dietary Practices

When developing health-focused recipes or any type of recipe for people following religious dietary practices, it's important to carefully review and understand these practices so your recipes will be sensitive and accurate. Following is a general overview of several religions that follow specific food practices.

Judaism

Jewish dietary laws, which are quite complex, include rules about which foods can and cannot be eaten and specifics on how kosher foods must be prepared in a properly kept kosher kitchen. Orthodox Jewish people follow these rules and restrictions. Some reform or conservative Jewish people may choose to observe a selection of the laws.

It is important to note that the term *kosher* applies to the types of food that a Jewish person may eat and the ways in which it may be prepared, but kosher is *not* a style of cooking. Any type of cuisine can be kosher if it is prepared according to Jewish dietary laws.

Tips on Developing Kosher Recipes
Keep these practices in mind when developing kosher recipes.

Prohibited foods (not kosher) include:

- Pork or products derived from pork, such as bacon and lard

- Shellfish (e.g., lobster, shrimp, crab), mollusks (e.g., oysters, clams, scallops), squid, octopus, and snails

- Fish that do *not* have scales and fins (e.g., eel, catfish, shark, swordfish, monkfish)

Meat and dairy products cannot be consumed together in the same recipe or in the same meal. For example, chicken Parmesan, buttermilk fried chicken, French onion soup (a meat stock and cheese are primary ingredients), cheeseburger, pepperoni pizza, and chocolate desserts eaten with a meat meal (if the chocolate contains milk) would not be kosher. If you are considering a recipe for a typically dairy-based side dish that will be served with a meat, use plant-based substitutions for the dairy. Recipe instructions should include direction on keeping pots, bowls, and utensils separate so meat and dairy do not mix.

Neutral (pareve) foods can be eaten or used in a recipe that also contains either meat or dairy. This includes fruit, vegetables, legumes, nuts, seeds, and grains (essentially, anything that grows from the ground), eggs, and fish. Produce must be washed and inspected for insects. Insects are not kosher.

Kosher foods (permitted for consumption) include:

- Fish that have scales and fins. There are no rules regarding ritual slaughter of fish.

- Land animals with split hooves that chew their cuds (e.g., antelope, bison, cows, deer, goats, sheep) and that are slaughtered by a trained and qualified kosher butcher in accordance with Jewish law.

- Birds (e.g., chicken, turkey, quail, pigeon) that are slaughtered by a trained and qualified kosher butcher in accordance with Jewish law.

- Milk and eggs from kosher animals.

- Wine bearing a kosher certification symbol (see the image below).

- Packaged foods bearing a kosher certification symbol. All processed foods, including bakery items, cereals, condiments, and any foods other than produce, must bear a kosher certification symbol to be considered kosher (see examples below). This certification verifies that the food was processed and packaged in a factory that complies with kosher rules and did not come in contact with nonkosher items or ingredients.

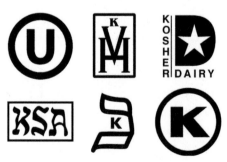

Islam

Muslims follow the Islam religion, which has various food restrictions according to Islamic dietary laws. *Halal* is an Arabic word meaning "lawful" or "permitted." When a halal claim is made on a food product, the word "halal" or equivalent terms or symbol should appear on the label. Here are examples of halal symbols:

 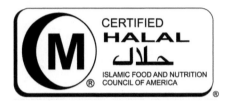

Foods or food products that are considered *haram*, an Arabic word that means "unlawful" or "prohibited," include:

- pork meat or pork products, including bacon and lard

- gelatin, rennet, or whey that is derived from pork

- any meat from animals that are not slaughtered and prepared in the correct halal way, meaning under Islamic law (Generally speaking, foods that are certified as kosher are also halal.)

- alcoholic drinks or alcohol-containing ingredients (Some people who follow a halal diet do not consume foods containing flavoring extracts, which contain very small amounts of alcohol, but others consider this permissible.)

A third Arabic term, *mashbooh,* means "doubtful." Mashbooh includes foods that contain enzymes, emulsifiers, and additives that could originate from haram foods.

Hindu

The Hindu religion encourages vegetarianism, but not all Hindus are vegetarians. Hindus do not eat beef, as the cow is considered to be a sacred animal, but some consume other animal products, including milk, yogurt, cheese, and butter. Many Hindus follow a lactovegetarian diet, which excludes meat, poultry, fish, and eggs but permits dairy products.

Buddhism

People who follow Buddhism, a religion with a diverse set of traditions and sects, have no set dietary restrictions or rules. Some Buddhists follow some variation of a vegetarian diet, but many don't. Much depends on the follower's individual choices and the sect and country they originate from.

Health- and Wellness-Focused Recipe Development Resources

In addition to the Recipe Development Resources listed in Chapter 1, consult some of these books and resources when developing recipes with a focus on nutrition and health.

Books

Academy of Nutrition and Dietetics Complete Food & Nutrition Guide, 5th edition, by Roberta L. Duyff. 2017. HarperCollins Books.

Culinary Nutrition: The Science and Practice of Healthy Cooking by Jacqueline Marcus. 2013. Academic Press.

Essentials of Nutrition for Chefs, 2nd edition, by Catharine Powers and Mary Abbott Hess. 2013. Culinary Nutrition Publishing.

Techniques of Healthy Cooking by the Culinary Institute of America. 2013. Wiley.

Government Websites and Resources

MyPlate:
myplate.gov

National Heart, Lung, and Blood Institute (NHLBI):
nhlbi.nih.gov/health-topics

National Institute of Diabetes and Digestive and Kidney Diseases (NIDDK), Health Information:
niddk.nih.gov/health-information

US Department of Agriculture, *Dietary Guidelines for Americans 2020–2025*:
dietaryguidelines.gov/resources /2020-2025-dietary-guidelines-online -materials

Other Websites

Academy of Nutrition and Dietetics:
eatright.org

American Diabetes Association:
diabetes.org

American Heart Association:
heart.org

Center for Mindful Eating:
thecenterformindfuleating.org

EatingWell:
EatingWell.com

Forks Over Knives:
forksoverknives.com

Harvard T.H. Chan School of Public health:
hsph.harvard.edu/nutritionsource

Oldways:
oldwayspt.org

Pulses:
pulses.org/us

Vegetarian Resource Group:
vrg.org

Whole Grain Council:
wholegrainscouncil.org

Religious Dietary Practices

Islamic Food and Nutrition Council of America (IFANCA): ifanca.org

Orthodox Union Kosher:
oukosher.org

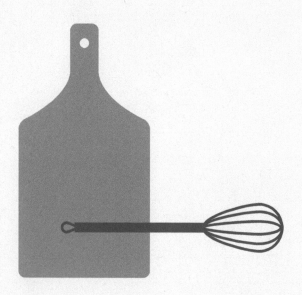

Bibliography

Agricultural Marketing Service. Grass fed small and very small producer program. Agricultural Marketing Service website. Accessed June 8, 2021. ams.usda.gov/services/auditing/grass-fed-SVS

Agricultural Marketing Service. Questions and answers—USDA shell egg grading service. FDA website Accessed June 8, 2021. ams.usda.gov/publications/qa-shell-eggs

Cattlemen's Beef Board and National Cattlemen's Beef Association. Grain-finished vs. grass finished beef. Beef It's What's For Dinner website. Accessed June 8, 2021. beefitswhatsfordinner.com/cuts/grass-vs-grain

DASH eating plan. National Heart, Lung, and Blood Institute website. Accessed May 7, 2021. nhlbi.nih.gov /health-topics/dash-eating-plan

Food Safety and Inspection Service. Meat and poultry labeling terms. Food Safety and Inspection Service website Accessed June 8, 2021. fsis.usda.gov/food-safety/safe-food-handling-and-preparation/food-safety-basics/meat -and-poultry-labeling-terms

Heart-check certified recipes. American Heart Association website. Accessed May 7, 2021. heart.org/en/healthy -living/company-collaboration/heart-check-certification/heart-check-certified-recipes

Heart-check recipe certification program nutrition requirements. American Heart Association website. May 1, 2018. Accessed May 7, 2021. heart.org/en/healthy-living/company-collaboration/heart-check-certification /heart-check-certified-recipes/heart-check-recipe-certification-program-nutrition-requirements

Mediterranean diet. Oldways Cultural Food Traditions website. Accessed May 7, 2021. oldwayspt.org/traditional -diets/mediterranean-diet

National Agricultural Library. Humane methods of Slaughter Act. Natural Agricultural Library website Accessed June 8, 2021. nal.usda.gov/animal-health-and-welfare/humane-methods-slaughter-act

National Agricultural Library. Local foods. Natural Agricultural Library website, Accessed June 8, 2021. nal.usda.gov/human-nutrition-and-food-safety/local-foods-and-communities

US Food and Drug Administration. Authorized health claims that meet the significant scientific agreement (SSA) standard. FDA website. Accessed May 7, 2021. fda.gov/food/food-labeling-nutrition/authorized-health-claimst -mee-significant-scientific-agreement-ssa-standard

US Food and Drug Administration. Food labeling guide: guidance for industry. 2013. FDA website Accessed May 7, 2021. fda.gov/regulatory-information/search-fda-guidance-documents/guidance-industry-food-labeling-guide

US Food and Drug Administration. Guidance for industry: use of the term "healthy" in the labeling of human food products. FDA website Accessed May 7, 2021. fda.gov/regulatory-information/search-fda-guidance -documents/guidance-industry-use-term-healthy-labeling-human-food-products

US Food and Drug Administration. Label claims for conventional foods and dietary supplements. FDA website Accessed May 7, 2021. fda.gov/food/food-labeling-nutrition/label-claims-conventional-foods-and-dietary -supplements

US Department of Agriculture. Sustainability definitions. USDA website. Accessed June 8, 2021. usda.gov/oce /sustainability/definitions

US Department of Agriculture and US Department of Health and Human Services. *Dietary Guidelines for Americans, 2020–2025*. 9th Edition. December 2020. Dietary Guidelines for Americans website. Accessed May 7, 2021. dietaryguidelines.gov

What is a healthy recipe? Food Network website. Accessed May 7, 2021. foodnetwork.com/healthy/packages /healthy-every-week/healthy-tips/what-is-a-healthy-recipe

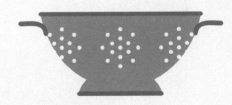

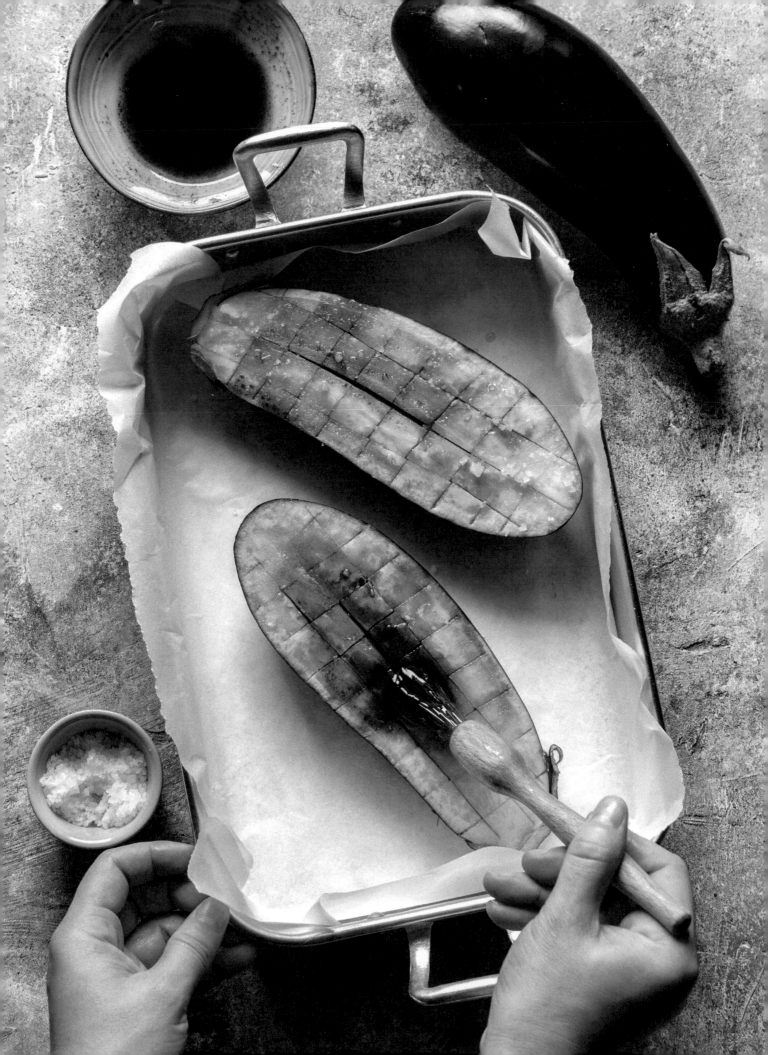

Chapter 3

Plant-Based Recipe Development

In this chapter, learn about:

- Plant-based nutrition and how a plant-based diet can support better health

- Developing plant-based recipes that optimize protein, vitamins, minerals, phytonutrients, dietary fiber, probiotics, and prebiotics

- Using plant foods as substitutes for egg, dairy, and meat in recipe development

- Identifying whole grain ingredients and how to cook and bake with them

Health and nutrition guidelines recommend a plant-based eating approach that emphasizes consuming mostly foods derived from plants, including vegetables, legumes (beans, peas, and lentils), fruits, whole grains, nuts, and seeds. Plant-based eating enhances health by supporting the immune system and reducing chronic inflammation in the body. This style of eating may help lower the risk for heart disease, some types of cancers, type 2 diabetes, and offers improvements in digestive, eye, and skin health. These advantages are likely a result of both the consistent consumption of health-promoting compounds found in plant foods, such as vitamins, mineral, phytonutrients, and dietary fiber, and a simultaneous reduction in the consumption of saturated fats found in processed and unprocessed meats and full-fat dairy foods.

Plant-based eating (sometimes referred to as plant-forward or plant-focused eating) is not synonymous with vegetarianism. Rather, it is interpreted to mean proportionately choosing and cooking foods from plant sources more frequently and, when choosing animal-based products, selecting moderate amounts of healthier choices, such as fish, seafood, lean meats, and nonfat or low-fat dairy products. An infinite number of recipes can be developed using combinations of plant foods. When including meats in a recipe, choose them wisely and use them in small amounts. Even a small amount of a flavorful cured meat (such as bacon, prosciutto, or salami) can add a lot of depth and flavor to dishes like grain salads and roasted vegetables.

This chapter addresses ways to optimize plant-based protein sources, dietary fiber, vitamins, minerals, phytonutrients, probiotics, and prebiotics when developing plant-centered recipes.

Plant-Based Nutrition

The belief that getting adequate nutrients with plant-based eating is difficult is simply not true. Plant-based diets can easily meet requirements for protein, fats, carbohydrates, vitamins, and minerals for optimal health when they are planned to include a variety of foods. And while plant-based foods differ from each other in their nutrient composition, there is no one "superfood" or "healthiest" fruit, vegetable, whole grain, nut, or seed to use when developing recipes. Using a variety of whole plant foods is best.

Quick Tip

"When developing plant-based and vegan recipes, it's important to understand the difference between these two terms. Plant-based eaters eat mostly plants and may or may not consume some animal products. Vegans consume no animal products at all and usually endeavor to avoid all animal products or their usage in alcoholic beverages, clothing, shoes, and more. Some wines and beers use animal products in the refining process, so vegans seek out vegan beverage brands. Same for sugar. Some conventional sugar is made using cow bone char in the refining process, so organic sugar should be used in vegan recipes." —Robin Asbell, plant-based chef and author of *Big Vegan*

A simple technique to improve a recipe's overall health profile is to use more fruits, vegetables, legumes (beans, peas, and lentils), soy foods, nuts, seeds, and whole grains. These plant-based foods are rich in vitamins, minerals, phytonutrients, dietary fiber, and water, yet are naturally low in saturated fat, sodium, and added sugars.

Fruits and vegetables supply many nutrients, including dietary fiber, potassium, vitamin A, vitamin C, folate, and phytochemicals. See page 63 for tips on using more fruits and vegetables in recipe development.

Beans, peas, and lentils are excellent sources of protein, dietary fiber, several B vitamins, iron, potassium, magnesium, zinc, and folate. Due to their nutrient density, they are considered either a protein or a vegetable by the Dietary Guidelines for Americans. Most meat substitutes are derived from beans, peas, and lentils. See page 68 for more on beans, peas, and lentils and using them in recipes. See page 83 for more information about dietary fiber.

Nuts and seeds provide protein as well as healthy monounsaturated and polyunsaturated fats.

Whole grains provide dietary fiber, B vitamins, antioxidants, and varying amounts of protein and minerals, including iron, selenium, and magnesium. See page 75 for information about using whole grains in recipes.

There is no single anti-inflammatory diet. Eating plans promoted as "anti-inflammatory" generally follow the tenets of the dietary approaches to stop hypertension (DASH) diet and Mediterranean diet (see Chapter 2 for more details on these guidelines for healthy eating). To develop recipes with a focus on fighting inflammation, incorporate more of these whole and minimally processed foods and ingredients:

- **Foods rich in antioxidant phytonutrients, antioxidants, and fiber:** Fruits (such as berries, apples, citrus), vegetables (such as onions, mushrooms, tomatoes), beans, peas, lentils, soybeans, whole grains, dark chocolate, tea, coffee, ginger, garlic, cinnamon, turmeric

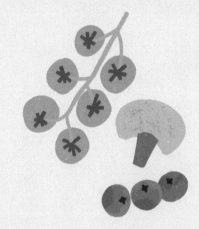

- **Foods that supply omega-3 fatty acids:** Oily fish (salmon, mackerel, sardines, and tuna), flaxseed and canola oil, walnuts, flaxseeds, and leafy green vegetables (such as spinach and kale)

- **Foods with unsaturated fats:** Nuts (such as almonds, pecans, walnuts), seeds (such as pumpkin, sesame, and flax), and plant oils (such as olive, peanut, canola)

While an anti-inflammatory diet emphasizes plant-based foods and healthy fats, it also limits processed and ultraprocessed foods that may promote inflammation. Food processing changes food from its natural state and often includes addition of manufactured ingredients, such as sugars, salt, *trans* fats, preservatives, and artificial colors and flavors. Examples of ultraprocessed foods: dehydrated soups and sauces, bottled sauces and dressings, processed meats, salty snacks, dessert mixes, and fried foods.

Phytonutrients in Plant Foods

Plant foods provide bioactive compounds called phytonutrients (or phytochemicals) that contribute to health promotion and disease prevention. Phytonutrients also contribute to a plant's color, taste, and aroma.

Some phytonutrients act as antioxidants, substances that prevent damage to cells from highly reactive molecules called free radicals. Other antioxidant nutrients (e.g., beta carotene, vitamins C and E, and selenium) along with antioxidant phytonutrients help fight inflammation in the body and offer protection in the development of chronic diseases like obesity, cardiovascular disease, and cancer.

Thousands of phytonutrients have been identified in vegetables, fruits, whole grains, beans, nuts, coffee, tea, and spices—and many more have yet to be identified. The main types of antioxidant phytonutrients are carotenoids, polyphenols, and organosulfur compounds, found in a variety of plant-based foods.

Carotenoids (lutein, beta carotene, and lycopene) are red, orange, and green pigments found in apricots, cantaloupe, pink grapefruit, peaches, mango, pumpkin, tangerines, watermelon, asparagus, beets, broccoli, carrots, corn, leafy dark green vegetables (kale, mustard greens, spinach, turnip greens), green peppers, sweet potatoes, and tomatoes.

Polyphenols (flavonoids: anthocyanidins, flavanols, flavones, and isoflavanones, resveratrol and curcumin) are found in red, blue, and purple berries, red and purple grapes, red wine, onions, scallions, kale, broccoli, apples, celery, hot peppers, citrus fruit and juices, soybeans, soy foods, legumes, teas, herbs like parsley and thyme.

Organosulfur compounds (allicin, glucosinolates, thiols, indoles) are found in broccoli, Brussels sprouts, cabbage, cauliflower, mushrooms, garlic, onion, and scallions.

NUTRIENTS IN PLANT FOODS

Nutrient	Examples of plant food sources
Protein	Legumes (beans, peas, and lentils), nuts, seeds, soy foods (tempeh, tofu), and whole grains, such as quinoa, sorghum, teff
Dietary fiber	Vegetables, fruits (berries, papayas, pears, dried fruits), avocados, legumes (beans, peas, and lentils), nuts, seeds, and whole grains
Omega-3 fats (as alpha-linolenic acid)	Seeds (chia, ground flax, hemp), soybeans, walnuts, wheat germ, and certain plant oils (canola, soybean, flax)
Calcium	Leafy green vegetables (kale, mustard greens, Swiss chard, collard greens, turnip greens), Brussels sprouts, beans, almonds, almond butter, sesame seeds, tahini, figs, blackstrap molasses, and fortified foods including some plant-based milks, juices, and tofu prepared with calcium
Iodine	Sea vegetables, seaweed (arame, dulse, nori, wakame), and iodized salt
Iron	Legumes (beans, peas, lentils, and peanuts), leafy green vegetables, soybeans, soy foods, quinoa, potatoes, dried fruit, dark chocolate, tahini, seeds (pumpkin, sesame, sunflower), sea vegetables, and seaweed (dulse, nori)
Magnesium	Leafy green vegetables, nuts, soybeans, potatoes, whole wheat, and quinoa
Potassium	Beans (kidney, black, adzuki), potatoes, soybeans, spinach, broccoli, bananas, oranges, cantaloupe, honeydew, apricots, grapefruit, and some dried fruits, such as prunes, raisins, and dates
Selenium	Brazil nuts, fortified breads, and other grain products
Zinc	Legumes ((beans, peas, lentils, and peanuts), soy foods, nuts, seeds, and oats
Choline	Legumes (beans, peas, lentils, and peanuts), bananas, broccoli, oats, quinoa, and soy foods
Folate	Leafy green vegetables, almonds, asparagus, avocado, beets, enriched grains (breads, pasta, rice), oranges, quinoa, and nutritional yeast
Vitamin A (beta carotene)	Sweet potatoes, carrots, winter squash, spinach, broccoli, red peppers, mangoes, cantaloupe, and pink/red grapefruit
Vitamin B12	Fortified foods, including nutritional yeast, plant-based milks, and some ready-to-eat breakfast cereals
Vitamin C	Berries, citrus fruits, cantaloupe, honeydew, kiwifruit, mango, papaya, pineapple, leafy green vegetables, potatoes, peas, broccoli, Brussels sprouts, bell peppers, cauliflower, chili peppers, and tomatoes
Vitamin D	Mushrooms grown under ultraviolet light, plant-based fortified milks, and some ready-to-eat breakfast cereals
Vitamin E	Seeds (sunflower), nuts (almonds, hazelnuts, peanuts), plant-based oils (sunflower, safflower, soybean), avocados, mangoes, pumpkins, red bell peppers, spinach, chard, mustard and turnip greens
Vitamin K	Leafy green vegetables, sea vegetables, seaweed, asparagus, avocado, broccoli, Brussels sprouts, cauliflower, peas, and natto (a traditional Japanese food made from fermented soybeans)

Source: Nutrient lists from standard reference legacy (2018) by USDA National Agricultural Library: nal.usda.gov/human-nutrition-and-food-safety/nutrient-lists-standard-reference-legacy-2018

ORGANIC VERSUS CONVENTIONAL PRODUCE

Using more fruits and vegetables in recipes, regardless of whether they are farmed organically or conventionally, will make them healthier. Any potential nutrient or health difference between organic or conventional produce is incremental and inconsistent. More importantly, very few Americans meet the recommended daily amounts for fruits and vegetables every day as it is. Now that organic produce is more widely available, consumers have more choices. Seeking out organic options is a lifestyle choice, but it doesn't mean that organic products are more healthful, nutritious, or always safer. See page 42 for more on organic labeling, which refers to a unique set of sourcing, growing, harvesting, and processing methods.

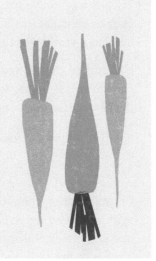

Types of Vegetarian Diets

Vegetarian eating styles can vary considerably: flexitarian (occasionally eating meat), pescatarian (eating fish), lacto-ovo vegetarian (eating dairy and eggs but no other animal products), and vegan (eliminating all animal products). Although it might be easier to meet daily nutrient requirements when dairy, eggs, and meats are included, vegetarian eating patterns that exclude all animal products can be nutritionally complete if a variety of plant foods are consumed. When developing vegan recipes, be mindful of the following nutrients (found in higher amounts in many animal products) that may be lacking in a vegan diet:

- protein
- vitamin B12
- calcium
- vitamin D
- iron
- zinc
- omega-3 fats

However, all of these nutrients can also be supplied by plant foods used in delicious and creative ways in recipes. For plant-based food sources of these nutrients, see Nutrients in Plant Foods.

Tips for Using Vegetables and Fruits in Recipe Development

There are myriad ways to include vegetables and fruits in recipes—whether fresh, canned, frozen, juiced, or dried. The following are just a few suggestions to help you get creative with plant-based recipe development.

- Replace some of the meat in burgers or loaves with vegetables and legumes. For example, mix shredded or chopped vegetables (e.g., zucchini, carrots, red pepper, onions, or spinach) into a meat loaf or turkey burgers. Dried mushrooms and bulgur make a meaty, richly flavored combination.

- Use more (think twice as much) fresh, canned, or frozen vegetables when developing a main or side dish recipe. For example, you can almost always find room for more vegetables in egg dishes, soups, hot pots, salads, grain bowls, noodle bowls, pastas, sandwiches, pizzas, pot pies, and casserole dishes. Focus on adding a variety of vegetables including dark green, red, and orange colors and choosing some that are starchy, such as winter squash.

- Use canned, frozen, and dried fruit options that are listed as "unsalted," "no salt added," "low sodium," or "no sugar added." Add salt and sugar to the recipe as needed.

- Add vegetables, such as zucchini or squash, to recipes where they're unexpected, such as pancake batter, smoothies, breads, muffins, desserts, and more.

- Try pasta products made with pureed vegetables, such as chickpeas, spinach, or zucchini, or simply add more vegetables to pasta dishes.

- Use pureed cooked vegetables, such as squash or cauliflower, as a base for dips and spreads and to thicken sauces and soups.

- Roast vegetables at high temperatures in the oven or in an open pan to obtain rich, concentrated flavor.

- Create recipes containing vegetable noodles or spirals or riced vegetables: options include jicama noodles or zucchini noodles ("zoodles"), riced cauliflower or broccoli, and more.

- Use a variety of lettuces as the exterior of a sandwich wrap.

- Re-create the traditional potato chip by using oven-baked beets, kale, and mustard greens instead.

- Try substituting jackfruit, which has a similar texture to pulled meat, in recipes for sloppy joes, tacos, and Asian curries. Jackfruit is available canned in brine or water at Asian grocery stores or online or in packages in a seasoned and flavored state (be sure to check the product's sodium content, as it can be quite high). Because jackfruit contains little protein, consider adding some beans, lentils, or peas to the recipe to boost protein content.

- Add fruit in unexpected ways—for example, add frozen, fresh, or dried fruits to salads, sandwiches, grain bowls, and braises.

- Focus on using a whole fruit versus only juice; if using juice, choose 100% juice.

- Add whole or pureed fresh or frozen fruits to baked goods.

- When they are slow roasted, moderately ripe bananas or plantains make a terrific side dish. Firm fruits, such as pineapple or peaches, are excellent grilled or roasted.

WHAT IS NUTRITIONAL YEAST?

Nutritional yeast—a dairy-free, low-sodium, and gluten-free savory food seasoning commonly used in vegetarian and vegan recipes—is a form of the yeast strain *Saccharomyces cerevisiae*, which is better known as baker's yeast. The difference between baker's yeast, used to leaven bread, and nutritional yeast is simple: baker's yeast is alive, and nutritional yeast is not.

Since a vegan diet is devoid of animal products, fortified nutritional yeast offers a non-animal source of vitamin B12 as well as other B vitamins (but do check the label since not all brands are fortified). It is also a source of protein and fiber. Nutritional yeast looks like dried yellow flakes, and it has a cheese-like flavor. Use it like salt and pepper to season foods, or use it like grated cheese in recipes. Sprinkle nutritional yeast over salads, roasted vegetables, and pasta, mix it into sauces, or incorporate it into a recipe to replace or reduce the amount of cheese, such as in mac and cheese, au gratin potatoes, or lasagna.

Plant-Based Protein Sources in Recipe Development

Protein needs can be easily met—including for vegetarian or vegan diets—by eating a variety of plant-based foods throughout the day while also getting sufficient calories. Twenty amino acids are used to produce proteins in the body; nine of these must come from food sources, and the remaining can be produced by the body. It was once believed that two incomplete plant proteins had to be eaten in a meal to create a "complete" protein, ensuring that all nine essential amino acids were provided. Research has since disproved the protein-combining theory; in fact, the human body maintains a pool of amino acids that can be used to create essential proteins.

Recipe Example: Using nutritional yeast as a plant-based alternative to cheese

Nutritional yeast, also referred to as *nooch*, is often used as a plant-based substitute in recipes that traditionally use a lot of cheese. In this recipe, nutritional yeast adds the necessary savory, umami-rich cheesy flavor as a replacement for the grated cheese used in a classic cheese sauce. You can use the cheese sauce for mac and cheese, nachos, as a sauce with vegetables, in soups, and more. Nutritional yeast is a versatile ingredient as it is nut-free, dairy-free, low-sodium or sodium-free (depending on the brand), and gluten-free. It also offers protein and fiber, and is often fortified with B vitamins, including vitamin B12.

Simple Vegan Cheese Sauce
By Raeanne Sarazen, MA, RDN

Preparation time: 15 minutes
Cooking time: 15 minutes
Yield: 8 servings (2 cups total; ¼ cup per serving)

1 large sweet potato, peeled and quartered
¾ teaspoon kosher salt, divided use
1 cup water
½ cup nutritional yeast
¼ cup olive oil
1 tablespoon apple cider vinegar
¼ teaspoon garlic powder

1. Place the sweet potato and ¼ teaspoon of the salt in a saucepan and add water to cover by about 1 inch. Heat to a boil; reduce the heat and simmer, uncovered, until the sweet potato is fork-tender, about 10 minutes. Drain.

2. Combine the sweet potato, water, yeast, olive oil, vinegar, garlic powder, and remaining ½ teaspoon salt in a high-power blender or food processor. Puree until smooth, occasionally stopping the blender or food processor to scrape down the sides.

3. Serve immediately or store in refrigerator for up to 1 week. When ready to use, reheat in the microwave or on the stovetop.

Nutrition per ¼-cup serving: 90 calories, 7 grams fat, 1 gram saturated fat, 200 milligrams sodium, 5 grams carbohydrate, 1 gram fiber, 1 gram total sugar, 3 grams protein

---

The amino acid profile of most plant proteins is less optimal than those of animal proteins found in meat, poultry, fish, eggs, and dairy. For example, levels of sulfur amino acids (methionine and cysteine) are lower in legumes, and the amino acid lysine is lower in cereal proteins. There are a few exceptions of plant foods that contain all nine essential amino acids, including soybean foods (tofu, edamame, and tempeh), quinoa, and pistachios. When two or more plant-based sources of protein are consumed, one or more of the foods can provide the essential amino acid(s) that the other(s) lack. Endless plant combinations are possible, but the following examples of complementary food pairings provide all of the essential amino acids, whether they are eaten at the same meal or throughout the day or week:

- **Beans, peas, or lentils *and* nuts, seeds, or whole grains.** Examples include rice and beans; black beans in quinoa chili; lentils, beans, or peas with pasta (e.g., escarole with beans over whole wheat pasta); hummus with whole wheat pita bread; a bean or lentil mushroom burger on a whole grain bun; a chickpea salad with tomatoes, cucumber, and sesame seeds; and a chopped vegetable salad with lentils and pistachios.

- **Whole grains *and* nuts or seeds.** Examples include millet with roasted vegetables and creamy cashew dressing, a peanut butter sandwich on whole wheat bread, and soba noodles with peanut sauce.

Both plant and animal protein sources can provide the protein needed to meet daily requirements, which vary based on age, gender, activity level, and other factors. See a nutritional comparison of common plant and animal sources on the next pages.

Nutritional Comparison of Protein, Calories, and Saturated Fat From Plant and Animal Sources

Grains (cooked)	Serving size	Protein (g)	Calories	Saturated fat (g)
Teff	1 cup	10	255	0
Wheat berries	1 cup	10	251	0
Quinoa	1 cup	8	222	0
Whole wheat pasta	1 cup	8	207	0
Pasta	1 cup	8	220	0
Bulgur	1 cup	6	151	0
Millet	1 cup	6	207	0
Oats	1 cup	6	166	0
Brown rice	1 cup	5	238	0.5
White rice	1 cup	4	204	0
Pearl barley	1 cup	4	193	0.5
Corn tortilla	1 (6-inch) tortilla	2	61	0

Legumes (beans, peas, lentils, soybeans, peanuts)	Serving size	Protein (g)	Calories	Saturated fat (g)
Miso	½ cup	17.5	272	1.5
	1 tablespoon	2	35	0
Tempeh	3 ounces	17	160	2
Tofu, firm	3 ounces	9	70	0.5
Edamame (soybeans in the pod), cooked and shelled	½ cup	9	94	0
Cannellini beans, canned or dried, cooked	½ cup	8	110	0
Lentils, dried, cooked	½ cup	8	103	0
Split peas, dried, cooked	½ cup	8	115	0
Peanut butter	2 tablespoons	8	191	3
Peanuts	1 ounce (about ¼ cup)	7	170	2
Chickpeas, canned or dried, cooked	½ cup	7	133	0
Black beans, canned or dried, cooked	½ cup	7	113	0
Soy milk	1 cup	7	101	0.5
Fresh peas, cooked	½ cup	4	66	0

Nuts	Serving size	Protein (g)	Calories	Saturated fat (g)
Almond butter	2 tablespoons	7	196	2
Almonds, roasted	1 ounce (about ¼ cup)	6	190	1
Pistachios	1 ounce (about ¼ cup)	6	170	1.5
Walnuts	1 ounce (about ¼ cup)	4	185	1.5
Pine nuts	1 ounce (about ¼ cup)	4	190	1.5
Almond milk	1 cup	1	90	0

Seeds	Serving size	Protein (g)	Calories	Saturated fat (g)
Hemp seeds	3 tablespoons (1 ounce)	10	180	1
Pumpkin seeds (pepitas)	¼ cup (1 ounce)	10	190	2
Sunflower seeds	¼ cup (1 ounce)	6	170	2
Sunflower butter	2 tablespoons	5.5	197	1.5
Chia seeds	2 tablespoons (1 ounce)	5	150	1
Flaxseed meal	3 tablespoons (1 ounce)	3	70	0.5
Sesame seeds	2 tablespoons	3	102	1

Animal protein	Serving size	Protein (g)	Calories	Saturated fat (g)
Boneless skinless chicken breast, grilled	3 ounces	26	128	1
New York strip steak, grilled	3 ounces (lean only)	25	160	2.5
	3 ounces (trimmed to ⅛-inch fat)	23	200	5
Pork chop, center loin, broiled	3 ounces	24	153	2
Cottage cheese, 2% milkfat	1 cup	23.5	183	3
Flank steak, grilled	3 ounces	23	172	2.5
Salmon, sockeye, baked	3 ounces	22.5	133	1
Pork tenderloin, roasted	3 ounces	22	125	1
Ground chuck (85% lean), broiled	3 ounces	22	212	5
Boneless skinless chicken thighs, grilled	3 ounces	20.5	163	2
Tuna, canned in water, drained	3 ounces	20	109	0.5
Greek yogurt, nonfat, plain	¾ cup	17	100	0
Yogurt, nonfat, plain	¾ cup	10	95	0
Milk, nonfat (0%)	1 cup	8	90	0
Milk, low-fat (1%)		8	110	1.5
Milk, reduced-fat (2%)		8	130	3
Milk, whole (3.25%)		8	150	5
Cheese, cheddar	1 ounce	7	110	5
Egg	1 large	6	75	1.5

Values rounded to nearest 0.5.

Sources: US Department of Agriculture, Agricultural Research Service, FoodData Central: fdc.nal.usda.gov | manufacturer data

Legumes and Pulses

Although the terms *legumes* and *pulses* are often used interchangeably, there are important distinctions. All plants that produce a pod containing edible seeds belong to the botanical Fabaceae family, commonly known as the legume family. The term *legume* is used to describe the entire plant, while the term *pulse* is used to describe the dried edible seed found in the legume plant's pod. These edible seeds (available dried or canned) are highly nutritious, provide both protein and dietary fiber, and are inexpensive and widely available.

In the *Dietary Guidelines for Americans 2020–2025*, pulses (referred to as "beans, peas, lentils") count as either a vegetable or a protein since they have a similar nutrient profile to foods found in both of these food groups. Soy foods (such as tofu) and peanuts, also classified as legumes, are only in the protein foods group because they contain higher amounts of fat. Fresh peas and fresh green beans are counted only as a vegetable because they are lower in protein.

Tips for Using More Beans, Peas, Lentils, Nuts, and Seeds

Beans, peas, lentils, nuts, and seeds are nutritious, flavorful, and versatile in recipe development and can be used in almost any type of recipe. Because they can be pureed, ground, or toasted, they can be simple (and secret) additions to boost nutrition, flavor, and texture in sweet or savory recipes, or they can be showcased in a dish. The following are just a few examples for using beans, peas, lentils, nuts, and seeds:

- Lentils, because of their color, can be a perfect substitution for some ground beef in a recipe, and chickpeas (whole or chopped) are an equally good match for ground chicken or turkey.

- Extend ground meat with tofu or meat substitute crumbles. Tofu mixed with a small amount of ground pork adds a delicious combination of flavor.

- Thicken soups with a bean puree by blending together a 1:1 ratio of cooked beans to liquid and adding it to the soup.

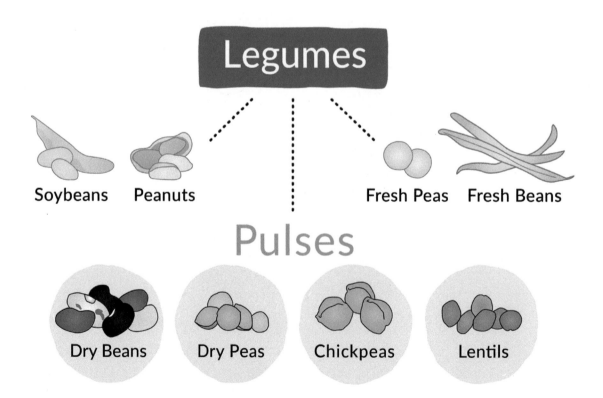

Courtesy of the USA Dry Pea & Lentil Council

- Use bean purees as a basis for dips and spreads or in quick breads, pancakes, or muffins.

- Experiment with pastas made from beans, lentils, or chickpeas.

- Add cooked beans, lentils, nut butters, or tofu to fruit or vegetable smoothies.

- Coat firm tofu with cornstarch before baking or stir-frying to crisp the exterior (use a seasoned cast iron or nonstick pan to prevent sticking).

- Think bold and acidic when developing marinades for tofu. Marinades for tofu need not be Asian-inspired, but soy sauce, miso, and fermented black beans add umami flavor.

- Blend soft silken tofu into salad dressings, desserts, and soups.

- Use soaked cashews, blended with a little water or plant-based milk, and nutritional yeast as a base for a cheese-like sauce. (See an alternate recipe for vegan cheese sauce on page 65.)

HOW TO COOK DRIED BEANS, PEAS, AND LENTILS

Before cooking pulses, rinse well and remove any broken pieces or debris. Dried beans and chickpeas require a two-step cooking process: soaking and then cooking at a simmer. Lentils and dry peas (e.g., split peas, black-eyed peas) do not need to be soaked.

Soak dried beans in salted water for at least 4 hours or up to 12 hours before cooking; drain and rinse well before cooking in salted water. Most beans require cooking times ranging from 45 minutes to 2 hours, and some must cook even longer depending on their variety, age, and size.

One pound (2 cups) of dry beans yields about 5 to 6 cups cooked beans, and one (15-ounce) can of beans, after draining, is equivalent to about 1¾ cups.

- Consider textured vegetable protein (pressure cooked and dried defatted soybean flour) or soy curls (protein strips made from whole soybeans) for a meat extender or meat substitute in tacos, meat loaf, chili, sloppy joes, stir-fries, or any other dish that uses ground meat. Rehydrate textured vegetable protein separately before adding it to a recipe to avoid oversaturation. Squeeze out excess water after rehydrating soy curls if cooking them in a pan of hot oil.

Reducing or Replacing Meat and Dairy

The simplest way to start reducing meat is by placing plant-based foods—vegetables, beans, chickpeas, peas, lentils, soybeans, tofu, or tempeh—in the center of the plate and using meat on the side or only as a flavoring. If animal protein is used occasionally as a main entrée, keep portions to no more than 3 to 4 ounces (after cooking) per serving. Choose fish and poultry more often than red meats and pork, and limit use of higher-fat beef and pork cuts and processed meats, such as bacon and sausage. Try the following tips to replace animal protein entirely:

- Pair a whole grain with a plant-based protein, such as beans, lentils, or soy foods. This helps fill in any nutritional gaps and also makes the dish more satisfying.

- Modify recipes for traditional casseroles, tacos, soups, or stews containing ground meat by replacing the meat with cooked whole grains, vegetables, beans, peas, or lentils. Start gradually by replacing a quarter to a half of the meat in these dishes.

- Try using dairy alternatives in recipes that call for milk, yogurt, and cheese. Use plant-based beverages fortified with vitamin A, vitamin D, and calcium. The nutrient composition of fortified soy milk is closest to cow's milk.

- Use nutritional yeast instead of grated cheese as a seasoning. Sprinkling it over salads, roasted vegetables, pasta, rice, or scrambled eggs provides a savory and cheesy flavor boost.

Recipe Example: Using grains, vegetables, and nuts as a plant-based alternative to meat

A traditional Bolognese meat sauce uses ground beef chuck (or 2 parts ground beef chuck and 1 part ground pork) and whole milk, while this meat-free cauliflower "Bolognese," adapted from a recipe from the Culinary Institute of America, uses a combination of riced cauliflower and walnuts as a meaty substitute. The addition of anchovies, a source of heart-healthy omega-3 fatty acids, adds a meaty, savory umami deliciousness that deepens the flavor of the lower-calorie and lower-saturated fat sauce. Serve the Bolognese over whole grain pasta or blanched vegetable noodles.

Cauliflower Bolognese Sauce
Adapted from the Culinary Institute of America at Greystone

Preparation time: 10 minutes
Cooking time: 1 hour 10 minutes
Yield: 6 servings (⅔ cup per serving, a total of 4 cups)

1 (16-ounce) bag fresh or frozen riced cauliflower (see Notes)
1 cup walnuts halves, finely chopped
4 anchovy fillets, finely chopped
5 garlic cloves, chopped
½ cup vermouth or dry white wine
1 (29-ounce) can tomato sauce
½ cup dried whole wheat breadcrumbs (see Notes)
½ teaspoon freshly ground black pepper
¼ teaspoon kosher salt
½ cup roughly chopped fresh basil
Freshly grated Parmesan cheese, optional

1. Heat a large nonstick skillet over medium heat. Add the cauliflower and spray with nonstick cooking spray. Cook, stirring frequently and spraying 5 or 6 more times with nonstick spray to prevent burning, until the cauliflower is caramelized and deep brown in color, about 35 minutes. Do not overspray the cauliflower as it will become soggy.

2. Add the walnuts and anchovies and cook, stirring, until the anchovies break down, about 2 minutes. Add the garlic and cook an additional 30 seconds.

3. Add the vermouth and cook over high heat, stirring once or twice with a wooden spoon, until the vermouth is absorbed, about 1 minute. Stir in the tomato sauce, breadcrumbs, pepper, and salt. Simmer over low heat until the flavors meld together, about 30 minutes. Stir in the basil. Garnish each serving with Parmesan cheese if desired.

Notes:
To rice whole cauliflower: Discard the core of one medium to large cauliflower and cut the remaining florets into chunks. Working in batches, process the chunks in a food processor into tiny pieces about the size of rice.

To make dried breadcrumbs: Heat the oven or toaster oven to 325° F. Grind fresh or stale bread slices (regular or gluten-free) in a food processor. Spread the crumbs in a single layer on a baking sheet and bake for about 10 minutes, until toasted and dry.

Nutrition per ⅔-cup serving: 263 calories, 13 grams fat, 1.5 grams saturated fat, 650 milligrams sodium, 24 grams carbohydrate, 6 grams fiber, 13 grams total sugar, 8 grams protein

Cooking With Plant-Based Meat Substitutes

Many meat substitutes are available in the refrigerated and frozen sections of grocery stores—from breakfast "meats," such as sausages and bacon, to bean or veggie burgers and other textured meat substitute products. Many of these packaged meat substitutes mimic the aromas, textures, and flavors of animal meat, making them good choices for people who are transitioning to a more plant-based diet. However, they are not necessarily more nutritious than animal products, so their Nutrition Facts label should be examined closely.

Meat substitutes usually have a lower or similar calorie content as their animal-based counterparts but often contain more sodium. While many are minimally processed and made with only plant-based main ingredients, such as quinoa, black beans, pea protein, mung beans, and sweet potatoes, some include ultra-processed ingredients, additives, and flavorings. Some meat substitutes contain coconut oil, which provides a similar mouthfeel to meat, making them also high in saturated fat. On the other hand, most meat substitutes contain dietary fiber, which animal products do not provide.

Success in cooking with a meat substitute depends on the recipe and the technique used to prepare it. In general, it's best to use quality ingredients and add flavor, since meat substitutes often contain less fat than their counterparts. When used correctly, a meat substitute can be a delicious alternative ingredient in a plant-based recipe.

Plant-Based Ground "Meat"

Made from plant-based ingredients, such as peas and brown rice or pea protein, a plant-based ground meat substitute works well in highly seasoned dishes, such as meatballs, meat loaf, chili, sloppy joes, and meat sauces. The most successful meat-substitute recipes use fresh herbs and spices or robust flavors like mushrooms, soy sauce, tomatoes, and aged cheeses—ingredients rich in glutamates, the chemical compounds responsible for the savory flavor known as umami. A sprinkle of monosodium glutamate (MSG) can work as well. When making burgers with a meat substitute, be aware that they cook more quickly than meat burgers.

When selecting a plant-based ground meat substitute for a recipe, read labels carefully. Look for one made with mostly whole food ingredients; beware of potential allergens (e.g., wheat, soy, and tree nuts), if applicable; and keep the overall sodium content of the recipe lower by being mindful of the amount of other high-sodium ingredients (e.g., barbecue sauce, soy sauce, or cheese). Remember that whole foods like beans, lentils, tofu, or vegetables can also serve as ground meat substitutes in health-focused recipes.

Tempeh

Tempeh is typically made of whole cooked soybeans (although just about any bean or grain can be used) that are cooled and inoculated with a fungal culture. During the fermentation process, the microorganisms of the culture grow a pale coating of mycelium around the soybeans, forming the tempeh into a firm cake.

Tempeh should never be eaten raw, as it must be cooked to deactivate the fungal culture. It's usually steamed first, which softens it and makes it more

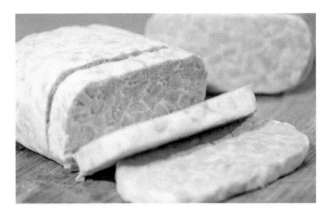

palatable by removing some of the bitterness. Steamed tempeh can be seasoned or marinated before stir-frying, panfrying, or baking. It works well as a ground beef substitute; simply cut the steamed tempeh into chunks and crumble it with your hands or mince it in a food processor. Tempeh crumbles can be used in countless ways and modified to fit any flavor profile, from tacos and burritos to pasta sauces and lasagnas.

Tofu

Tofu is made by boiling, curdling, and pressing whole soybeans. First, the soybeans are made into soy milk by being soaked, ground into a slurry, warmed with water, and strained. Next, a coagulant (e.g., nigari or calcium sulfate) is added, and the mixture simmers until it separates into curds and whey. The curds are placed in cloth-lined molds and pressed into solid blocks—the longer they are pressed, the firmer the tofu will be. Soft tofu contains the most water, and extra-firm tofu has the least. Silken tofu does not have separate curds and whey, resulting in a smooth, custard-like texture.

Tofu is neutral tasting. This quality makes it a blank slate for taking on any flavor it is paired with. The following are tips for using different types of tofu in recipes:

- Before using soft block tofu, drain off any excess liquid. Silken tofu, which is available in soft, firm, and extra-firm types, should not be pressed. These products are best used in delicate dishes and purees; they're great for salad dressings, smoothies, dips, miso soup, sauces, and desserts. Silken tofu is also a good substitute for soy milk, eggs, or dairy products like cream.

- Medium block tofu should be pressed and drained for about 20 to 30 minutes. It can be baked, simmered in soups, or incorporated into puddings or pie fillings.

- Firm or extra firm block tofu should also be pressed and drained for about 20 to 30 minutes. This type of tofu, sliced or cubed, is best suited for heartier dishes—kebabs, stews, rice dishes, stir-fries, sandwiches, and more. Season the tofu in a marinade for at least 30 minutes or as long as overnight before using. Alternatively, if baking or panfrying and serving warm, toss the tofu in cornstarch for added exterior crispiness and then add marinade to glaze the fried exterior. If scrambling, smash the tofu with a potato masher, cook, and season. If there is time, freezing tofu overnight before pressing it can help give it a chewier texture and increase its ability to absorb flavors.

Seitan

Seitan, a mildly flavored, high protein meat substitute, is made by rinsing away the starch in wheat dough, leaving only the high-protein wheat gluten behind. It is the base for many commercial vegetarian products, including alternatives to bacon and hot dogs. Cooked seitan is similar in look and texture to meat. It is marinated before cooking and can be sautéed, stir-fried, roasted, or grilled; it can also be cut into chunks and braised in soups, chilis, or stews.

Recipe Example: Using soy-based products as a plant-based alternative to meat

Tempeh is a versatile meat substitute in plant-based cooking as it takes on the flavor of whatever it is marinated or cooked in. Plus, it's a great source of protein (with 17 grams per 3-ounce serving) and has a naturally firm texture and nutty flavor that is enhanced by steaming or boiling—a process that also helps remove some of the bitterness and aids the absorption of marinades and sauces. It makes for a great substitute for chicken in this salad, which can be made vegan by using vegan mayonnaise. Serve the tempeh salad between two slices of bread as a sandwich, on top of salad greens, or stuffed into a tomato.

Tempeh Mock Chicken Salad

By Jill Nussinow, MS, RDN

Preparation time: 20 minutes
Cooking time: 15 minutes
Marinating time: 20 minutes
Yield: 3 servings (¾ cup per serving)

1 (8-ounce) package tempeh, cut into ½-inch cubes
¼ cup water
1 tablespoon vegan bouillon powder or vegan broth base and seasoning
¼ teaspoon freshly ground black pepper, plus more to taste
¼ cup mayonnaise or vegan mayonnaise
1 stalk celery, chopped
3 tablespoons minced onion
1 tablespoon minced fresh parsley
1 tablespoon nutritional yeast
1 teaspoon Dijon mustard
Pinch kosher salt

1. Place the tempeh in a saucepan, cover with water, and bring to a boil. Reduce the heat and simmer for 15 minutes. Drain tempeh.

2. Stir together the water, bouillon powder, and pepper in a medium bowl. Add the tempeh and let marinate at room temperature for 20 minutes.

3. Mix the mayonnaise, celery, onion, parsley, yeast, mustard, and salt and pepper to taste in a medium bowl. Add the tempeh and mix until the tempeh is evenly coated.

Note: *To make a curried mock chicken salad, add ¼ cup raisins or sliced grapes, ¼ cup slivered almonds, and ½ teaspoon curry powder to the mayonnaise mixture.*

Nutrition per ¾-cup serving: 297 calories, 22 grams fat, 4 grams saturated fat, 600 milligrams sodium, 9 grams carbohydrate, 1 gram fiber, 1 gram total sugar, 17 grams protein

Recipe Example: Using soy-based products as a plant-based alternative to egg and dairy

This plant-based mousse uses silken tofu to replace both the eggs and cream, reducing the calories, fat, and saturated fat and making it a perfect dessert for a plant-based, egg-free, or dairy-free diet. Tofu's smooth, creamy texture whips up easily, and its mild flavor naturally picks up the chocolate and orange flavors.

Dark Chocolate Orange Mousse

By Laura M. Ali, MS, RDN

Preparation time: 10 minutes
Chilling time: 3 hours
Yield: 6 servings (½ cup per serving)

MOUSSE

3½ ounces dark chocolate (see Note), chopped

1 (16-ounce) package silken tofu

1 tablespoon agave syrup

1 tablespoon Cointreau (or other orange liqueur)

2 teaspoons grated orange zest

¼ teaspoon kosher salt

MACERATED STRAWBERRIES

½ cup sliced strawberries

2 tablespoons Cointreau (or other orange liqueur)

1 teaspoon grated orange zest

1. For the mousse, place the chocolate in the top of a double boiler and melt slowly. Alternatively, place chocolate in a glass bowl and melt in the microwave in 20- to 30-second intervals, stirring the chocolate each time to ensure even melting.

2. Whip the tofu in the bowl of a food processor until smooth. Add the agave syrup, Cointreau, orange zest, and salt and whip until combined and smooth. Add the melted chocolate and blend until combined. Divide the mixture among six glasses or ramekins and refrigerate for at least 3 hours or overnight.

3. For the macerated strawberries, place the strawberries in a small bowl and mix with the Cointreau and orange zest. Allow to sit at room temperature for 30 minutes, tossing occasionally.

4. When ready to serve, garnish the mousse with the macerated strawberries.

Note: *You can find a variety of dark chocolate bars with varying amounts of cocoa, from 60% to 90%. The lower percentage cocoa bar will be less bitter and sweeter while the higher percentage bar will be less sweet and have a little more bite to it. A 78% cocoa bar works well in this recipe.*

Nutrition per ½-cup serving: 150 calories, 7 grams total fat, 3.5 grams saturated fat, 85 milligrams sodium, 15 grams carbohydrate, 1 gram fiber, 11 grams total sugar, 4 grams protein

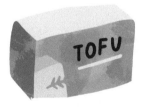

Quick Tip

"Look at your favorite foods—the dishes you love to create time and time again—and give them a plant-based makeover. Making easy swaps such as trading out beef for lentils in spaghetti sauce, using black beans in place of ground beef in tacos, or substituting cubed tofu for chicken in a stir-fry will make plant-based eating more accessible and familiar for the whole family." —Sharon Palmer, MSFS, RDN, The Plant-Powered Dietitian

Plant-Based Milks

Plant-based milks are nondairy alternative beverages made from plant ingredients, such as rice, soy, nuts, seeds, coconut, oats, peas, or blends of these ingredients. Many plant-based milks come in both sweetened and unsweetened varieties. Fortified soy milk and soy yogurt are included as part of the dairy group because their nutrient content is similar to that of dairy milk and yogurt when they are fortified with calcium and vitamins A and D. Other plant-based products sold as "milk" may contain added calcium and other nutrients, but they typically lack some of the nutrients found in dairy milk.

To make plant-based milks, the raw plant materials, whether they are cereals (e.g., oats), legumes (e.g., peas, soybeans), or nuts (e.g., almonds), are soaked in water (or sometimes ground and then soaked), rinsed, drained, and ground into a smooth paste or puree. The resulting slurry is strained to remove all solids, and then flavorings, sweeteners, nutrients, thickening agents, and stabilizers are added.

Reasons for using a plant-based milk in recipes might be to address a milk allergy or lactose intolerance, for vegan diets, and for health conditions such as Crohn's disease or irritable bowel syndrome.

Nutritional Comparison of Dairy and Plant-Based Milks

Per 1 cup (8 fl oz) serving	Calories	Protein (g)	Total fat (g)	Saturated fat (g)	Carbohydrate (g)	Fiber (g)	Calcium (mg)*	Vitamin D (mcg)*	Vitamin B12 (mcg)*
Whole milk	146	8	8	5	11	0	300	3	1
2% milk	122	8	5	3	12	0	307	3	1
1% milk	105	8	2	2	13	0	307	3	2
Skim milk	83	0	0	0	12	0	322	3	1
Soy milk	105	6	4	0	12	1	300–450	3	2
Unsweetened soy milk	79	7	4	0	3	2	300	0	3
Oat milk	120	3	5	0–1	16	2	350	0–4	1
Unsweetened oat milk	79	4	2	0–1	14	2	20–460	0–4	0
Almond milk	73	1	2	0	13	1	432	2	0
Unsweetened almond milk	37	1	2	0	3	1	430–450	0–5	0
Pea milk	70	8	5	0	0	0	450–465	3–6	0
Hemp milk**	50–60	2–3	5	0–1	0–1	0–1	255–300	2	0–1
Rice milk	115	1	2	0	22	1	280–290	2	2
Unsweetened rice milk	113	1	2	0	22	1	280–325	1	2
Cashew milk	156	5	11	0–2	11	2	20–450	0	0
Unsweetened cashew milk	130	4	10	0–1	7	0	15–450	0	0
Macadamia milk	55	1	5	1	1	1	180–470	0–4	0–6
Coconut milk	76	1	5	3–5	7	0	459	3	2
Unsweetened coconut milk	45	0	4	5	2	1	130–470	0–3	0–3
Unsweetened flax milk**	25	0	3	0	1	0	280	2	1
Unsweetened quinoa milk beverage**	40	1	0	0	8	0	390	5	0

Source: Unless otherwise noted, data obtained from US Department of Agriculture, Agricultural Research Service, FoodData Central: fdc.nal.usda.gov

* Values may vary due to differences in fortification.

** Information obtained from manufacturers.

Whole Grains in Recipe Development

All grains start out whole, but they do not all end up on grocery store shelves as whole grains. When a grain is milled, the bran and germ are removed from the grain kernel, which reduces the grain's dietary fiber, B vitamins, iron, healthy fats, and other nutrients. The end result is a grain with a finer texture and longer shelf life. While most refined grains are subsequently enriched—meaning that specific B vitamins (thiamin, riboflavin, niacin, folic acid) and iron are added back after processing—the dietary fiber, other minerals (e.g., magnesium, selenium, and copper), and antioxidant-rich phytochemicals that are lost to the refining process are not added back. By definition, a whole grain must be the entire kernel—germ, bran, and endosperm.

Grains may be milled and ground into flours, or they may be harvested and eaten as whole grains. Whole Grain Options for Recipe Development provides a list of grains and the forms in which they are typically available.

The Whole Grains Council considers amaranth, quinoa, and buckwheat to be "pseudo-grains" because they are not in the same botanical family as other cereal grains. However, these pseudo-grains, which are naturally gluten-free, are normally categorized as whole grains because of the similarity of their nutritional profiles, preparation, and uses. Although there

---

WHOLE GRAIN OPTIONS FOR RECIPE DEVELOPMENT

Amaranth: available as a whole grain or as whole grain flour; can be popped like popcorn

Barley: available as whole barley, hulled barley (with the tough outer hull removed), or hull-less barley; also available as whole barley flour or pearled (polished to remove the bran; not a whole grain but still provides fiber)

Buckwheat: available as groats, kasha (roasted buckwheat), or whole grain flour

Corn: whole grain corn products include cornmeal, popcorn, and corn tortillas made with whole grain corn or masa flour

Millet: available as a whole grain or as whole grain flour

Oats: available as whole oats in many forms: rolled, old fashioned, quick cooking, or steel cut; also available as whole oat flour

Quinoa: available as a whole grain or as whole grain flour

Rice: brown, black, red, or purple rice are whole grain; white rice is refined; also available as brown rice flour

Rye: available as whole berries or as whole rye flour or rye meal

Sorghum: available as a whole grain or as whole grain flour

Teff: a type of millet; all varieties are whole grain because the kernel is too small to mill easily; available as teff flour

Wheat
- **Flour:** whole wheat flour
- **Bulgur:** available as parboiled, dried, and cracked
- **Einkorn:** available as a whole grain or as whole grain flour
- **Farro/emmer:** while farro/emmer is whole grain, note that semi-pearled and pearled farro are not whole grain
- **Freekeh:** available as roasted and cracked
- **Kamut:** available as flakes, berries, and hot cereal or porridge
- **Spelt:** available as flakes, berries, and flour
- **Triticale:** (a cross between wheat and rye) available as flakes or flour
- **Wheat berries:** whole kernels of wheat

Wild rice: technically a grass but is considered a whole grain; it is naturally gluten-free

Source: Whole grains A to Z by Whole Grains Council: wholegrainscouncil.org/whole-grains-101/whole-grains-z

is no official definition for "ancient grains," the Whole Grains Council shares that ancient grains are loosely defined as grains that have been largely unchanged over the last several hundred years. Einkorn, emmer/farro, Khorasan wheat (brand name is Kamut), and spelt are considered ancient grains in the wheat family. Heirloom varieties of other common ancient grains include sorghum, teff, millet, quinoa, buckwheat, and amaranth.

Identifying a Whole Grain Food

Foods labeled with the terms "multigrain," "stone ground," "100% wheat," "cracked wheat," "seven grain," or "bran" are usually not whole grain products. Check to make sure "whole" followed by the name of the grain is the first item in the product's ingredient list. If a product contains two grain ingredients and only the second ingredient listed is a whole grain, the product may have as little as 1% or as much as 49% whole grain content, according to the Whole Grains Council.

Color is not an indication of the presence of whole grains. For example, a bread may have a brown color because molasses or other ingredients have been added. Always check the ingredient list to verify whether a food is whole grain. Use the product's Nutrition Facts label to choose whole grain products with a higher percentage of the Daily Value (DV) for dietary fiber. (20% DV or more per serving of dietary fiber is considered high.) Many, but not all, whole grain products are good or excellent sources of dietary fiber—and be aware that some high-fiber products sometimes contain bran or other added fiber but don't have much, if any, whole grain content.

FORMS OF GRAINS

Whole grain: Includes the entire grain seed (kernel). Each component of a grain (bran, germ, and endosperm) contains health-promoting nutrients.

Refined grain: A grain that is milled to remove its bran and germ.

Enriched grain*: A milled grain enriched with certain B vitamins (thiamin, riboflavin, niacin, folic acid) and iron after processing.

* Examples of enriched refined grain products and refined grains: white bread, refined grain cereal and crackers, corn grits, cream of rice, cream of wheat, pearled barley, masa, pasta, and white rice.

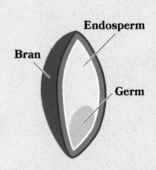

Tips for Using Whole Grains in Savory Recipes

Whole grains are great in salads, soups, and casseroles; as a base for stews, roasted vegetable dishes, and stir-fries; or in recipes containing ground meat or meat substitutes. They can also be prepared pilaf style or cooked and drained like pasta. Whole grains are versatile enough to be used in many different types of recipes. For example:

- Use rolled oats, crushed whole wheat cereal, or any whole grain crumb in place of white breadcrumbs in meat loaves, meatballs, and burgers. Start with ¾ cup dry oats per pound of raw meat.

- Use whole grains in side dishes or as a texture enhancer in soups, stews, chilies, and casseroles.

- Use whole grains like bulgur, brown rice, barley, or millet in stuffing mixtures to fill acorn squash, bell peppers, and other hollowed vegetables.

- Use whole grain bread when making sandwiches, panini, croutons, French toast, or avocado toast.

- Use farro instead of arborio rice as the grain of choice in a risotto-type dish ("farrotto").

- Use colored rice (brown, black, red, or purple), barley, bulgur, millet, wheat berries, wild rice, or other whole grains in place of white rice.

- Use whole wheat or another whole grain pasta in place of regular pasta.

- Develop "bowl" recipes using the following formula: whole grain + pulse + vegetable and/or fruit + nuts/seeds + savory sauce.

See Guide to Cooking Whole Grains on page 78.

> *Quick Tip*
>
> "Consider the sauce you use with whole wheat pastas. The slight bitterness of whole wheat may be heightened by acidic sauces, like tomato sauce or lemony sauces. Whole wheat pasta pairs wonderfully with mushrooms and other earthy ingredients (carrots, peas), which bring out the sweetness in the whole grain."
> —Sanna Delmonico, MS, RDN, Associate Professor, Culinary Institute of America at Greystone

KNOW THE DIFFERENCE: CORNMEAL, CORN FLOUR, POLENTA, AND GRITS

Cornmeal	Cornmeal is made from milled, dried white or yellow dent (also known as field) corn; it is coarsely ground, producing a gritty texture. It is available in a degerminated form, meaning that the germ and bran are removed during processing, making it more shelf stable, or it can be purchased in a stone ground form, where the germ and bran remain ("whole grain" in the ingredient list).
Corn flour	Corn flour is made from milled, dried dent corn that produces a fine and smooth texture.
Polenta	Polenta is a dish, rather than a type of cornmeal, that is usually made with medium-grind cornmeal. It is traditionally made from flint corn, which retains a distinctive texture and flavor when cooked.
Grits	Grits are made from dent corn or hominy (corn treated with lime), like cornmeal, but with a coarser grind.
Masa harina	This corn flour is made from dried dent corn kernels soaked in a lime water solution and then dried and finely ground. It is used to make dough for tamales and tortillas.
Cornstarch	This is a fine and powdery starch made from the endosperm of the corn kernel.

GUIDE TO COOKING WHOLE GRAINS

Use the following guidelines for quick-cooking grains and longer-cooking grains when developing and writing recipes with different types of whole grains.

Quick-Cooking Grains

Grain (1 cup)	Water/liquid (cups)	Salt (teaspoons)*	Cooking time (minutes)	Approximate cooked yield (cups)**
Absorption method				
Polenta (precooked medium-ground cornmeal), instant or quick cooking	4	1	2–5	4
Couscous, fine	1¼	¼	5–10	3
Teff (pilaf) Teff (cereal)	1½ 3–4	½	8–10 15–20	2½
Barley, quick cooking	2	¼	10–12	3
Bulgur	1¾–2	¼–½	12–15	3
Quinoa	1¾	¼	15	3
Millet	1¾–2	½	15–20	3
Amaranth (pilaf) Amaranth (cereal)	1½ 2½	¼ ½	20 25	2½
Corn grits	4–4½	1	20–25 (60 if stone ground)	4
Oats, steel cut	3½–4	¼–½	20–30 (depending on preferred chewiness)	3
Cornmeal	3½–4	1	25–30	4
Boiled/drained method				
Buckwheat groats	2	½	15	3
Farro (semipearled; pearled/Italian; outer bran layer removed)	8	1	20–30	3

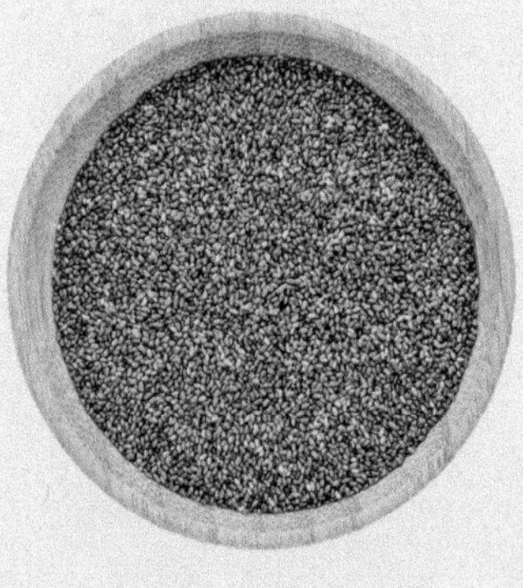

Teff

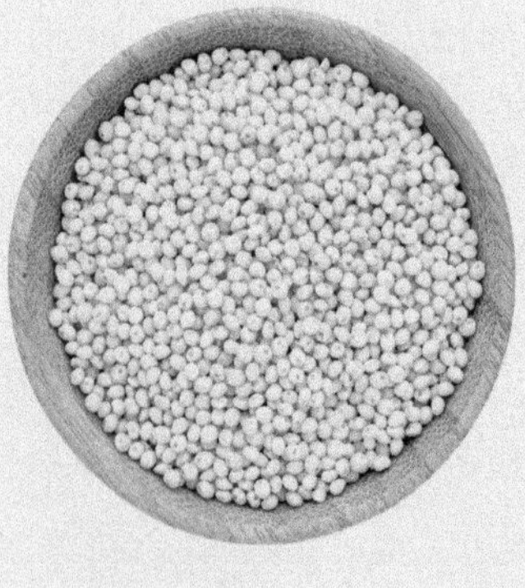

Millet

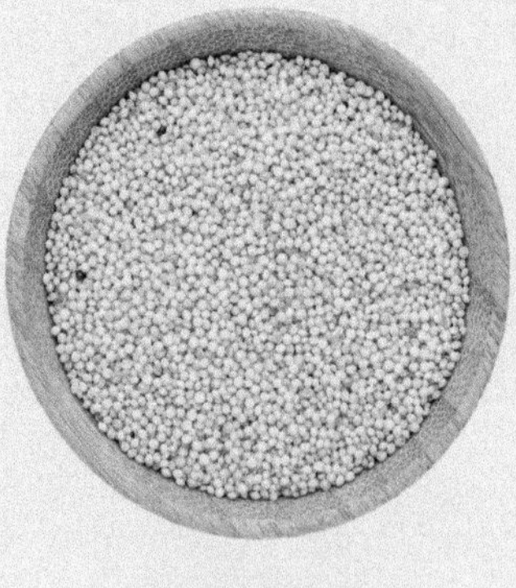

Amaranth

Longer-Cooking Grains

Grain (1 cup)	Water/liquid (cups)	Salt (teaspoons)*	Cooking time (minutes)	Approximate cooked yield (cups)**
Absorption method				
Brown rice	2½	¼	25–45	3
Black or purple rice	1¾ (or 6 if boiled/drained method is preferred)	¼	30–35	3
Polenta (medium-ground cornmeal)	3	1	30	3
Barley, hulled (whole)	3	½	45–60	3½
Wild rice	3	1	45–50	3½
Boiled/drained method				
Oat berries (whole or groats)	8	1	30–35	2½
Barley (pearl)	8	2	45–60	3½
Spelt berries	4–8	1	Soak overnight + 45–60	3
Kamut berries	8	1	Soak overnight + 40–60	3
Farro (whole grain)	8	1	Soak overnight + 45–60	3
Sorghum	8	1	50–60	2½
Wheat berries (hard)	4	½	Soak overnight + 60	2½

* Use less salt if cooking liquid contains salt.

** Yields may vary due to age of grain, changes in the recipe ratio, soaking, and cooking times.

Sources: *Book of Yields*, 8th Edition, by Francis T. Lynch. 2010. Wiley. | *Joy of Cooking* by Irma Rombauer, 2019. Scribner | *Ancient Grains for Modern Meals* by Maria Speck. 2011. Penguin Random House | Whole Grains Council | Bob's Red Mill product directions

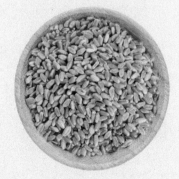

Wheat berries

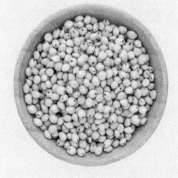

Sorghum

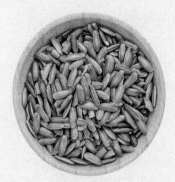

Brown Rice

Recipe Example: Using grains, beans, seeds, and vegetables as a plant-based alternative to meat

This recipe uses a blend of old-fashioned oats, white beans, hemp seeds, chia seeds, and a medley of vegetables to create a high-quality plant-based alternative to meat that has lots of protein and fiber. Incorporating tomato paste and soy sauce adds an extra umami layer of flavor. Serve the burgers alone or on a bun with condiments and toppings of your choice.

Curried White Bean and Oat Veggie Burgers
By Sharon Palmer, MSFS, RDN

Preparation time: 35 minutes
Chilling time: 1 hour
Cooking time: 45 minutes
Yield: 8 patties

2 medium carrots, roughly chopped
2 stalks celery, roughly chopped
1 small onion, roughly chopped
2 garlic cloves, peeled
1 (1-inch) piece fresh ginger, peeled
1 jalapeño pepper, stemmed and quartered
½ cup cilantro leaves
1 teaspoon dried ground turmeric
1 (15-ounce) can white beans (such as navy or cannellini), drained and rinsed
1 cup old-fashioned oats
¼ cup hemp seeds
3 tablespoons tomato paste
2 tablespoons chia seeds
1 tablespoon ground cumin
1 tablespoon regular or gluten-free soy sauce
Juice of 1 lemon

1. Place the carrots, celery, onion, garlic, ginger, jalapeño, cilantro, and turmeric in the container of a food processor. Process until the vegetables are chopped finely but not pureed or liquefied.

2. Add the beans, oats, hemp seeds, tomato paste, chia seeds, cumin, soy sauce, and lemon juice. Process until the mixture is smooth and well combined but not liquefied. Chill the mixture for 1 hour so that it is easier to shape into burgers.

3. Heat the oven to 375° F. Spray a baking sheet with nonstick cooking spray. Scoop up some of the veggie burger mixture using a ½-cup measuring cup and shape into a round patty, about 1 inch thick. Place on the baking sheet and repeat to make eight patties.

4. Bake the patties until golden brown and firm, 45 to 50 minutes.

Nutrition per patty: 142 calories, 3 grams total fat, 0 grams saturated fat, 229 milligrams sodium, 22 grams carbohydrate, 6 grams fiber, 2 grams total sugar, 7 grams protein

HOW TO STORE WHOLE GRAIN FLOURS

Since whole grains, by definition, include the oil-rich germ of the grain, they don't keep as long as their refined counterparts. When stored at room temperature, whole grains start to deteriorate quickly. It's best to store whole grains sealed in an airtight container or bag in the freezer; the next best option is to store in an airtight container in the refrigerator or pantry. An exception to this is oats, which are shelf-stable due to the processing they undergo.

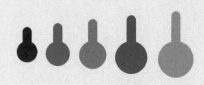

Baking With Whole Grains

Baking with whole grain flours in place of all or some all-purpose flour is not straightforward. The balance depends on the type of recipe (e.g., yeast breads, quick breads, cookies, or pancakes) and the type of whole grain flour used (traditional whole wheat or specialty flours like buckwheat, millet, sorghum, or spelt). To better understand the science of whole grain baking, experiment in the kitchen and use guidance from baking experts (see Recipe Development Resources in Chapter 1).

All-purpose flour's gluten-forming proteins make it the most commonly used flour for baking. These gluten-forming proteins determine the structure and volume of baked goods. Many of the specialty flours contain the same amount of protein and may be nutritionally similar, but the proteins in them form little to no gluten. As a result, whole wheat flour is the easiest whole grain flour to start with when developing whole grain baking recipes.

Baked goods made with whole wheat flour in place of all-purpose flour often have reduced volume, a darker color, and a coarser texture, but they also have a flavor profile that is nuttier and more nuanced. Whole wheat flour is high in gluten-forming proteins, but the bran and germ present in whole wheat flour interferes with the gluten's formation, making yeast breads denser. For information on whole grain gluten-free flours and baking, see Chapter 6.

Types of Wheat Flour

The quantity and quality of the protein found in wheat flour, also known as the gluten-forming protein, determine how to choose a type of flour for baking. The higher the protein the more gluten development, making it a good choice for chewier breads; the lower the protein content, such as in cake flour and pastry flour, the softer and more tender the baked good. All-purpose flour contains an average protein content, which makes it the most versatile and commonly used flour choice.

All-purpose flour is available in bleached or unbleached forms that can be used interchangeably in many recipes. Be aware, however, that the bleaching process changes the flour's starch granules, enabling water and other liquids to enter more easily and inhibiting gluten formation. Bleaching can also destroy some of the protein, which is why unbleached all-purpose flour is slightly higher in protein (the amount varies by brand). For these reasons, baked goods such as cookies and pie crust made with unbleached flour

TYPES OF AND USES FOR WHEAT FLOUR

Flour type	% Protein	Suggested uses
High gluten	14%–15%	Yeast baking: pizza dough, bagels, extra-chewy breads; often mixed with other flours
Whole wheat	13%–14%	Flavorful, hearty breads; often mixed with other flours
White whole wheat	13%	Use in place of all-purpose flour for extra fiber
Bread	12%–13%	Yeast baking: pizza dough, bagels, sandwich breads
All-purpose	10%–12%	Most versatile: cakes, cookies, muffins, quick breads, pie crusts, breads, scones
Double zero (00)	8%–12%	Preferred for thin-crust pizza; produces a crisp crust that is chewy on the inside
Self-rising	9%–11%	Gives a light and airy texture due to the added baking powder; biscuits, scones, pancakes
Pastry	8%–9%	Pie crusts, pastries, cookies, scones
Cake	7%–9%	Extra-light and extra-fluffy cakes; a more tender crumb in cookies

Sources: How do you choose the right flour by Posie Brien: kingarthurbaking.com/blog/2019/07/12/types-of-flour | Wheat Foods Council, Flour 101, wheatfoods.org/wheat-101/flour-and-baking/flour-101

may be less tender and may brown more quickly. If a recipe test using bleached all-purpose flour produces a tender and flaky product—specify "bleached all-purpose flour" in the ingredient list. Otherwise, assume that a home cook will use one of the available varieties of bleached or unbleached all-purpose flour.

Tips for Using Whole Grains in Baking

Baked Goods

Experiment with whole grain flours when modifying recipes for cookies, brownies, scones, pancakes, muffins, and quick breads, and see what suits your taste. A small amount of additional liquid may be needed when substituting with whole grain flour. Other tips include the following:

- Start by replacing ¼ to ⅓ of the all-purpose flour with whole wheat flour or another whole grain flour. Experiment and increase the proportion up to a 50:50 ratio.

- Whole grain flour works best in naturally darker and denser baked goods, such as banana bread or oatmeal cookies. The whole wheat flavor will come through and the color and texture will be altered. Some may find the results undesirable, but others find it delicious.

- Replace all of the all-purpose flour called for in a recipe with white whole wheat flour, which is made from a special variety of white wheat. It is nutritionally equivalent to whole wheat flour but lighter in color and milder in flavor.

- Replace all of the all-purpose flour with whole wheat pastry flour, which is milled from a low-protein soft wheat, in a 1:1 ratio. Whole wheat pastry flour has less gluten-forming potential than regular whole wheat flour, ensuring a more tender result in baked goods.

Bread

The effects of whole wheat flour in yeast-raised doughs are more nuanced because the bran and germ interfere with gluten formation. Some experts suggest adding 2% to 5% vital wheat gluten (gluten flour)

for strengthening or to use a wheat flour with a higher gluten content to compensate for the gluten deficit of whole wheat flour. Other tips include the following:

- Substitute up to 30% whole wheat flour or other whole grain flour when baking breads.

- Some whole grains milled into flours, such as brown rice, corn, oats, buckwheat, and sorghum, form little to no gluten, which is why they are often blended with other wheat flours in recipes. (They contain other proteins, but no gluten-forming ones.) Tips for using these specialty flours in gluten-free baking are discussed in Chapter 6. Rye is a special case: it has some gluten, but not the kind that creates the network necessary for a light and airy bread. As a result, rye breads are heavy and dense.

- Experiment with adding unprocessed wheat bran, flaxseed meal, hemp seeds, or chia seeds to baked goods. These ingredients can add desirable texture and additional dietary fiber and other nutrients.

Quick Tip

"I find that 20% whole grain flour—whether it's whole wheat flour or an alternate whole grain flour—and 80% all-purpose flour or bread flour is a good starting point when developing whole grain baked goods or bread. The whole grain flour adds a complex and earthy flavor, but there is still enough of the functional properties from the all-purpose or bread flour. You might experiment and go up to 50% whole wheat or whole grain, but you'll need to consider adding more liquid to the recipe, especially with bread baking. The bran and germ in whole wheat flour absorbs more water, so adding about ½ ounce of water (1 tablespoon) to each 2 ounces of whole wheat flour (about ½ cup) will help a dough become more supple." —Peter Reinhart, faculty member at Johnson and Wales University and author of six books on bread baking

Dietary Fiber, Prebiotics, and Probiotics in Recipe Development

Plant-based recipes are generally higher in dietary fiber, which offers health benefits including helping to lower risk of cardiovascular disease and improving gut health and blood sugar control, and it may play a role in managing weight. Different types of fiber have different physiological effects and health benefits. In general, dietary fiber is categorized into two main types, soluble and insoluble, and most foods contain a combination of these types.

Soluble fiber absorbs water during digestion. It produces a thick gel in the gastrointestinal tract that blunts the body's normal blood sugar spikes that occur after eating. Soluble fibers are found in a variety of foods, including beans, peas, apples, pears, strawberries, citrus, carrots, potatoes, shiitake mushrooms, oats, and barley.

Insoluble fiber remains unchanged during digestion. This helps encourage bowel regularity by adding bulk to stools and speeding intestinal passage, which limits the time that potential carcinogens remain in contact with the intestinal wall. Insoluble fiber is found in a variety of foods, such as wheat bran, whole grain foods (e.g., brown rice), broccoli, cauliflower, cabbage, and kale.

Prebiotics, Probiotics, and Resistant Starch

Developing recipes that contain sources of prebiotics, probiotics, or resistant starches is another approach for health-focused recipe development. These specific functional components of foods affect the type and amount of healthy bacteria in the gastrointestinal tract and can help improve gut health. They are found in a variety of high-fiber foods, some dairy products, and fermented foods.

The community of bacteria living in and on the human body, which is known as the microbiome, is a living dynamic environment where the abundance of bacteria may fluctuate on a daily, weekly, and monthly basis depending on diet, medication, exercise, and

Understanding Prebiotics, Fiber, and Probiotics

Prebiotics	Fiber	Probiotics
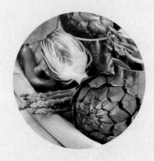	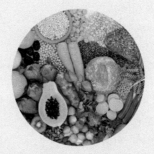	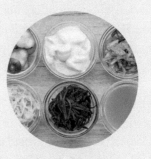
▪ Found in a variety of high fiber foods, such as asparagus, artichokes, leeks, onions, beans, and whole grains ▪ Serves as the "food" for health-promoting probiotics	▪ Found in fruits, vegetables, legumes, and whole grains ▪ Regulates and maintains bowel health, helps to lower blood cholesterol and blood glucose	▪ Found in yogurts and fermented foods and beverages ▪ Provides healthy bacteria to improve gut health
Try to pair prebiotics with probiotics.	**Aim for 25–38 grams per day.**	**Consume probiotics at least once per day.**

a host of other environmental exposures. Naturally occurring beneficial bacteria are not only important for a healthy gut but also for overall health and well-being.

Prebiotics

Some insoluble fibers act as a prebiotic—a nondigestible food component—that feeds friendly bacteria in the gut. These prebiotics can stimulate the growth and balance of healthy bacteria in the gut and potentially enhance calcium absorption as well. Although all prebiotics are fiber, not all fiber is prebiotic. Prebiotics are naturally found in many fruits, vegetables, and whole grains, such as asparagus, Jerusalem artichokes (sunchokes), bananas, leeks, garlic, onions, beans, peas, lentils, soybeans, whole wheat foods, and oats.

Resistant starch, which acts as a prebiotic, is a group of low-viscosity fibers that resist digestion in the small intestine and ferment in the large intestine. As the fibers ferment, they act as a prebiotic and feed the good bacteria in the gut.

When regular starches are digested, they typically break down into glucose, but because resistant starch is not digested in the small intestine, it doesn't raise glucose levels in the blood. Gut health is improved thanks to the fermentation occurring in the large intestine that makes more good bacteria and reduces bad bacteria in the gut. Increased healthy gut bacteria may improve blood sugar control. Other benefits of resistant starch include an increased feeling of fullness, treatment and prevention of constipation, and reduced risk of colon cancer. Resistant starch is found in plantains, green bananas, beans, peas, lentils, whole grains (e.g., oats, barley), and cooked and cooled white rice.

Probiotics

Probiotics are live bacteria that naturally live in the gut. When consumed regularly, they confer such health benefits as breaking down indigestible components of the diet, aiding in nutrient absorption, and ridding the body of potentially harmful bacteria. The live cultures found in certain foods help supplement and foster the development of healthy bacteria already present in the gastrointestinal system.

Probiotics may also help boost immunity, assist in the management of irritable bowel syndrome symptoms, and improve overall health. To be considered a probiotic, a bacteria strain must have benefits

PROBIOTICS AND FERMENTED FOODS

Not all fermented foods and beverages contain probiotics. Fermentation is when carbohydrates (sugars) are broken down by bacteria or yeast into end products like alcohol or lactic acid. Beer and wine are produced through fermentation, but they undergo additional processing after fermentation that eliminates the helpful bacteria. When fermented foods are pasteurized, both harmful and beneficial bacteria are destroyed. In other fermented foods, the live active cultures used for fermentation produce a natural source of healthy, live probiotics. The words "contains live cultures" on the label are a good indication that the food has live microorganisms. Foods that contain probiotics include:

- yogurt
- kefir
- acidophilus milk (cultured low-fat milk that is fermented with bacteria)
- buttermilk
- sauerkraut (unpasteurized fermented cabbage)
- kimchi (Korean fermented cabbage)
- miso or miso soup (fermented soybeans)
- tempeh (fermented soybeans)
- kombucha (fermented green tea–based beverage)
- pickles (only naturally fermented ones, not those pickled using vinegar)
- natto (Japanese fermented soybeans)
- cheeses (that have been aged, but not heated afterwards), including Gouda, Edam, Gruyère, provolone, Swiss, mozzarella, and cheddar

supported by scientific research and must be delivered in a sufficient quantity to confer health benefits.

Prebiotics and probiotics work together. Prebiotics offer long-term nourishment for gut bacteria, and probiotics provide a quick influx of good bacteria. Regular intake of prebiotics is necessary for the good bacteria found in probiotics to thrive in the gut.

Boosting Fiber in Recipes

Using more plant-based foods in recipes will increase their dietary fiber content, and the closer a grain, legume, fruit, or vegetable is to its original state, the more dietary fiber it generally contains. For example:

- An apple with skin (1 medium apple = 4.4 grams fiber) compared to apple juice (½ cup = 0 grams fiber)

- Soybeans (½ cup = 5 grams fiber) compared to tofu (3 ounces = 0.8 grams fiber)

- Cooked lentils (½ cup cooked = 8 grams fiber) compared to lentil "chips" (1 ounce = 0 grams fiber)

When comparing food products to increase a recipe's dietary fiber, read the product's Nutrition Facts label and look for those that are high in fiber (at least 6 grams per serving) or a "good source" of fiber (at least 3 grams per serving). You can also reference the % DV of dietary fiber on the label to choose ingredients with a higher DV for fiber (the DV for fiber is 28 grams per day):

- 5% DV or less of dietary fiber per serving is low
- 20% DV or more of dietary fiber per serving is high

Dietary Fiber in Common Plant-Based Foods

Food	Amount	Dietary fiber (grams)*
Grains		
Wheat berries, cooked	1 cup	9.5
Sorghum, cooked	1 cup	9
Bulgur, cooked	1 cup	8
Teff, cooked	1 cup	7
Pearl barley, cooked	1 cup	6
Whole wheat pasta, cooked	1 cup	5
Quinoa, cooked	1 cup	5
Oats, cooked	1 cup	4
Brown rice, cooked	1 cup	3
Pasta, cooked	1 cup	2.5
Millet, cooked	1 cup	2
Corn tortilla	1 (6-inch) tortilla	1.5
White rice, cooked	1 cup	0.5
Flours		
Amaranth flour	½ cup	8
Spelt flour	½ cup	8
Whole wheat pastry flour	½ cup	8
Barley flour	½ cup	6
Whole wheat flour	½ cup	6
Buckwheat flour	½ cup	6

TABLE CONTINUES >

Dietary Fiber in Common Plant-Based Foods (continued)

Food	Amount	Dietary fiber (grams)*
Corn flour (cornmeal)	½ cup	4
Oat flour	½ cup	4
Gluten-free flour	½ cup	0–4 (varies by brand)
Brown rice flour	½ cup	3.5
Almond flour	½ cup	2
All-purpose flour	½ cup	2
Millet flour	½ cup	2
Rice flour (white)	½ cup	0
Bran and germ		
Wheat bran, raw	2 tablespoons	3
Wheat germ, raw	2 tablespoons	2
Oat bran, raw	2 tablespoons	2
Legumes (beans, peas, lentils, soybeans, peanuts)		
Pinto beans, canned or dried, cooked	½ cup	8
Cannellini beans, canned or dried, cooked	½ cup	8
Lentils, cooked	½ cup	8
Split peas, dried, cooked	½ cup	8
Black beans, canned or dried, cooked	½ cup	7
Tempeh	3 ounces (85 grams)	7
Chickpeas, canned or dried, cooked	½ cup	6
Fresh peas, cooked	½ cup	4.5
Edamame (soybeans in pod), cooked, shelled	½ cup	4
Peanuts	1 ounce (¼ cup)	3
Peanut butter	2 tablespoons	2
Tofu	3 ounces (85 grams)	1
Nuts		
Almond butter	2 tablespoons	3
Almonds, roasted	1 ounce (about ¼ cup)	3
Pistachios, pecans, hazelnuts	1 ounce (about ¼ cup)	3
Walnuts	1 ounce (about ¼ cup)	2
Sunflower butter	2 tablespoons	2
Pine nuts	1 ounce (about ¼ cup)	1
Seeds		
Chia seeds	2 tablespoons	10
Flaxseed meal	2 tablespoons	3
Sunflower seeds	2 tablespoons	2
Hemp seeds	2 tablespoons	0.5
Pumpkin seeds (pepitas)	2 tablespoons	0.5

TABLE CONTINUES >

Food	Amount	Dietary fiber (grams)*
Vegetables		
Brussels sprouts, cooked	1 cup	6
Artichoke hearts	1 cup	6
Broccoli, cooked	1 cup	5
Sweet potato, skin on	1 medium	5
Cauliflower, cooked	1 cup	5
Potato, skin on	1 medium	4.5
Spinach, frozen and cooked	½ cup	3.5
Kale, cooked	½ cup	2.5
Carrots	½ cup sliced cooked or 1 (7-inch) carrot	2.5 2
Eggplant, cooked	1 cup	2.5
Corn, canned or frozen	½ cup	2
Cabbage, cooked	½ cup	1.5
Spinach, raw	1 cup	0.5
Fruit		
Pear	1 medium	5.5
Avocado	½ medium	5
Dried figs	5	5
Apple	1 medium	4.5
Raspberries	½ cup	4
Blackberries	½ cup	4
Dried dates	5	3.5
Orange	1 medium	3
Banana	1 medium	3
Peach	1 medium	2.5
Pineapple	½ cup (chunks)	1
Kiwi	1 medium	2
Strawberries	½ cup (halved)	2
Blueberries	½ cup	2
Melon (cantaloupe/honeydew)	½ cup (cubes)	1

* Values are rounded to the nearest 0.5 grams.

Source: US Department of Agriculture, Agricultural Research Service, FoodData Central: fdc.nal.usda.gov

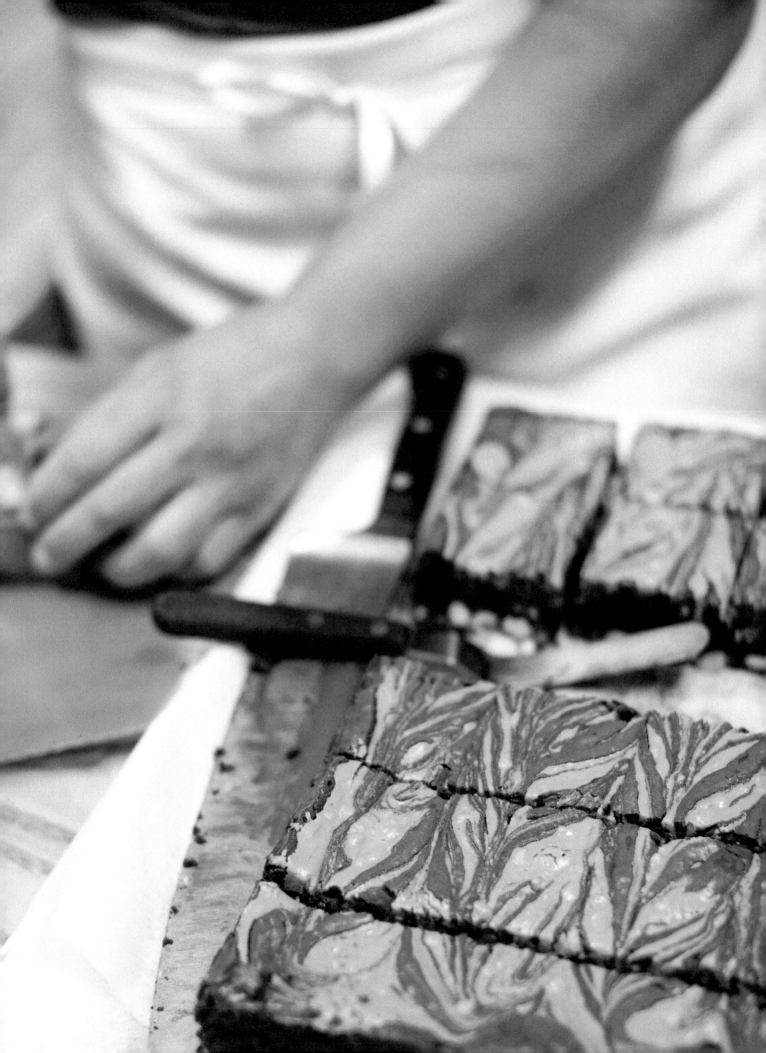

Chapter 4

Modifying Fat, Sodium, and Sugar in Recipe Development

IN THIS CHAPTER, LEARN ABOUT:

- The reasons for modifying fat, sodium, and sugar in recipe development

- Fat and its culinary functions in recipes, and how to modify total amount and types of fat in cooking or baking

- Sodium and its culinary functions in recipes, and how to modify recipes to reduce sodium

- Sugar and its culinary functions in recipes, and how to reduce or replace sugar in recipes

Recipe developers are often asked to develop recipes with limits on calories, while also modifying or limiting the amount of saturated fat, salt, and sugar. In turn, this can help people manage their diet-related health conditions and achieve their health and wellness goals. This chapter addresses the nutritional rationale for making these modifications, the functional roles of fat, salt, and sugar in recipes, and offers culinary techniques and tips for making these recipe modifications—with a focus on taste and flavor. The modifications in this chapter are meant to be paired with the tips and examples found in Chapters 2 and 3 for using nutrient-rich ingredients in recipes.

Modifying Total Fat or Type of Fat in Recipes

Reducing the total amount of fat or changing the type of fat in a recipe is often an objective in creating "healthier" recipes. Fat, an essential nutrient, provides fatty acids that the body cannot make itself, assists with the absorption of fat-soluble vitamins, and serves as an important source of energy. But dietary fat is also relatively high in calories, which is why it's referred to as being calorie or energy dense, supplying more calories (9 calories per gram) than either carbohydrate or protein (both contain 4 calories per gram).

The *Dietary Guidelines for Americans, 2020–2025* recommend that saturated fats should comprise no more than 10% of total daily calories starting at age 2. For those at risk of heart disease, the American Heart Association advises that no more than 6% of total daily calories should come from saturated fat—about 13 grams per day for a 2,000-calorie diet.

Developing recipes using less fat is one way to lower a recipe's calories, which can help support weight loss efforts. Modifying fat in a recipe might also mean addressing the type of fat used. In general, health-focused recipes use more monounsaturated and polyunsaturated fats, such as plant oils (e.g., corn, safflower, sunflower, avocado, olive, canola, peanut, sesame) and foods including nuts, seeds, and fish in place of fats containing high levels of saturated fats (e.g., butter, coconut oil, lard, and palm oil; full-fat dairy and fattier cuts of beef and

pork). Replacing saturated fats with monounsaturated and polyunsaturated fats can help reduce the risk of heart disease and stroke.

Which Fat to Choose?

When choosing which fat to use in cooking and baking, consider the smoke point, flavor, and fatty acid profile (i.e., healthfulness) of the fat. See Fatty Acid Comparison of Common Fats.

Smoke Point

The smoke point is the temperature when a fat or oil breaks down and begins to smoke, releasing free radicals and a substance called acrolein, the chemical that gives burnt foods an acrid flavor and aroma. Foods cooked in fats that have a higher smoke point can be cooked at higher temperatures without ruining the flavor of the food.

Flavor

Many fats are neutral in flavor. Others bring their own flavors and aromas to a recipe, such as a stir-fry dish finished with a touch of toasted sesame seed oil; a vinaigrette made with extra-virgin olive oil; and croissants or pie dough made with butter.

Fatty Acid Profile

Fats and oils (as well as foods that contain fat) are made up of a mix of fatty acids, the scientific name for the building blocks of fats. These fatty acids are classified as monounsaturated, polyunsaturated, or saturated depending on their chemical structure. Foods that contain fats, including fats and oils used in cooking, are often categorized based on the predominant type of fatty acid they contain. For example, oils and nuts contain predominately unsaturated fats, but they also have some saturated fat, too.

Unsaturated fats (monounsaturated and polyunsaturated) are considered healthier. They can help reduce total and low-density lipoprotein (LDL) blood cholesterol levels when they replace saturated fats, thus helping to lower the risk of heart disease and stroke.

Monounsaturated fats are found in higher concentrations in:

- olive, peanut, safflower, sesame, avocado, and canola oils
- nuts, such as almonds, pecans, and hazelnuts
- seeds, such as pumpkin and sesame seeds
- avocados

Polyunsaturated fats are found in higher concentrations in:

- corn, sunflower, soybean, and flaxseed oils
- walnuts
- flaxseeds
- fish

Omega-3 fats are an important type of polyunsaturated fat found in fish, including salmon, mackerel, and sardines. A plant form called alpha-linolenic acid (ALA) found in flaxseeds, walnuts, and canola and soybean oils is converted to forms of omega-3 fats in the body. See Omega-3 Fats Naturally Found in Selected Fish and Plant Sources on page 93.

Saturated fats, which are less healthful, are found in higher concentrations in:

- butter
- coconut oil
- meat products, such as sausage, bacon, beef, pork, lamb, and poultry with skin
- full-fat dairy foods including whole and reduced-fat milk, cheese, whipping cream, and dairy desserts, such as ice cream

Fatty Acid Comparison of Common Fats

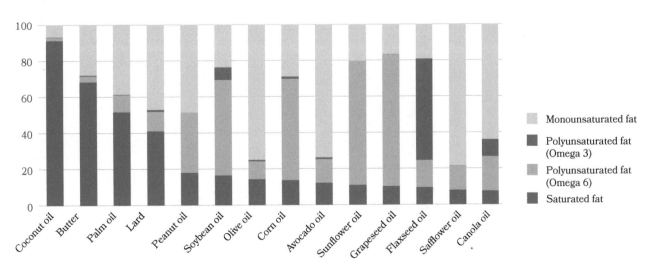

COMPARISON OF COOKING FATS AND OILS

Fat	Smoke point*	Flavor	Suggested use
Safflower oil	510° F	Neutral	High heat Searing, panfrying, deep-frying, sautéing
Camellia (tea seed) oil	485° F	Neutral	Stir-frying (often used in Chinese cooking), searing, panfrying, deep-frying, sautéing, roasting
Light olive oil**	465° F	Neutral	High heat Searing, panfrying, deep-frying, sautéing
Soybean oil	450° F	Neutral	High heat Searing, panfrying, deep-frying, sautéing
Peanut oil	450° F	Neutral to nutty	High heat Searing, panfrying, deep-frying, sautéing
Clarified butter	450° F	Silkier, richer, and more butter-like flavor than butter because the water and milk solids are removed in the clarifying process	High heat Searing, panfrying, sautéing; good in sauces and dips
Corn oil	450° F	Neutral	High heat Searing, panfrying, deep-frying, sautéing
Sunflower oil	440° F	Neutral	High heat Searing, panfrying, deep-frying, sautéing
Vegetable oil	400° F–450° F	Neutral	High heat Searing, panfrying, deep-frying, sautéing
Avocado oil	480° F–520° F	Neutral	High heat Searing, panfrying, sautéing; good in dressings
Canola oil	400° F	Neutral	High heat Searing, panfrying, deep-frying, sautéing
Grapeseed oil	390° F	Neutral	High heat Searing, panfrying, sautéing
Sesame oil	350° F–410° F	Neutral	Medium heat Sautéing
Toasted sesame oil	—	Nutty flavor and aroma	A finishing oil; flavor may change if used in cooking
Butter	350° F	Sweet, buttery, creamy	Medium heat Sautéing
Coconut oil	350° F	Neutral; less refined oil has plenty of coconut flavor	Medium heat Sautéing
Extra-virgin olive oil	325° F–375° F	Spicy, fruity, grassy	Medium to medium-high heat Sautéing; good in dressings and dips
Walnut	320° F	Nutty	Good in dressings and dips
Flaxseed	225° F	Mildly nutty	Good in dressings and dips or as a finishing oil

* Approximate, as variations and types of processing can influence the smoke point. High smoke point fats smoke around 400° F and above; medium smoke point fats smoke around 350° F; and low smoke point fats smoke around 320° F and below.

** Light olive oil is a refined oil that has a higher smoke point than extra-virgin olive oil. It is not light in terms of calorie or fat content.

Omega-3 Fats Naturally Found in Selected Fish and Plant Sources

The *Dietary Guidelines for Americans, 2020–2025* recommends two or more servings of cooked seafood per week for heart health, with an emphasis on choosing seafood species higher in omega-3 fats. When developing heart-healthy recipes, consider using these fish, or, alternatively, plant-based ingredients that naturally contain omega-3 fats.

Fish, cooked (3-ounce serving)	Omega-3 fats (grams)	Total fat (grams)
Pacific herring	2	15
Atlantic salmon, farmed	2	10.5
Atlantic salmon, wild	1.9	7
Atlantic herring	1.8	10
Atlantic mackerel	1.6	15
Rainbow trout, farmed	1	6
Halibut	1	2
Rainbow trout, wild	0.8	5
Tuna, white, canned in water, drained	0.8	2.5
Anchovy, canned in oil, drained	0.6	8
Flounder or sole	0.4	2
Tuna, light, canned in water, drained	0.3	1
Tuna, white, canned in oil, drained	0.2	7
Catfish, wild	0.2	2
Atlantic cod	0.2	1
Catfish, farmed	0.2	6
Tilapia	0.2	2
Pacific cod	0.1	0.5

Plant-based foods	Omega-3 fats (grams) as alpha-linolenic acid	Total fat (grams)
Chia seed (2 tablespoons)	5	8
Ground flaxseed (2 tablespoons)	2.9	6
Walnuts (1 ounce, about 12–14 halves, or ¼ cup)	2.5	18
Flaxseed oil (1 tablespoon)	2.4	14
Canola oil (1 tablespoon)	1.3	14
Soybean oil (1 tablespoon)	0.9	14
Edamame (½ cup)	0.3	5
Kidney beans, canned (½ cup)	0.1	0

Sources: US Department of Agriculture, Agricultural Research Service, FoodData Central: fdc.nal.usda.gov | Omega-3 fatty acids fact sheet for professionals by National Institutes of Health: ods.od.nih.gov/factsheets/Omega3FattyAcids-HealthProfessional/#en29

Tips for Modifying the Fat in Savory Recipes

To decrease the amount of total fat or modify the type of fat in a recipe, start by incrementally decreasing the amount of fat to determine how much fat is necessary to maintain the quality of the dish. This may take several rounds of experimentation, depending on the recipe. Another technique is to alter the cooking technique, such as the following:

- Instead of deep-frying or panfrying, try cooking methods that require little or no fat, such as grilling, broiling, flat-top grilling (a la plancha), roasting, steaming, poaching, boiling, baking, stir-frying, air frying, and sous vide.
- Use a rack when roasting meat so that the fat drips into the pan.
- After browning meat or poultry, drain the fat from the pan before adding other ingredients.
- To use less fat for sautéing, add a little water, broth, or even unsweetened green tea to a skillet, get it hot, and use it to sauté vegetables, meat, or fish.
- Stick-resistant cookware, such as well-seasoned or enameled cast iron or nonstick, requires less oil or butter to prevent sticking.
- When greasing a dish, use a nonstick cooking spray. For high-heat cooking, use a spray with a high smoke point, such as a canola or avocado oil spray.

VEGETABLE OILS

The category or term, *vegetable oil* generally refers to any oil that comes from a plant source, so it includes oils pressed from the seeds, nuts, grains, or fruits of plants. Oils can come from a variety of plant sources—including sesame seeds, flaxseeds, corn, peanuts, walnuts, olives, and more. An oil that is labeled vegetable oil on a supermarket shelf is often a single oil (most often soybean oil), but it can also be a blend of different plant oils (e.g., soybean, corn, safflower, sunflower). Most vegetable oils are refined and filtered to create clear, neutral-tasting oils for cooking, frying, and baking.

TRANS FATS

Trans fats were once common in many prepared foods, formed through an industrial process called hydrogenation, which involved converting a vegetable oil into a solid fat. After evidence surfaced linking these artificial *trans* fats to increased risk for heart disease, stroke, and type 2 diabetes, *trans* fats were banned from all foods sold in grocery stores and restaurants in the United States.

Although the amount of *trans* fat is required to be included in a Nutrition Facts label, the amounts are generally very small or listed as zero (an amount less than 0.5 grams is rounded to zero). Be aware that small amounts of *trans* fats are found naturally in some meat and dairy products, including beef, lamb, and butterfat. At this time, the evidence is lacking on whether these naturally occurring *trans* fats have the same negative effects on blood cholesterol levels and heart disease risk as artificial *trans* fats.

- Spray food with nonstick cooking spray before placing it in the pan.
- Use parchment paper or nonstick aluminum foil on baking sheets or jelly roll pans to prevent food from sticking when using less fat (this also makes cleanup a breeze).
- When cooking soups, stews, and other braises, skim off and discard fat from the top regularly or refrigerate the cooked dish overnight (as it chills, the fat will rise to the top and solidify, making it easier to remove).

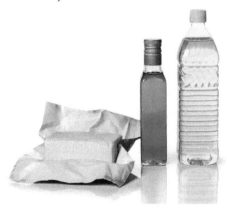

Solid fats, oils, nuts, and seeds

Replace saturated fats (e.g., butter, bacon fat, lard, coconut oil) with more heart-friendly vegetable oils that contain monounsaturated and polyunsaturated fats:

- Use monounsaturated fats like olive, peanut, canola, avocado, safflower, or other nut oils to sauté, stir-fry, or panfry.
- Cook or bake with polyunsaturated fats (e.g., corn, sunflower, or walnut oil) instead of butter.

To incorporate healthy fats into recipes for flavor and texture:

- Use ground nuts or seeds in place of breadcrumbs in breaded dishes (e.g., bread chicken with ground pistachio "breadcrumbs" or fish with walnut "breadcrumbs").
- Add nuts and seeds to salads, pastas, oatmeal, or smoothies.
- Add nuts and flaxseed meal to baked goods.
- Use tahini in dressings, dips, and sauces.
- Make marinades and dressing with healthy oils.

Fruits, vegetables, legumes (beans, peas, lentils)

- Use more of these flavorful plant-based foods that are naturally low in fat or contain healthy fats.
- Add them whole or pureed into recipes in place of a higher saturated fat ingredient such as heavy cream or cheese in a cream-based soup or sauce.
- Revise the ratio of the ingredients (e.g., add more cooked beans and/or vegetables and less meat).
- Boost the dish's flavor by using horseradish, flavored mustards, and homemade chutneys, salsas, sauces, dressings, or dips to anchor a variety of different dishes.

Packaged products

- To reduce the amount of total and saturated fat, use a lower-fat version of the original ingredient (e.g., light versus full-fat coconut milk or reduced-fat versus regular mayonnaise) and bump up the flavor if needed (e.g., sauté curry paste and then add light coconut milk).
- Another option if you cannot maintain the texture and flavor of a dish in a lower-fat version is to reduce the total amount of the full-fat product.

Milk, cheese, and yogurt

Whole-milk dairy is higher in both total fat and saturated fat. Use nonfat, low-fat, or reduced-fat dairy products, if appropriate. Or use smaller amounts of full-fat milk, cheese, or yogurt when it makes a difference in flavor in a recipe. Other options:

- Try using nonfat, low-fat, or reduced-fat cream cheese, cheddar, mozzarella, ricotta, cottage cheese, sour cream.
- Use less of the full-fat versions of highly flavorful cheeses, such as feta, goat, or sharp cheddar (e.g., use a vegetable peeler to slice cheese very thin).
- In place of heavy cream, try evaporated skim or 2% milk, whole milk, half-and-half, or fat-free half-and-half. Or use a combination of these to help lower the amount of total fat and saturated fat.

Eggs

Substitute 1 whole egg with:

- 2 egg whites or a commercial egg replacer or substitute
- flax "eggs" (mix 1 tablespoon flaxseed meal with 3 tablespoons water)
- chia "eggs" (mix 2 teaspoons chia seeds with ¼ cup water)

BOX CONTINUES >

Meat

- Use meat, poultry, and fish that meets the definition of lean or extra lean (see Defining Lean and Extra-Lean Meat Cuts).
- To reduce the fat content of poultry and meat, remove the skin from poultry and trim all visible fat from meat. Use beef that is graded as choice or select, as these cuts have less internal marbling than prime cuts.
- Use chicken, turkey, or plant-based sausage in place of pork or beef sausage. Be sure to read the Nutrition Facts label of these products to compare their calories and saturated fat content.
- Use Canadian bacon or turkey bacon instead of regular bacon, or make "bacon" using portobello mushrooms.
- Use whole grains, vegetables, beans, or plant-based options (e.g., jackfruit, seitan, tofu, tempeh products) to replace some or all of the meat in a recipe.

Meat Serving Sizes

The serving size used for the labeling of meat and poultry is generally 4 ounces raw or 3 ounces cooked. This allows food manufacturers to create uniform nutrition information and labeling, permitting consumers to compare similar amounts. However, consumers sometimes find it confusing that cuts sold in grocery stores or butcher shops differ from the standard serving sizes used on Nutrition Facts labels. For example, consider the retail size of the following meat and poultry cuts:

- New York strip steak: 12 to 16 ounces
- filet mignon: 8 to 10 ounces
- pork chop, center loin: 9 to 12 ounces
- pork chop, blade: 8 to 9 ounces (bone in)
- chicken breast: 6 to 12 ounces (boneless, skinless)
- chicken thigh: 4 to 6 ounces (boneless, skinless)

When developing recipes, consider the raw-to-cooked amounts for serving size. In general, meat, fish, and poultry will shrink by about 25% when cooked. For example, 1 pound (16 ounces) of raw boneless and skinless chicken breast will yield about 12 ounces of cooked chicken. When testing recipes, be sure to record the meat's weight before and after cooking, since the exact amount of shrinkage is dependent on how much fat and moisture the meat, fish, or poultry contains, how long it cooks, and its cooking temperature. See Chapter 8 for more on recipe testing and page 381 for more on meat cuts for recipe development.

DEFINING LEAN AND EXTRA-LEAN MEAT CUTS

In general, lean cuts of meat have the word "round" or "loin" in their name. According to the USDA, a lean cut of meat is defined based on a Reference Amount Customarily Consumed (RACC) of 3 ounces of cooked meat.

- **Lean:** Less than 10 grams total fat, 4.5 grams or less saturated fat, and less than 95 milligrams cholesterol per 3-ounce cooked serving (and per 100 grams or 3.5 ounces)

- **Extra lean:** Less than 5 grams total fat, 2 grams or less saturated fat, and less than 95 milligrams cholesterol per 3-ounce cooked serving (and per 100 grams or 3.5 ounces)

This "oven-fried" recipe modifies both the ingredients and cooking technique to create a lower-fat and lower-calorie dish than a traditional fried chicken recipe. Replacing some of the traditional flour coating used in fried chicken with whole wheat panko breadcrumbs adds a natural crispy texture. (Other ideas for adding natural crunch include crushed melba toast and crushed corn flakes.) To help achieve crispiness without a lot of fat, deep-frying is replaced by oven frying at a high temperature (450° F or higher), with the breaded chicken tenders cooking on a wire rack placed in a baking sheet to prevent soggy bottoms.

Pecan-Crusted Chicken Tenders with Yogurt Dill Dip
By Michelle Dudash, RDN

Preparation time: 25 minutes
Cooking time: 8 minutes
Yield: 4 servings (2 to 3 tenders and 2 tablespoons dip per serving)

CHICKEN

½ cup pecan halves
⅓ cup whole wheat flour
2 teaspoons paprika
2 teaspoons dry mustard
2 teaspoons garlic powder
1 teaspoon onion powder
½ teaspoon kosher salt
½ teaspoon freshly ground black pepper
1 tablespoon canola or avocado oil
½ cup whole wheat panko breadcrumbs
1 egg
1 pound chicken tenders, larger pieces cut in half lengthwise

YOGURT DILL DIP

¼ cup nonfat plain Greek yogurt
¼ cup avocado oil or light mayonnaise
1 teaspoon fresh lemon juice
¼ teaspoon dried dill
¼ teaspoon garlic powder
¼ teaspoon onion powder
1 pinch kosher salt
Freshly ground black pepper to taste

1. Heat the oven to 475° F. Line a sheet pan with parchment paper and place a wire rack on top. Spray rack with nonstick cooking spray.

2. For the chicken, whir the pecans, flour, paprika, dry mustard, garlic powder, onion powder, salt, and pepper in a bowl of a food processor until the pecans are ground to a powder, about 30 seconds. With the motor running, drizzle in the oil, blending completely. Transfer the mixture to a shallow dish and stir in the panko.

3. Beat the egg in a second shallow dish. Add the chicken to the egg, turning to coat completely. Transfer each tender to the breading mixture and turn to coat evenly. Arrange the chicken on the rack. Bake until golden brown and nearly firm, about 8 minutes.

4. For the dip, stir all the ingredients together in a small bowl. Enjoy the cooked chicken with the dip.

Notes: *Chicken tenders come from the undersides of chicken breasts and are naturally portioned into strips, saving you time in cutting them. If you don't have chicken tenders, substitute chicken breasts cut into 4- by 1-inch strips.*

Reheat leftovers in a toaster oven or conventional oven for best results.

Nutrition per serving: 418 calories, 20 grams fat, 3 grams saturated fat, 380 milligrams sodium, 23 grams carbohydrate, 4 grams fiber, 4 grams total sugar, 34 grams protein

Comparison of Calories and Fat in Common Ingredients

Fats	Calories	Fat (g)*	Saturated fat (g)*
Avocado oil (1 tablespoon [15 milliliters])	124	14	1.5
Butter (1 tablespoon [14 grams])	102	11.5	7
Canola oil (1 tablespoon [15 milliliters])	120	14	1
Coconut oil (1 tablespoon [15 milliliters])	121	13.5	11
Olive oil, extra-virgin (1 tablespoon [15 milliliters])	120	14	2.5
Olive oil, light (1 tablespoon [15 milliliters])	120	14	2
Vegan butter sticks (1 tablespoon [14 grams])	90–100	10–11	3.5–8

Fat-containing products	Calories	Fat (g)*	Saturated fat (g)*
Canned coconut milk, unsweetened, full fat (⅓ cup [79 milliliters])	140	14	12
Canned coconut milk, unsweetened, lite/light (⅓ cup [79 milliliters])	50	5	4
Mayonnaise (1 tablespoon [13 grams])	90	10	1.5
Mayonnaise, light (1 tablespoon [13 grams])	35	3.5	0.5
Mayonnaise, low fat (1 tablespoon [13 grams])	15	1	0

Eggs and dairy products	Calories	Fat (g)*	Saturated fat (g)*
Egg (1 large whole)	75	5	1.5
Buttermilk, low fat (1 cup [240 milliliters])	100	2.5	1.5
Crème fraîche (2 tablespoons [28 grams])	110	11	7
Cream cheese (2 tablespoons [30 grams])	100	10	6
Cream cheese, reduced fat (Neufchatel) (2 tablespoons [30 grams])	70	6	4
Evaporated milk (2 tablespoons [30 milliliters])	40	2	1.5
Evaporated milk, nonfat (2 tablespoons [30 milliliters])	25	0	0
Mascarpone cheese (2 tablespoon [28 grams])	120	12	9
Milk, whole (1 cup [240 milliliters])	150	8	4.5
Milk reduced fat (2%) (1 cup [240 milliliters])	120	5	3
Milk, low fat (1%) (1 cup [240 milliliters])	102	2.5	1.5
Milk, nonfat or skim (1 cup [240 milliliters])	80	0	0
Sharp cheddar cheese (1 ounce [28 grams])	110	9	6
Sharp cheddar cheese, light (1 ounce [28 grams])	70	4.5	3
Sour cream, full fat (2 tablespoons [30 grams])	60	5	3.5
Sour cream, reduced fat/light (2 tablespoons [30 grams])	40	2.5	1.5
Yogurt, Greek, plain, whole milk (¾ cup; 6 ounces [170 grams])	165	8.5	4
Yogurt, Greek, plain, nonfat (¾ cup; 6 ounces [170 grams])	100	0.5	0
Yogurt, plain, whole milk (¾ cup; 6 ounces [170 grams])	130	6	4
Yogurt, plain, low fat (¾ cup; 6 ounces [170 grams])	107	2.5	1.5
Yogurt, plain, nonfat (¾ cup; 6 ounces [170 grams])	95	0	0

Plant-based milks (1 cup [240 milliliters])	Calories	Fat (g)*	Saturated fat (g)*
Almond milk	75	2	0
Cashew milk	155	11	0–2
Oat milk	120	5	0
Pea milk	70	5	0
Soy milk	105	4	0.5

Source: US Department of Agriculture, Agricultural Research Service, FoodData Central: fdc.nal.usda.gov

Comparison of Calories and Fat in Beef, Pork, and Poultry

Beef (3 ounces [85 grams] cooked)	Calories	Fat (g)*	Saturated fat (g)*
Rib roast (fat trimmed to ⅛≈inch; prime rib)	340	29	12
Brisket, point cut (fat trimmed to 0 inches)	302	24	9.5
Strip steak, boneless (fat trimmed to ⅛ inch)	200	14	6
Strip steak, boneless (lean only)	160	6	2.5
Chuck roast, chuck eye roast, chuck pot roast, boneless (for pot roast and cubed for stew meat) (fat trimmed to 0 inches)	241	15	6
Hanger steak	190	12	4.5
Tri-tip roast	188	11	4
Skirt steak (fat trimmed to 0 inches)	187	10	4
Ribeye steak, boneless	190	10	4
London broil (top round)	190	9	4
Flat iron steak (top blade)	180	9	4
Flank steak (fat trimmed to 0 inch)	172	8	3
Strip loin roast (top loin roast)	163	7.5	2.5
Beef tenderloin (lean only)	170	7	3
Beef top round (fat trimmed to 0 inches)	140	3.5	1.5
Beef shank (whole or meat off bone; fat trimmed to ⅛ inch)	171	5.5	2
Rump roast (bottom round roast; fat trimmed to 0 inches)	144	4.5	1.5
Beef, ground (70%–75% lean)	237	16	6
Beef, ground (80%–85% lean)	212	13	5
Beef, ground (93% lean)	164	7.5	3
Bison, ground	121	2	1

Pork (3 ounces [85 grams] cooked)	Calories	Fat (g)*	Saturated fat (g)*
Pork, ground	251	17.5	6.5
Pork shoulder (Boston butt)	227	15	5.5
Pork rib chops, bone-in	189	11	4
Blade chops, bone-in	196	12	4
Pork loin roast	147	5.5	1.5
Pork tenderloin	120	3.0	1.0

Poultry (3 ounces [85 grams] cooked)	Calories	Fat (g)*	Saturated fat (g)*
Chicken thigh/leg, bone-in, with skin	183	11	3
Chicken thigh, boneless, skinless	149	7	2
Chicken breast, bone-in, with skin (rotisserie)	149	6.5	1.5
Chicken breast, boneless, skinless; grilled	128	3	1
Turkey breast (meat only, roasted)	125	2	0.5

* Numbers rounded to closest 0.5 grams. Averages used when a range is provided.

Sources: US Department of Agriculture, Agricultural Research Service, FoodData Central: fdc.nal.usda.gov | commodity boards | product packaging

Risotto is a creamy dish of short-grain arborio or carnaroli rice and onions that are "toasted" in olive oil, deglazed with dry white wine, cooked slowly with stock, and finished with Parmesan cheese and butter; sometimes, heavy cream is added to provide an even richer and creamier consistency. Traditional risotto is prepared using the risotto method, which means hot stock is added gradually to the rice as it cooks, slowly releasing the natural starch in the rice, and ultimately achieving a creamy consistency and al dente cooked rice. Classic risotto is often high in calories, saturated fat, and sodium while providing few vitamins and minerals.

To create a healthier take on risotto, culinary nutritionist Kristy Del Coro used the techniques of modifying an ingredient and the cooking method. The recipe achieves a creamy grain-based dish by replacing rice with sorghum, a whole grain containing dietary fiber, vitamins, and minerals; using a cooking liquid of either water or a homemade corn stock with no added salt; and adding a corn puree to provide creaminess and nutrients without additional butter or cream. As a result, the risotto is significantly lower in saturated fat than traditional recipes.

The method differs because the sorghum is cooked ahead of time, and the rich and creamy mouthfeel that makes traditional risotto so appealing is provided by the silky-smooth corn puree. Other whole grains and vegetables can be used with the same technique; for example, farro and mushroom puree, brown rice and butternut squash puree, or barley and pea puree.

Corn Sorghum "Risotto"

By Kristy Del Coro, MS, RDN

Preparation time: 20 minutes
Cooking time: 1 hour 15 minutes
Yield: 4 servings (1 cup per serving)

SORGHUM

1 cup uncooked sorghum, rinsed
3 cups water or corn stock (see Note)
½ teaspoon kosher salt

CORN PUREE

1 tablespoon extra-virgin olive oil
4 ears of corn, shucked and kernels removed (or 2 cups fresh or frozen kernels)
1 small onion, diced
½ teaspoon kosher salt
1 cup water or corn stock (see Note)

GARNISH

2 teaspoons extra-virgin olive oil
2 ears of corn, shucked and kernels removed (or 1¼ cups fresh or frozen kernels)
⅛ teaspoon kosher salt
½ cup grated Parmesan cheese
2 tablespoons thinly sliced basil leaves
Drizzle of olive oil, optional

1. For the sorghum, combine the sorghum, water or corn stock, and salt in medium pot. Bring to a boil over medium-high heat. Reduce the heat to low, cover, and simmer until chewy and tender, 50 to 60 minutes. Drain, reserving 1 cup of the cooking liquid. Return the sorghum to the pot and set aside.

2. While the sorghum is cooking, prepare the corn puree. Heat the oil in a medium saucepan over medium heat. Stir in the corn kernels, onion, and salt. Reduce the heat to medium-low and gently cook, stirring occasionally, until the vegetables are softened but not browned, 2 to 3 minutes. Add the water and simmer, uncovered, until the liquid is reduced by half, 15 to 20 minutes. Remove from the heat and let cool slightly.

3. Pour the corn mixture into a blender, allowing steam to escape before putting on the lid. Blend on low speed, gradually increasing to high speed, until the mixture is smooth with a consistency of regular yogurt. If desired, strain the corn puree through a fine mesh strainer for an extra smooth puree.

4. For the garnish, heat the oil in a medium nonstick skillet over medium-high heat. When the oil starts to shimmer, add the corn kernels and salt and stir to combine. Cook, stirring occasionally to prevent burning, until the corn begins to caramelize and brown, about 5 minutes. Remove from the heat and set aside.

RECIPE CONTINUES >

5. To make the risotto, add the corn puree and ½ cup of the reserved sorghum cooking liquid to the cooked sorghum. Bring to a simmer over medium heat and cook, stirring frequently, until the texture is creamy and looks similar to a traditional risotto, about 5 minutes. If the risotto seems too thick, adjust with more cooking liquid; if it's too thin, simmer an additional few minutes. If needed, turn the heat to low to prevent splattering and any browning or sticking due to the natural sugar from the corn. Remove the risotto from the heat and stir in the Parmesan.

6. To serve, ladle the risotto into bowls and garnish with the sautéed corn, basil, and a drizzle of olive oil, if using. Serve immediately.

Note: *You can easily make a corn stock to add a more intense corn flavor to the dish if you're using fresh corn for the risotto: After the kernels have been removed from the cobs, combine four of the bare cobs and enough water to just cover them in a medium pot. Simmer over medium heat until the liquid is infused with corn flavor, about 45 minutes. Strain the stock into another pot or large bowl; discard the cobs. The corn stock can be made ahead and refrigerated for 3 to 4 days or frozen for 4 to 6 months.*

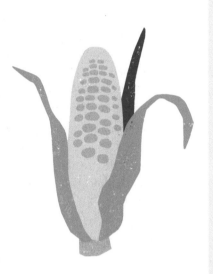

Nutrition per 1-cup serving (without optional drizzle of olive oil): 380 calories, 11 grams fat, 3 grams saturated fat, 730 milligrams sodium, 68 grams carbohydrate, 7 grams fiber, 0 grams total sugar, 12 grams protein

Recipe Example: Reducing calories using lower-fat and lower-calorie packaged products

When a reduced-calorie recipe is the goal, using a lower-fat version of a packaged product can save calories. With salad dressings, it's easy to pour on the calories. In this homemade salad dressing, the little bit of fat in the low-fat products helps make this dressing creamy and more satisfying. And when paired with healthy salad greens or fresh vegetables it delivers plenty of nutrient-rich benefits with fewer calories and fat.

Green Goddess Dressing
By Jill Melton, MS, RD

Preparation time: 15 minutes
Yield: 1½ cups (2 tablespoons per serving)

½ cup light mayonnaise
½ cup low-fat sour cream
½ cup low-fat plain Greek yogurt
¼ cup chopped fresh parsley
¼ cup minced fresh chives
2 tablespoons minced fresh tarragon
2 teaspoons sugar
1 tablespoon lemon juice

Whisk all the ingredients together in a small bowl. Transfer to an airtight container and refrigerate for up to 1 week.

Note: *If salt is not an issue for you, add a pinch of salt and 1 teaspoon anchovy paste for a punch of umami.*

Nutrition per 2-tablespoon serving: 64 calories, 4 grams fat, 2 grams saturated fat, 8 milligrams sodium, 2 grams carbohydrate, 0 grams fiber, 2 grams total sugar, 2 grams protein

Recipe used with the permission of *Food & Nutrition Magazine®.*

USING COCONUT PRODUCTS IN RECIPES

Coconut oil is fat pressed from coconut meat. It has been popular in health-focused recipe development, but many of the health claims for coconut oil are based on studies that use a formulation of coconut oil made mostly of medium-chain triglycerides (MCTs), rather than the coconut oil available at most supermarkets.

The *Dietary Guidelines for Americans, 2020–2025* considers coconut oil to be a solid fat that is high in saturated fat. One tablespoon of coconut oil provides about 13 grams of saturated fat. Coconut oil can be used as a periodic alternative to other vegetable oils, such as olive or canola, and it works well as an alternative to butter in vegan desserts. However, evidence is lacking that coconut oil should be viewed any differently from other sources of saturated fat.

It is also important to know the differences between coconut milk, coconut cream, and coconut water. Coconut milk products can vary considerably in their nutrient content depending on the relative amount of coconut and water they contain, and they may be packaged in cans or cartons.

Coconut milk: blended and grated mature coconut is combined with hot water and then strained; the resulting liquid is thick and white

Light coconut milk: coconut milk diluted with additional water

Coconut cream: the thick substance that floats to the top of coconut milk and can be spooned off

Coconut water: a clear and slightly sweet liquid found inside young, green coconuts

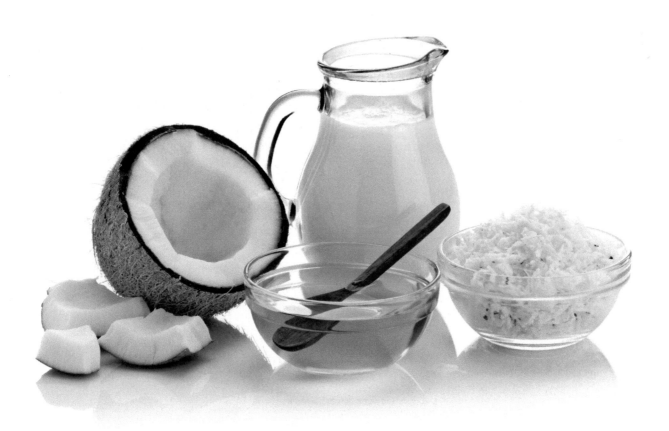

Tips for Modifying the Fat in Baked Goods

Modifying fat in baked goods is more difficult than modifying it in savory dishes, and substitutions can be tricky because baking recipes are formulated based on specific ratios of ingredients and chemical interactions. In general, first determine what function the fat is providing in the recipe, then use trial and error to determine which modifications work. Take care not to remove too much fat in a baked good, since fat's functional role of providing tenderness, a fine texture, or lightness will be diminished or absent altogether. It may be helpful during this process to reference culinary and food science resources to get a deeper understanding of the role ingredients play in baking.

If choosing to use an alternative ingredient to replace the fat, such as pureed fresh or dried fruit, canned pumpkin, pureed cooked or canned beans, or yogurt, it's important to understand that these ingredients generally add moisture but do not provide the functional role of leavening. Most fat replacer ingredients don't trap air like butter and other solid fats do when beaten with sugar, and, as a result, the end product could be very dense.

While there are no hard and fast rules for reducing or replacing fat in baked goods, there are some general suggestions and tips, such as the following:

- To reduce total fat, start by decreasing the fat in the recipe by about 10%.

- If you intend to cut more fat from the recipe (say, 25%–50%), replace the amount removed with a similar amount of a fat replacement ingredient like pureed fresh or dried fruit (e.g., applesauce, apple butter, mashed bananas); canned pumpkin; or pureed cooked or canned beans. For example, try replacing ½ cup of fat with ½ cup of a moist fat replacement, such as pureed cooked beans, pureed pumpkin, pureed prunes, or mashed bananas. Use pureed black beans and prune purees with chocolate cake or brownies, and cannellini beans and applesauce with lighter colored baked goods. It might be necessary to thin out the puree with a little water or vegetable oil or cut flour down by 25%.

- Replace ½ cup butter with ½ cup full-fat Greek yogurt; reduced-fat sour cream; or reduced-fat cream cheese, cottage cheese, or low-fat buttermilk. In general, make the replacement in a 1:1 ratio, but do not use more than 1 cup of an alternative.

- Experiment with healthy fat alternatives like nut butters or mashed avocado. For example, replace half the amount of butter in a recipe with an equal amount of mashed or pureed avocado (if the recipe calls for 1 cup of butter, use ½ cup butter and ½ cup mashed avocado). Reduce the oven temperature by 25° F to prevent the baked good from browning too quickly and increase the baking time a bit.

- When making whipped cream, in place of whipping or heavy cream, try aquafaba (chickpea liquid) or evaporated fat-free milk. The evaporated milk must be well chilled before whipping, and gelatin or cream of tartar may be needed to stabilize it after whipping.

- Use cacao nibs or dried fruit in place of chocolate chips.

SUBSTITUTING BUTTER WITH OIL IN BAKING

Butter is often preferred for baking, but when recipes call for melted butter, consider replacing it with vegetable oil to reduce the saturated fat. Since both are liquid fats, they will perform in a similar way in the baked good, with the exception of the butter's flavor.

Oil is not a good choice for substitution if a recipe requires the butter and sugar to be creamed together; creaming is necessary to trap air and help with leavening. In recipes where the fat isn't needed for leavening, such as in baked goods like quick breads and muffins, oil can work well in place of butter. The primary difference is that the crumb will have more moistness and will be denser and coarser.

Start by using about 25% less oil than the amount of butter called for in a recipe. For example, if a recipe calls for ½ cup butter (8 tablespoons), substitute 6 tablespoons oil. There are no hard and fast rules, so testing and tasting is necessary. See Chapter 8 for more on recipe testing.

Recipe Example: Using moist ingredients in place of butter in baked goods to reduce saturated fat and calories

Inspired by the popular Venezuelan dessert *negro en camisa*, this healthier version of a decadent chocolate cake reduces saturated fat, sugar, and calories by using avocado in place of butter, dried plums in place of sugar, and shredded coconut as a garnish instead of the traditional topping of English cream.

Coconut-Topped Chocolate Cake
By Ashley Thomas, MS, RDN, LDN

Preparation time: 25 minutes
Cooking time: 45 minutes
Yield: 12 servings (one 9- by 13-inch cake)

2 avocados, peeled and pitted
½ cup plus 2 tablespoons water, divided use
1⅓ cups pitted dried plums
½ cup 1% milk
2½ cups bittersweet chocolate chips (70% cacao)
6 large eggs, yolks and whites separated
¾ cup whole wheat flour
2 tablespoons shredded unsweetened coconut

1. Heat the oven to 350° F. Grease a 9- by 13-inch baking dish with nonstick cooking spray.

2. Puree the avocado with the 2 tablespoons water in a blender. Transfer to a bowl. Puree the plums with the remaining ½ cup water and transfer to the bowl with the avocado. Set aside.

3. Fill a medium pot with 1 to 2 inches of water; place a heatproof bowl (tempered glass or stainless-steel) inside the pot (or use a double boiler). Heat the milk in the bowl (or top of double boiler) and bring to a simmer. Reduce the heat to low, add the chocolate chips, and melt, stirring frequently with a heat-proof rubber spatula, until the chocolate becomes silky smooth. Stir in the avocado and plum purees. Transfer the mixture to a large bowl.

4. Add the egg yolks to the chocolate mixture and stir until well combined. Add the flour and mix until just combined.

5. In a clean (grease-free) medium bowl, beat the egg whites until stiff peaks form. Gently fold the egg whites into the chocolate mixture.

6. Transfer the mixture to the prepared baking dish. Bake until a toothpick inserted in the center comes out clean, about 45 minutes. Let cool in the pan for about 10 minutes. To serve, cut into 3-inch squares and sprinkle each piece with ½ teaspoon shredded coconut.

Nutrition per 3-inch square and ½ teaspoon coconut: 296 calories, 13 grams fat, 6 grams saturated fat, 45 milligrams sodium, 45 grams carbohydrate, 7 grams fiber, 29 grams total sugar, 7 grams protein

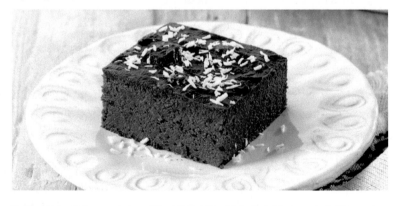

Recipe used with the permission of *Food & Nutrition Magazine*®. Photography by Kate Cauffiel; Food styling by Christina Zerkis; Prop styling by Lindsey Parker

Reducing Sodium in Recipes

Sodium, an essential mineral with a recommended average daily intake, is primarily consumed as salt (sodium chloride). Consuming too much sodium (and too little potassium) may increase the risk of high blood pressure, heart disease, and stroke. The *Dietary Guidelines for Americans, 2020–2025* recommends that adults consume less than 2,300 milligrams of sodium per day—the equivalent of about 1 teaspoon of table salt—and lesser amounts for children under the age of 14. The average daily intake of sodium among US individuals aged 1 year and older is around 3,400 milligrams. Estimates vary, but around 70% of the sodium we consume comes from packaged and prepared foods, including restaurant foods, rather than from the salt added during cooking and eating.

Foods considered to be high in sodium contain 20% or more of the percent Daily Value (%DV) per serving, or more than 460 milligrams per serving (%DV is based on 2,300 milligrams of sodium per day). But they don't always taste salty, so it's important to read the Nutrition Facts label when using packaged foods and condiments in recipes, making note of higher-sodium products, such as canned tomato products, processed meats such as bacon and sausage, and soy sauce. Look at the quantity of sodium in milligrams and the %DV on the Nutrition Facts label of ingredients to help make the best selections. A nutrient content claim on the front of a product's label can also be used as a quick and general guide.

When looking at the sodium content in potential recipe ingredients, it's easy to understand how the sodium per serving can add up quickly in a recipe. For example, consider the sodium amounts in these commonly used recipe ingredients:

- one (17.6-ounce) package of potato gnocchi contains 2,220 milligrams sodium (740 milligrams per 1-cup serving).
- ¼ cup tomato sauce contains 220 to 320 milligrams sodium.
- ¼ cup Parmesan cheese contains about 360 milligrams sodium.
- four ounces of fresh, boneless, skinless chicken breast contains 40 to 330 milligrams sodium depending on if it's injected with a sodium solution.

CULINARY FUNCTIONS OF SALT

Salt enhances and deepens flavors in food, which is often considered its primary function in recipes. Yet salt serves other key roles, including to:

- cure meats
- stabilize yeast fermentation in baking
- enhance gluten structure and even browning in baked goods
- serve as a preservative
- help foods retain moisture

SODIUM LABELING

What it says	What it means
Salt/Sodium Free	Less than 5 milligrams of sodium per serving
Very Low Sodium	35 milligrams of sodium or less per serving
Low Sodium	140 milligrams of sodium or less per serving
Reduced Sodium	At least 25% less sodium than the regular product
Light in Sodium or Lightly Salted	At least 50% less sodium than the regular product
No Salt Added or Unsalted	No salt is added during processing—but these products may not be salt-free

- one (15-ounce) can of black beans contains about 1,350 milligrams sodium (450 milligrams per ½-cup serving).
- one (15.25-ounce) can of whole sweet corn contains about 900 milligrams sodium (300 milligrams per ½-cup serving).
- one tablespoon of fish sauce contains about 1,400 milligrams sodium.
- one tablespoon of soy sauce contains about 920 milligrams sodium.

THE ROLE OF POTASSIUM IN A HEALTHY DIET

Increasing potassium in the diet can counterbalance some of sodium's harmful effects by helping to decrease blood pressure and, according to some studies, improve bone health. Since potassium is classified as a nutrient of public health concern, the amount of potassium per serving is now required on the Nutrition Facts label. Most health experts recommend that sodium intake be decreased *and* potassium intake be increased to see the benefits.

Sources of potassium include vegetables (e.g., potatoes, tomatoes, leafy greens), fresh and dried fruits (e.g., avocado, bananas, strawberries, cantaloupe, kiwi, figs), beans (e.g., kidney, white, pinto, lima), fish/seafood (e.g., salmon, clams), and dairy (e.g., yogurt, milk).

Tips for Reducing Sodium in Recipes

Because salt is an essential ingredient in many recipes, reducing (or replacing) it will require careful testing. From a flavor perspective, this means tasting food each time salt is reduced while testing a recipe, during the cooking process (tasting as you go as appropriate), and in the final dish. If possible, recommend a baseline amount in recipes that is essential for salt to serve its necessary functions. Any additional salt might be considered "to taste," which could be noted as optional.

- Start by cutting the salt in a recipe by 20% to 25% from a starting point. From a flavor perspective, sensory research suggests that tasters usually do not detect 10% to 20% reductions in sodium.

- Track the amount of salt used while developing a recipe by filling a ramekin with a specific amount of salt and measuring the amount left over after testing the recipe.

- If a recipe is developed using table salt or a specific brand of kosher salt, be sure to note it since the amount of sodium in equivalent amounts of different types of kosher salts and table salt varies.

See page 53 in Chapter 1 for more on the various types of salt and salting guidelines for different types of dishes.

- If available, read the Nutrition Facts label on the ingredient being used to determine if it is high (20% DV or more) or low (5% DV or less) in sodium and to compare the sodium content to similar food products under consideration.

- Be aware of the sodium content of canned, jarred, and packaged food products and condiments. Use them sparingly or choose reduced-sodium, low-sodium, or no-salt-added versions and consider adding salt to taste, if needed.

- Drain and rinse canned beans and vegetables. Doing so can reduce their sodium content by as much as 40%.

- Limit the use of prepackaged sauces, mixes, and "instant" products, including flavored rice, instant noodles, and salad dressings. Processed foods generally contain more sodium.

- Use fresh, naturally low-sodium foods like fruits, vegetables, whole grains, unsalted or lightly salted nuts, and eggs.

- Use fresh poultry, seafood, pork, and lean meats instead of processed meat and poultry. Be aware that some fresh meat products are sold with added seasoning or brine injection for flavor.

When Reducing Salt, Add Extra Flavor

A key skill for developing lower sodium recipes is knowing how to choose among similar types of ingredients, selecting those that are naturally lower in sodium without sacrificing taste and using alternate cooking techniques that intensify flavor without using more salt. For example:

- Extract more flavor from a dried whole or ground spice by heating a small amount of oil in a skillet, adding the spice, and cooking it until fragrant. This technique, known as blooming, brings out the spice's flavor by extracting its natural aromatic compounds. Alternatively, toast a whole or ground spice in a dry sauté pan over medium-low heat as this also serves a similar purpose.

- Use a salt-free spice rub on meats and poultry.

- Grill, roast, or pan sear meats, poultry, and fish to intensify their flavor; grill or roast vegetables to caramelize them and sweeten their natural flavors.

- Use bold and flavorful ingredients, where a small amount can go a long way in terms of flavor (e.g., horseradish, chipotle peppers, hot sauces, salsas, chutneys, sun-dried tomatoes).

- Use nutritional yeast to enhance natural flavors and mimic the flavor of cheese in risottos, mashed potatoes, popcorn, salads, and roasted vegetables. See pages 64 and 65 for more on nutritional yeast.

- Use flavorful ingredients like dried mushroom powder or dried tomato powder in stews, sauces, and soups to add a layer of flavor.

- Finish the dish with a splash of vinegar or citrus juice or zest at the end of cooking to brighten the natural flavors of the food.

- Use small amounts of umami-rich ingredients (e.g., anchovies, Parmesan cheese, fish sauce, miso, seaweed like nori or kelp, or bacon) when reducing added salt in recipes, as this can result in a dish with less total sodium but similar flavor to the original.

- Use small amounts of flavorful condiments and spice blends (e.g., yuzu kosho, gomashio, togarashi) with soba or udon noodles, salads, soups, grilled meat, chicken, or fish.

- As appropriate, finish the dish with a small amount of large-granule finishing salt for a final, noticeable layer of flavor.

Recipe Example: Using a bold sauce to add flavor with less sodium

This variation of chimichurri, a South American sauce and marinade, provides an abundance of flavor with its bold ingredients and has a hint of Mexican-inspired flavor with the addition of cilantro, jalapeño, and cumin. It is a perfect accompaniment to steak, chicken, fish, or to any dish where you want to add a zesty and bright flavor—along with some heart-friendly monounsaturated fats. Because it's packed with flavor, a small amount can go a long way and replace the need for salty seasonings or sauces. Unlike pesto, chimichurri does not use nuts or cheese, making it a good alternative for individuals with nut and dairy allergies.

Mexican-Inspired Chimichurri Sauce
By Jill Melton, MS, RD

Preparation time: 20 minutes
Yield: about 2 cups (2 tablespoons per serving)

2 cloves garlic, peeled
1 cup firmly packed cilantro leaves (about 1 bunch)
1 cup firmly packed parsley leaves (about 1 bunch)
¼ cup extra-virgin olive oil
Juice of 1 lime
1 jalapeño, stemmed and chopped
1 teaspoon ground cumin
1 teaspoon red wine vinegar
½ teaspoon kosher salt

Pulse the garlic in a food processor until minced. Add the cilantro and parsley and pulse until chopped. Add the oil, lime juice, jalapeño, cumin, vinegar, and salt and process until the sauce comes together. Serve immediately or store in refrigerator up to 2 weeks.

Nutrition per 2-tablespoon serving: 35 calories, 3.5 grams fat, 0.5 grams saturated fat, 60 milligrams sodium, 1 gram carbohydrate, 0 grams fiber, 0 grams total sugar, 0 grams protein

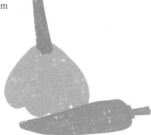

UMAMI INGREDIENTS

Umami ingredients can help lower a recipe's total sodium content without sacrificing flavor when they are used *sparingly* in combination with a reduction of table or kosher salt in the recipe. Some of these ingredients are high in sodium, but small amounts of them can be used to provide umami, which adds a savory boost to a dish while enhancing the perception of saltiness. Examples of these ingredients include:

- soy sauce
- oyster sauce
- liquid aminos
- fish sauce
- black bean sauce
- miso
- MSG (monosodium glutamate)

- tomato-based products (e.g., tomato sauce, ketchup, tomato paste)
- anchovies
- olives
- capers
- aged cheese, such as Parmesan
- brined or cured meats

- pickles and pickled vegetables
- kimchi
- salted nuts
- steak, barbecue, or Worcestershire sauce
- canned broths, dried soup mixes, and bouillon cubes

USING MSG IN RECIPE DEVELOPMENT

Monosodium glutamate (MSG) is a flavor enhancer that contains about one-third the amount of sodium compared to salt. It is derived from an amino acid called glutamic acid, which occurs naturally in such foods as mushrooms, aged Parmesan cheese, and fermented soybean products like soy sauce. Glutamic acid belongs to a broad category of compounds called glutamates, which are the source of the fifth taste known as umami. MSG has been said to trigger headaches and nausea in some people, but research has revealed no clear evidence or explanation for this phenomenon. Adding MSG, a synthetic glutamate, to food adds umami flavor and enhances other flavors by imparting depth, fullness, and an increased perception of saltiness. You can find MSG in the spice and seasonings section at most grocery stores. It is gluten-free.

Tips for cooking with MSG

- Do not swap out 100% of the salt in a recipe with MSG. Instead, experiment with MSG in cooking to get a dish to taste exactly as you'd like. Over seasoning with MSG will result in an undesirable taste. MSG does not work well in sweet recipes.

- When developing recipes, start by cutting back on the total salt while adding a sprinkle of MSG. Taste the dish, and ask yourself, "Does it taste better?" Adjust the seasoning from there.
- When swapping in MSG for the total amount of salt in a recipe, experiment using either half kosher salt and half MSG or two-thirds kosher salt and one-third MSG. For example, in a soup recipe, if using 1 teaspoon of kosher salt, try ½ teaspoon of kosher salt and ½ teaspoon of MSG. (This change would result in a 900 milligrams savings of sodium.)
- While it is possible to season food with MSG at the table, it's best to add MSG to foods before or during cooking for even distribution. For example, with meats, poultry, and seafood, sprinkle it on before cooking; for casseroles, soups, vegetable or egg dishes, gravies, and sauces, add MSG during the cooking process. An estimated amount to enhance the flavor: approximately ½ teaspoon of MSG is enough for 1 pound of meat or 4 to 6 servings of vegetables, casseroles, or soups.
- Some chefs like using table salt versus kosher salt when creating an MSG and salt blend due to the similarity in grain size.

Recipe Example: Using MSG to reduce sodium

Chef and registered dietitian nutritionist Michele Redmond uses MSG to replace some of the salt in her quinoa salad. This ingredient modification helps reduce the sodium by almost 40% while also adding MSG's unique flavor-enhancing properties. With one-third of the sodium found in salt, MSG can be used as a key ingredient when developing lower sodium recipes.

Quinoa Spiced Cucumber Salad

By Michele Redmond, MS, RDN, FAND

Preparation time: 15 minutes
Cooking time: 20 minutes
Yield: 4 servings (1⅓ cups per serving)

SALAD

1 cup dry quinoa
1¾ cups water
¼ teaspoon table salt
¼ teaspoon MSG (see Notes)
6 baby or 2 medium cucumbers (about 1 pound), cut into bite-sized pieces
6 green onions, thinly sliced
1 cup grape tomatoes (8 ounces), cut in half

DRESSING

1 teaspoon cumin seeds (see Notes)
¼ cup extra-virgin olive oil
3 tablespoons fresh lemon juice
1 teaspoon ground coriander
½ teaspoon ground allspice
½ teaspoon crushed red pepper
¼ teaspoon table salt
¼ teaspoon MSG

1. For the salad, toast the quinoa in a dry medium pot over medium-high heat, shaking the pan several times, until the quinoa is toasted, 4 to 5 minutes. Add the water, salt, and MSG and stir. Bring to a boil, reduce the heat to low, and cover. Cook until the water is absorbed, about 20 minutes. Remove from the heat and let sit, covered, for about 5 minutes.

2. Uncover the quinoa and fluff using a fork. Transfer to a large bowl and cool. Add the cucumbers, green onions, and tomatoes to the quinoa and toss to combine. Set aside.

3. For the dressing, toast the cumin seeds in a dry small pan over medium heat until you notice a toasted aroma, about 3 minutes. Transfer the toasted cumin seeds to a small bowl and add the olive oil, lemon juice, coriander, allspice, crushed red pepper, salt, and MSG; whisk to combine the dressing.

4. Toss the quinoa salad with the dressing. Allow the salad to absorb the dressing for 10 to 15 minutes. Serve at room temperature.

Notes: *MSG is sold under brand names such as Ac'cent and AJI-NO-MOTO. If table salt is used in place of MSG in this recipe, the amount of sodium per serving is about 600 milligrams versus 360 milligrams.*

If ground cumin in the dressing is preferred, pulverize the cumin seeds with a mortar and pestle or coffee grinder after toasting.

Nutrition per 1⅓-cup serving: 330 calories, 17 grams fat, 2.5 grams saturated fat, 360 milligrams sodium, 37 grams carbohydrate, 6 grams fiber, 0 grams added sugar, 8 grams protein

---

Quick Tip

"The presence of ingredients and products high in glutamic acid can increase the perception of salt but at lower sodium levels and without flavor loss. I make my own 50/50 blend of MSG crystals and salt. When used in my recipes, it reduces sodium by about 40%."

—Michele Redmond, MS, RDN, FAND

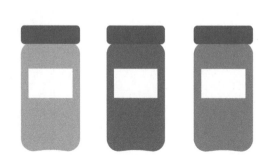

Recipe Example: Using no-salt-added or reduced-sodium products to reduce sodium

Chef and registered dietitian nutritionist Garrett Berdan controls the amount of sodium in this tomato sauce by using no-salt-added canned whole tomatoes and adding just the necessary amount of salt to draw out the natural tomato flavor. Tomatoes are an umami-rich ingredient, and using no-salt-added or reduced-sodium canned tomato products when developing lower-sodium recipes provides a sodium reduction ranging from 100 milligrams to 400 milligrams less per serving. In this recipe, using no-salt-added tomatoes provides a reduction of just over 400 milligrams of sodium per serving. The recipe also offers a tip to roast the tomatoes for a more concentrated and intense flavor.

Basic Tomato Sauce
By Chef Garrett Berdan, RDN

Preparation time: 5 minutes
Cooking time: 20 minutes
Yield: 2½ cups (4 servings, about ⅔ cup per serving)

1 tablespoon extra-virgin olive oil
1 clove garlic, minced
1 (28-ounce) can no-salt-added whole plum tomatoes
½ teaspoon sugar
½ teaspoon kosher salt
⅛ teaspoon ground black pepper

1. Heat the olive oil in a medium saucepan over medium heat. Add the garlic and sauté until fragrant, about 30 seconds. Add the tomatoes with their juice and break the tomatoes into smaller chunks using the side of a spoon. Stir in the sugar, salt, and pepper.

2. Heat the sauce to a simmer. Cook, uncovered, until thickened, about 15 minutes. Remove from the heat. For a smoother sauce, puree with a food mill, blender, or immersion blender.

Note: *For a more concentrated tomato flavor, drain the tomatoes and reserve the juice. Arrange the whole tomatoes on a baking sheet, drizzle with 2 teaspoons olive oil, and toss to coat. Roast in a 375° F oven until the tomatoes start to caramelize, 15 to 20 minutes. Proceed with the basic tomato sauce recipe, adding the oven-roasted tomatoes and the reserved tomato juice.*

Nutrition per ⅔-cup serving: 80 calories, 3.5 grams fat, 0.5 grams saturated fat, 260 milligrams sodium, 7 grams carbohydrates, 2 grams fiber, 2 grams total sugar, 2 grams protein

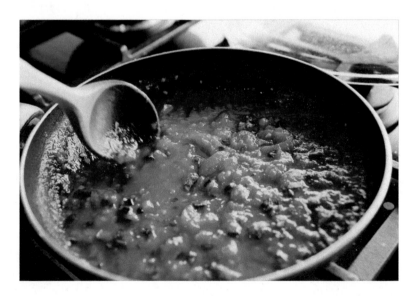

Reducing Sugar in Recipes

Consuming too much added sugar contributes to an eating pattern with excess calories. This in turn may be linked to weight gain and health problems associated with overweight and obesity, including type 2 diabetes and heart disease. The *Dietary Guidelines for Americans, 2020–2025* recommends limiting added sugars to less than 10% of calories per day starting at age 2, or no more than 50 grams added sugars in a 2,000-calorie diet. The American Heart Association recommends 25 grams or less added sugar for women (about 6 teaspoons) and 36 grams or less for men (about 9 teaspoons). One gram of sugar contains 4 calories; a teaspoon of sugar weighs 4 grams and contains 16 calories.

Sugars can naturally occur in foods—such as fruits, nuts, vegetables, dairy products—or it can be included as an added sugar from such sources as sugar beets, sugar cane, syrups, nectars, and honey. The primary difference is that the sugars naturally found in fruits and vegetables are accompanied by other healthy nutrients like vitamins, minerals, and dietary fiber. All added sugars are considered simple carbohydrates and concentrated sources of calories with little or no other nutrients. Both naturally occurring and added sugars provide the same amount of calories (4 calories per grams), and the body digests and uses them in the same manner.

Reducing added sugars can reduce the total amount of carbohydrate in a recipe and can possibly lower the calories, depending on the modification. When developing recipes for people with diabetes, or for anyone trying to reduce carbohydrates from sugars, both the total amount of carbohydrate and the type of carbohydrate should be considered. See Developing Recipes for People With Diabetes on page 117 for more information.

Tips for Reducing Sugar in Savory Recipes

In savory recipes, sugar is typically added to balance flavors, and the amount is often relatively small. Limiting the use of food products that contain hidden sugars, even some that may not taste sweet, can help to reduce added sugars. Check the Nutrition Facts label to confirm if there are added sugars (in grams) and the %DV.

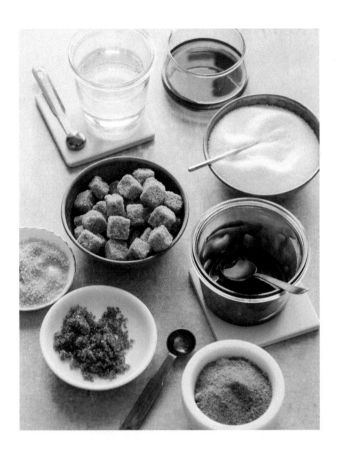

Note that single-ingredient sugars such as pure honey, pure maple syrup, granulated sugar, and other pure sugars and syrups are required to include the amount of total sugar they contribute per serving. An added sugar amount is not required on the label for single-ingredient sugars.

Examples of packaged food products with added sugars that might be used in savory recipes include ketchup and barbecue sauce, salad dressing, jarred sauces, salsa, chutney, fruit preserves, and fruit juice. The ingredient list is another place to check for added sugars. Examples of ingredients that are considered added sugars include the following:

- agave nectar
- brown sugar
- brown rice syrup
- coconut sugar/syrup
- corn sweetener
- corn syrup
- date sugar
- fruit juice concentrates
- granulated sugar
- high-fructose corn syrup
- honey
- invert sugar
- malt sugar
- maple syrup
- molasses
- raw sugar
- sugar cane
- sugars ending in "ose" (e.g., dextrose, fructose, glucose, lactose, maltose, sucrose)

TYPES OF CARBOHYDRATES IN FOOD

Three types of carbohydrate are in food: starches, sugars, and fiber. Many foods, such as fruits and vegetables, contain a mixture of all three.

Type of carbohydrate	Key food sources
Starches (complex carbohydrate)*	**Grain-based foods,** such as breads, cereals, pasta, oatmeal, and single grain foods (e.g., rice, quinoa, barley, spelt) **Starchy vegetables,** such as corn, potatoes, peas, and butternut and acorn squash
Sugars (simple carbohydrate)**	**Naturally occurring sugars** found in fruits, some vegetables, and dairy products **Added sugars*** - **From sugar cane and sugar beets:** Granulated sugar, brown sugar, confectioners' sugar/powdered sugar, invert sugar, golden syrup, turbinado sugar, demerara sugar, molasses, and caster sugar/superfine sugar - **From corn:** High-fructose corn syrup, corn syrup, dextrose, glucose, and high-maltose corn syrup - **From other sources:** Agave syrup, coconut sugar, coconut syrup, date sugar, date syrup, fruit juice concentrate, honey, maple syrup, rice syrup, sweet sorghum syrup/juice
Fiber (the part of plants that the body cannot digest or absorb)	Whole grains, fruits, vegetables, beans, peas, lentils, soybeans, nuts, and seeds
Resistant starches (resists digestion in the small intestine and ferments in the large intestine; considered a dietary fiber because it behaves like soluble fiber)	Plantains and green bananas (as a banana ripens, resistant starch changes to regular starch); beans, peas, and lentils (white beans and lentils are highest in resistant starch); whole grains, including oats and barley; and cooked and cooled white rice

* Complex carbohydrates that are refined, such as white flour, are generally less nutritious because nutrients are lost in processing.

** Sugars can be classified by their chemical structure as monosaccharides (a single sugar) or disaccharides (two sugars linked together). Some sugars, such as fructose, glucose, and sucrose, impart a sweet taste, and other sugars, such as the lactose in dairy products, do not.

*** The term "added sugars" refers to any caloric sweetener added to a food during processing, cooking, or at the table.

Quick Tip

"When developing recipes and deciding whether to eliminate sugar, reduce sugar, or replace sugar with a sugar substitute, ask yourself, 'Why is the change needed?' Are you developing a recipe for general health and wellness, calorie reduction, total carbohydrate reduction, blood sugar management, heart health, bariatric diet, FODMAP diet, or another diet? Knowing your 'why' can help you focus on choosing the type of sweetener."

—Marlene Koch, RDN, cookbook author and diabetes expert

CULINARY FUNCTIONS OF SUGARS

Provides sweetness and enhances taste: The most recognized function of sugar is sweetness, but sugar can also heighten flavor or depress the perception of other flavors (e.g., sugar can help change the perception of acidity in a tomato sauce).

Tenderizes: Sugar provides bulk, which affects the mouthfeel and texture of baked goods. In cakes, the ratios of ingredients to each other are important: sugar and fat tenderize the structure, and flour and egg affect structure.

Provides moisture and preserves: Sugar is hydroscopic, which means that it attracts and holds moisture. This helps preserve and extend a baked good's shelf life.

Aerates: Sugar is integral to the creaming process, which incorporates air into a batter and makes the texture of the baked good lighter and more tender.

Allows for spreading: When it is heated, sugar melts, causing the baked good to spread.

Helps with browning and flavor: When heated to around 340° F, sugar begins to caramelize and darken in color. This contributes new qualities of flavor, such as nuttiness and caramelization. During baking and browning, sugar recrystallizes as the moisture evaporates, resulting in a crisp texture.

Provides food for yeast: In small amounts, sugar helps yeast begin to produce the gas necessary to raise yeast dough. In large amounts, it slows down yeast fermentation (i.e., the rise time for a sweet dough is longer).

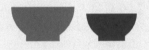

Tips for Reducing Sugar in Baking

When developing baked-good recipes with reduced sugar, plan to approach each recipe individually. This requires quite a bit of experimentation and testing, all while keeping in mind the functional role of sugar in the recipe and the best way to modify it. In general, it's easier to reduce sugar in quick breads, cakes, no-bake bars, and some cookies. Slightly reducing the sugar content of these types of recipes should not significantly affect the final product; on the other hand, reducing sugar in recipes for candy, meringue, custard, ice cream, and frozen desserts can be more difficult and require more testing.

- Start by reducing the sugar (e.g., corn syrup, granulated white sugar, brown sugar, coconut sugar, honey, agave nectar, maple syrup, or molasses) in the original recipe by ¼ of the amount used. If a recipe typically uses 1 cup of sugar, try ¾ cup instead. If the reduction by a quarter produces favorable results, try cutting the amount by a third and use ⅔ cup instead.

- Further reduction in sugar content will require more testing and adjusting, as doing so is more likely to yield negative effects. Try other ingredients that can provide moisture, bulk, and sweetness, such as apple sauce, fruit puree, or yogurt.

- Reduce the baking time, or at least check for doneness earlier than usually required. Sugar helps keep baked goods moist, and overbaking will dry them out.

- Use more brown sugar than white sugar to provide more moistness. Brown sugar makes baked goods a bit moister and chewier than granulated sugar because of the hydroscopic nature of molasses. Light brown sugar is about 10% molasses; dark brown sugar, about 20%.

- When sugar functions in a recipe primarily to add sweetness, such as in a topping for a coffee cake or muffins, it's easier to reduce the total amount.

- To enhance flavor and make up for reduced sweetness, consider adding extracts (e.g., vanilla, lemon, orange, almond, coconut); fresh citrus juice or zest; or spices (e.g., cinnamon, cardamom, nutmeg).

Using Alternatives to Granulated Sugar in Recipes

Choosing to use other sugars, such as honey, maple syrup, coconut sugar, or agave syrup, instead of white or brown sugar is more about personal taste than better health. From a calorie and carbohydrate perspective, they are all very similar. The American Diabetes Association and the Dietary Guidelines for Americans both recommend limiting added sugars, regardless of their source. Some sugars contain trace amounts of vitamins and minerals, but in the amounts these sugars are typically consumed, these would be negligible. For culinary purposes, a liquid sweetener may be desirable when altering flavor or texture in a recipe.

Honey

Honey is best in quick breads, puddings, ice cream, yeast breads, muffins, pancakes, and waffles. It can also be a nice alternative to regular sugar in vinaigrettes and glazes or any savory recipe that needs a bit of sweetness to balance flavors. Honey also acts as an emulsifier, making it ideal for salad dressings.

The color and flavor of honey differs depending on the honeybees' nectar source (blossoms). Honey color and flavor range from almost colorless with mild flavor to dark brown with a distinctively bold flavor. If the unique flavor of honey matters in a recipe, be sure to recommend a specific kind. Honey is sweeter than sugar, so less may be needed to achieve the same amount of sweetness; however, it is more calorie dense, so reducing the quantity of it may not reduce the total calories.

Tips for substituting honey for granulated sugar:

- To achieve the same level of sweetness, replace each 1 cup of sugar with about ¾ cup of honey.

- Honey is about 20% water, so if it is used as a substitute for granulated sugar, reduce the liquid in the recipe by about a quarter. If the recipe includes no other liquid, add a bit more flour (this will likely require some experimentation).

- In baked-good recipes where butter is creamed with granulated sugar, which incorporates air pockets that help create a lighter texture, substitute no more than ⅓ to ½ of the sugar with honey.

- Honey is naturally acidic, so if the recipe does not include an ingredient to help neutralize its acidity, such as sour cream or buttermilk, add a pinch of baking soda (about ¼ teaspoon of baking soda per 1 cup of honey).

- Honey has a higher sugar content and burns more easily than granulated sugar, so reduce the baking temperature by about 25° F.

Maple Syrup

Maple syrup is made by boiling the sap from maple trees until some of the liquid evaporates and the sugars condense into a thick syrup. The darker the maple syrup is, the more intense and complex its flavor will be. Maple syrup has about the same level of sweetness as granulated sugar, and it's best used in recipes for ice creams, puddings, candies, caramels, and some cookies.

Tips for substituting maple syrup for granulated sugar:

- Replace the sugar with an equal amount of maple syrup.

- When using maple syrup instead of sugar, slightly reduce (by 20%–25%) the liquid in a recipe (for example, if using ½ cup of maple syrup, reduce the liquid by 2 tablespoons) or add 20% to 25% more flour if the recipe includes no other liquid (e.g., if using ½ cup of maple syrup, add 2 tablespoons of flour).

- Due to its higher water content, maple syrup is usually not a good choice for baked goods that require creaming butter and sugar together.

Molasses

Molasses is the dark, thick, and sweet syrup that remains after sugar beets or sugar cane is processed to make white sugar. The type of molasses depends on the maturity of the sugar beet or sugar cane, the amount of sugar that is removed, and the extraction process, and different types vary in color and sweetness. The three types of molasses are light, dark, and blackstrap. Light molasses is lightest in color and has the highest sugar content, and it is the least viscous type. Dark molasses is darker and more viscous than light molasses, and blackstrap molasses is darkest in color, very viscous, and has a spicy and almost bitter flavor because it is highly concentrated. Use molasses sparingly in baked goods unless its intense flavor is desired; it can easily overpower other flavors.

Tips for substituting molasses for granulated sugar:

- Molasses is less sweet than sugar; however, you should start experimenting by substituting a small amount of molasses for part of the recipe's sugar in a 1:1 ratio (for example, if a recipe calls for 2 tablespoons of granulated sugar, try 2 tablespoons of molasses). Depending on the recipe, the molasses flavor may be too robust to add more in order to obtain the same level of sweetness.

- Since molasses is acidic, it should be neutralized in a recipe for a baked good. Add a bit of baking soda to neutralize the molasses if it's not already present in the recipe.

- When substituting molasses for sugar in a recipe that contains another liquid, reduce the liquid amount by about a third. If the recipe includes no other liquid, add 1 tablespoon of flour for every ¼ cup of molasses.

Coconut Sugar

Coconut sugar, also known as coconut palm sugar, is made from the flower-bud sap (or nectar) of the coconut palm tree rather than from coconuts themselves. To make coconut nectar, the sap is mixed with water and boiled down to a syrup. Granulated coconut sugar is made by drying out the nectar until it crystallizes. The dried chunks are broken down into granulated coconut sugar.

Coconut sugar, which has a mild caramel flavor, provides the same calorie and carbohydrate content as regular sugar: about 15 calories and 4 grams of carbohydrate in each teaspoon.

Tips for substituting coconut sugar for granulated sugar:

- Use a 1:1 ratio when replacing brown or granulated white sugar.
- Some bakers say it produces a denser and drier texture in baked goods, requiring a bit more fat or pureed fruit to compensate.

HEALTHY-SOUNDING SUGARS

Choosing to use a "natural," "unrefined," or "raw" sugar instead of granulated white or brown sugar might sound healthier, but these labeling terms are defined loosely or not at all.

- **Natural:** According to the US Food and Drug Administration (FDA), all sweeteners are natural if they are derived from a "natural source." The FDA's designation does not address processing and manufacturing methods, which means that any highly processed or refined sweetener or sugar that is synthetically produced by enzymes or fermentation can be labeled "natural."
- **Raw:** To make raw sugar, liquid is removed from sugar cane crystals, creating an intermediate raw sugar product that still contains molasses and impurities.
- **Unrefined:** An unrefined sugar contains impurities; sugars are refined to remove impurities.

All added sugars supply calories with little or no additional nutrient differences. While some sugars, such as agave or coconut, have a lower glycemic index (GI)—a measure of how quickly a food affects blood sugar levels and the body's insulin response—than white granulated sugar, these sugars still provide the same 4 calories per gram. Also, these sugars and the recipes they are used in are often eaten with other foods at the same time, so a lower GI for one sugar ingredient may not be very relevant. Reducing the total amount of sugar in a recipe will have a greater impact on health than simply changing the type of sugar.

Agave Syrup or Nectar

Agave syrup, commonly labeled as agave nectar, is a processed sweetener from the agave plant. Agave syrup has a lower glycemic index than granulated sugar due to a higher fructose percentage, but any evidence suggesting this offers health benefits is lacking.

Tips for substituting agave syrup for granulated sugar:

- Replace 1 cup of sugar with ⅔ to ¾ cup agave nectar.
- If the recipe includes an additional liquid, reduce its amount by a third or add extra flour.
- Reduce the baking temperature by 25° F.
- Agave syrup, a vegan alternative to honey, is about 1½ times sweeter than sugar.
- Due to its higher water content, agave syrup is usually not a good choice for baked goods that require creaming butter and sugar together.

Turbinado Sugar

Turbinado sugar, which is also called raw sugar, is cane sugar that is minimally processed so it retains some of its naturally present molasses content. It is light brown in color and has slightly larger crystals than granulated or brown sugar, and it provides the same level of sweetness as granulated sugar so it can be used in a 1:1 ratio. Turbinado sugar may retain very small amounts of some vitamins and minerals, which makes it appear to be a slightly healthier option, but its calorie and carbohydrate content are the same as granulated sugar. Turbinado sugar is not exposed to bone char, an animal product often used to refine sugar, so it's suitable for vegan recipes.

NUTRITIONAL COMPARISON OF ADDED SUGARS

Sugar	Calories per tablespoon	Carbohydrate (or added sugar) per tablespoon (grams)
Granulated sugar	48	12
Brown sugar	51	12
Honey	63	17
Maple syrup	54	14
Molasses	60	14
Coconut sugar	54	15
Agave	60	16
Turbinado (raw sugar)	55	14

Source: US Department of Agriculture, Agricultural Research Service, FoodData Central: fdc.nal.usda.gov

LOW-CARBOHYDRATE AND KETOGENIC DIETS

Low-carbohydrate diets (often called low-carb diets) are used as a strategy for weight loss, however, study findings vary as to whether a low-carb diet can help with weight maintenance in the long term. A low-carb diet generally restricts carbohydrates to less than 45% of daily calories or less than 225 grams of carbohydrates based on a 2,000-calorie diet. A standard recommendation for carbohydrates is 45% to 65% of daily calories or 225 to 325 grams of carbohydrates based on a 2,000-calorie diet.

The focus of a low-carb diet, sometimes referred to as the Paleo, South Beach, or Atkins diet, is on protein. While a keto diet is also considered a low-carb diet, it is much lower in carbohydrates and the diet's focus is on fat. The keto diet restricts carbohydrates to less than 5% of daily calories or less than 50 grams of carbohydrates per day with 70% to 80% of calories coming from fat. When developing recipes for people who follow a low-carb or keto diet, eliminating added sugars is usually the first step, but to keep carbohydrates to a minimum, many nutrient-rich sources of carbohydrates, such as fruits, starchy vegetables, whole grains, milk, and yogurt must also be restricted.

To decrease the carbohydrate amount in recipes, try using:

- vegetable noodles instead of pasta
- cauliflower rice instead of rice
- mashed cauliflower instead of mashed potatoes
- mixture of half almond flour and half Parmesan cheese instead of breading on proteins
- leaf lettuce instead of buns and tortillas, and cut vegetables instead of crackers

DEVELOPING RECIPES FOR PEOPLE WITH DIABETES

There are very few differences between a diet for people with diabetes and a healthy diet, except that people with diabetes must watch their total carbohydrate intake to control blood glucose levels. The American Diabetes Association recommends that people with diabetes consume nutrient-dense carbohydrate sources that are high in fiber and minimally processed.

In addition to watching the type and total amount of carbohydrate by focusing on portion size and meal-planning methods like carbohydrate counting, people with diabetes may be interested in recipes that control calories to promote weight loss, limit saturated fat to help prevent heart disease, or reduce sodium to help lower blood pressure.

Since there is no one "diet for diabetes," approach developing recipes for people with diabetes in the same manner as developing any health-focused recipe, keeping the following tips in mind:

- Ensure a recipe's total carbohydrate and added sugar levels are moderate and the nutrition information is provided. (For example, you might aim for about 40–60 grams carbohydrate per serving for an entrée or combination meal; 30 grams per side dish or dessert.)

- Reduce or eliminate carbohydrate-rich foods or liquids that aren't essential to the recipe when possible.

- Develop diabetes-friendly dessert recipes by using fruit instead of added sugar as a source of sweetness, and include whole grains, nuts, or seeds in the recipes to increase dietary fiber.

- Create recipes using low-calorie or zero-calorie sweeteners so that people can choose for themselves if they want this option.

- Increase dietary fiber by:
  - focusing on nonstarchy vegetables (starchy vegetables include peas, corn, lima beans, winter squash, and potatoes)
  - including whole grains and legumes, such as beans, peas, and lentils.
- Use lean protein foods (e.g., lean meat, fish, poultry, plant-based protein sources) and reduced-fat dairy products.

- Add less salt and use reduced-sodium packaged foods as ingredients to help reduce a recipe's total sodium content (recommended daily intake: 2,300 milligrams or less per day for adults and lower amounts for children younger than 14). For example, you might aim for about 360 to 600 milligrams sodium per serving for an entrée or combination meal; 240 milligrams per side dish or dessert.

- Use modest amounts of fat for calorie control and keep the focus on monounsaturated and polyunsaturated fats (e.g., canola oil, olive oil, peanut oil, avocados, walnuts, almonds, pecans) instead of saturated fat (e.g., butter).

- Be mindful of appropriate portion sizes for meals, snacks, and desserts.

- Use cooking techniques that reduce calories, such as baking, broiling, grilling, or poaching, instead of frying.

Meal Planning Methods for People With Diabetes

Carbohydrate counting involves keeping track of the grams of carbohydrate contained in meals and snacks. Compared with protein and fat, carbohydrate has the most significant effect on blood glucose. In this meal-planning approach, a defined serving equals 15 grams of carbohydrate; most meal plans include 3 to 4 carbohydrate servings per meal, depending on the total calories.

The plate method helps limit total carbohydrate intake by filling about half the plate with nonstarchy vegetables, a quarter of it with lean protein foods, and limiting carbohydrate (starchy vegetables, grains, fruit, milk, yogurt) to only a quarter of the plate. For recipe development, these basic proportions can be used in recipes for combination entrées (i.e., stir-fry, soups, salads, bowls, pastas): 2 parts nonstarchy vegetables, 1 part lean protein, 1 part carbohydrate.:

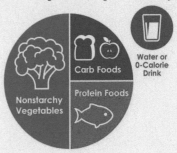

Image reproduced from the Centers for Disease Control and Prevention. cdc.gov/diabetes/managing/eat-well/meal-plan-method.html

Recipe example: Reducing added sugars in a traditional holiday dish

Instead of a traditional marshmallow or crumble topping, this sweet potato casserole is topped with a crunchy layer of pecans coated with a small amount of honey. The natural sweetness of sweet potatoes shines, with canned peaches replacing most of the added sugar for a naturally sweet flavor. These small changes result in a decadent side dish with less than half the calories and sugar of a traditional sweet potato casserole.

Peachy Sweet Potato Casserole
By Charmaine Jones, MS, RDN, LDN

Preparation time: 25 minutes
Cooking time: 35 minutes
Yield: 6 servings (¾ cup per serving)

2 large sweet potatoes (about 1¾ pounds), peeled and cut into chunks
1 tablespoon ground cinnamon
1½ teaspoons vanilla extract, divided use
½ teaspoon ground nutmeg
1 (15-ounce) can sliced no-sugar-added peaches, drained
3 tablespoons honey (see Note), divided use
2 tablespoons unsalted butter, melted
1 teaspoon fresh lemon juice
¼ teaspoon kosher salt
¼ cup pecan halves, chopped

1. Heat the oven to 325° F. Grease an 8-inch square baking dish with nonstick cooking spray.

2. Combine the sweet potatoes, cinnamon, 1 teaspoon of the vanilla, and the nutmeg in a medium saucepan and add water to cover by about 1 inch. Heat to a boil, reduce the heat, and simmer, uncovered, for about 10 minutes. Add the peaches and cook until the sweet potatoes are very tender, about 5 minutes. Drain the sweet potatoes and peaches, saving ½ cup of the cooking liquid.

3. Transfer the sweet potatoes and peaches to a large bowl or back to the pot. Mash or puree them using a potato masher or an electric mixer. Add the reserved cooking liquid, remaining ½ teaspoon vanilla, 2 tablespoons of the honey, butter, lemon juice, and salt. Mix until smooth. Spread the mixture into the prepared dish.

4. Mix the remaining 1 tablespoon honey with the pecans in a small bowl. Sprinkle the top of the casserole evenly with the pecans. Bake until hot, about 20 minutes. Serve warm.

Note: *If desired, use a sugar-free honey alternative to cut part or all the added sugar.*

Nutrition per ¾-cup serving: 210 calories, 7 grams total fat, 2.5 grams saturated fat, 280 milligrams sodium, 37 grams carbohydrate, 5 grams fiber, 20 grams total sugar (9 grams added sugar), 3 grams protein

Recipe Development with Sugar Substitutes

If more significant sugar (or calorie) reduction is the goal of a new or modified recipe, a sugar substitute may be in order. Sugar substitutes, also referred to as high-intensity sweeteners, nonnutritive sweeteners, artificial sweeteners, or zero- or low-calorie sweeteners, can significantly decrease a recipe's total number of calories, total carbohydrate, and added sugars. Since they have little or no effect on blood sugar, they are popular among people with diabetes.

Sugar substitutes are typically 200 times sweeter (or more) than sugar and provide the key function of adding sweetness. A zero- or low-calorie sugar substitute is best used when additional sweetness is desired, while a sugar blend (part sugar substitute and part regular sugar or another bulking agent) is best used in baking. Using zero- or low-calorie sweeteners as the only sweetener in baked goods is generally not recommended, since most baked goods rely on sugar for other functions than sweetness. Some factors to consider are listed below.

Color Sugar substitutes tend to lack the browning effects of sugar.

Volume Baked products made with sugar substitutes tend to be denser and may lack the desired height.

Texture Sugar substitutes generally do not have the moisture-retaining properties of sugar, so the result may be dry.

Taste Depending on the sugar substitute used, some people report an undesirable aftertaste.

Quick Tip

"When developing diabetes-friendly recipes, be mindful of including certain carb-rich foods if they are not essential to a recipe. The American Diabetes Association does not ban any ingredients but recommends reducing amounts of certain ingredients whenever possible. For example, when developing a diabetes-friendly chicken salad, you might leave out the raisins or find a lower carb ingredient that can add the same pop of sweetness, like a small amount of chopped apple or pomegranate seeds. Or is it really necessary to add corn to a chili recipe? Or a sugary glaze to a protein dish? These types of changes in a recipe can be very helpful to people with diabetes who are trying to trim carbs wherever they can."

—Jaclyn Konich, MPH, RDN, former editor, ADA Books, American Diabetes Association

CHOOSING FRUIT JUICES IN RECIPE DEVELOPMENT

Some fruit juices on supermarket shelves appear to be 100% fruit juice but are not—even if the label includes the fruit's name. Many juice products contain added sugars and other ingredients—sometimes even sugar substitutes. Check the label on the bottle for the percentage of juice and make sure the Nutrition Facts label lists 0 grams added sugar. Ingredient names that indicate the presence of a sugar substitute include sucralose, acesulfame potassium, neotame, stevia, or aspartame.

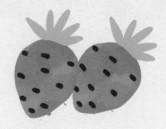

Tips for Using Sugar Substitutes in Recipes

Start by replacing a quarter of the sugar called for in a recipe with the same amount of zero-calorie sweetener; continue testing up to half granulated sugar and half zero-calorie sweetener. Tasting and testing are equally important, as each sugar substitute tastes and functions differently.

Try experimenting with one or two of the adjustments listed below when developing recipes for baked goods with sugar substitutes to help modify the end result's texture, volume, or browning:

- Use a smaller pan to achieve a better rise.
- Decrease the baking time slightly—3 to 5 minutes for cookies, 5 minutes for muffins and quick breads, and 7 to 10 minutes for cakes.
- Slightly decrease the amount of flour used.
- Add an extra egg or egg white.
- Replace part of the butter called for in the recipe with vegetable oil.
- Add a small amount of honey or molasses to provide flavor and moistness.
- Slightly increase the amount of liquid in the recipe, anywhere from an additional 2 tablespoons to ¼ cup.
- Add slightly more baking soda or baking powder to increase leavening and improve the volume of cakes and muffins.
- Lightly spray the batter or dough with cooking spray just before placing the pan in the oven to achieve a more golden color.
- Zero-calorie sweeteners do not activate yeast, so add a bit of sugar or honey for this function.

See Sugar Substitutes on page 122 for detailed information on several common types of sugar substitutes.

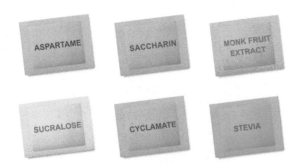

"Do NOT think of low- or no-calorie sweeteners as interchangeable. Each of these sweeteners is unique in its structure and taste profile and [its] ability to withstand high temperatures (e.g., aspartame breaks down and loses its sweetness at high temperatures). The more roles you are trying to have the low- or no-calorie sweeteners fulfill, the more challenging replacement will be. Study how brands use the sweeteners and how they change recipes for optimal results. They have a vested interest in serving up recipes that turn out well and taste good."

—Hope Warshaw, MMSc, RD, CDCES, BC-ADM, author and consultant focused on diabetes and nutrition

WHAT ARE SUGAR ALCOHOLS?

Sugar alcohols, a type of carbohydrate, are partially resistant to digestion, so they provide fewer calories compared to other regular sugars. Their chemical structure is a cross between sugar and alcohol—hence the name—but they do not contain any ethanol (the intoxicant found in alcoholic beverages).

A key benefit of sugar alcohols other than being lower in calories is that they have a negligible effect on blood glucose levels (and a low or zero score on the Glycemic Index). The downside to sugar alcohols is that they can cause stomach upset and bloating. Commonly used sugar alcohols in foods include xylitol, mannitol, sorbitol, malitol, and erythritol.

Italian cheesecake is made with ricotta cheese, so it differs from the familiar New York–style cheesecake that uses cream cheese only. In this recipe, a one-to-one replacement of granulated sugar with sucralose reduces calories and added sugars, and it cuts the total carbohydrate per serving in half—from 45 grams to 22 grams—while still retaining the delicious flavor and creamy texture of a traditional Italian cheesecake.

Italian Cheesecake

By Raeanne Sarazen, MA, RDN

Preparation time: 35 minutes
Cooking time: 1 hour, 25 minutes
Chilling time: 8½ hours
Yield: 12 servings (one 9-inch cheesecake)

CRUST
10 whole graham crackers (see Note)
½ cup packed dark brown sugar
3 tablespoons unsalted butter, melted

FILLING
1 (15-ounce) container part-skim ricotta cheese
2 (8-ounce) packages ⅓-less-fat cream cheese, softened
1½ cups sucralose sugar substitute (such as Splenda granulated sweetener)
4 large eggs
1 teaspoon vanilla extract
3 tablespoons cornstarch
3 tablespoons all-purpose flour
1 (16-ounce) container reduced-fat sour cream

1. Heat the oven to 325° F. Grease a 9-inch springform pan with nonstick cooking spray.

2. For the crust, place the graham crackers in a plastic bag and crush into fine crumbs with a rolling pin (alternatively, pulse into crumbs using a food processor). Mix the crumbs and brown sugar in small bowl and stir in the butter. Press the crumbs onto the bottom and about 1 inch up the side of the springform pan. Refrigerate until ready to use.

3. For the filling, beat the ricotta in the bowl of an electric mixer until fluffy, about 2 minutes. Add the cream cheese and sugar substitute and beat until fluffy and smooth. Slowly add the eggs and vanilla, mixing until well blended. Mix in the cornstarch and flour until well combined. Beat in the sour cream until just blended.

4. Pour the batter into the crust. Bake on a baking sheet until lightly golden and just set, about 1 hour, 25 minutes. Run a knife around edge of pan to release the side and help prevent cracking. Cool completely on wire rack. Refrigerate for 8 hours or overnight before serving.

Note: *You can also use packaged crushed graham cracker crumbs. You'll need 1⅓ cups.*

Nutrition per serving (¹⁄₁₂ of cheesecake): 340 calories, 23 grams total fat, 13 grams saturated fat, 330 milligrams sodium, 22 grams carbohydrate, 0 grams fiber, 14 grams total sugar, 12 grams protein

SUGAR SUBSTITUTES

Recipe development with sugar substitutes requires extensive trial-and-error testing, all while keeping in mind the functional properties that sugar provides. Each sugar substitute is unique. For that reason, it's wise to consult the website for a sugar substitute to find recommendations and tips on how best to use that product.

Sweetener and description	Brand name examples	Calories	Sweetness compared to table sugar	How to use	Good to know
Sugar blends Blend of regular sugar (cane, coconut, or fructose) and a sugar substitute	• Splenda Sugar Blend • Pure Via Stevia Turbinado Cane Sugar Blend • SugarLeaf Cane Sugar Blend • Truvia Cane Sugar Blend	10 to 20 calories per teaspoon	Equal to sugar or 3 times sweeter	Most sugar blend brands recommend replacing 1 cup sugar with ½ to ⅓ cup sugar blend. Check the label instructions.	Sugar blends tend to work best for reduced-sugar baking because they mimic the properties of sugar more closely than sugar substitutes alone.
Sucralose Made from regular sugar (sucrose) through a multi-step chemical process that allows most of it to pass through the body without being metabolized or providing energy (as calories)	• Splenda	Zero calories	400 to 600 times sweeter	Use a mixture of half sucralose and half regular sugar for best structure and browning results. Alternatively, use a packaged sugar blend like Splenda Sugar Blend that combines sucralose and regular sugar.	Sucralose contains maltodextrin, a bulking agent, and remains stable at high temperatures, which helps achieve some of the usual functions of sugar.
Stevia Sweet tasting components of stevia are steviol glycosides, which are extracted from the leaves of the *Stevia rebaudiana* Bertoni plant; stevia found on grocery shelves contains the rebaudioside A and rebaudioside D leaf extract (also known as Reb A or Reb D)	• Truvia Stevia • Pure Via Stevia • Pyure Stevia • Splenda Naturals Stevia • Sweetleaf Stevia	Zero calories	200 to 400 times sweeter	Liquid product: ¼ teaspoon in place of 2 teaspoons of sugar in hot or cold beverages. Granulated product: Most are used as a one-to-one replacement for sugar; bakes and browns in recipes.	Most stevia brands contain erythritol (sugar alcohol), maltodextrin, or dextrose, bulking agents that provide some of sugar's functions. Some report that baked goods made with stevia have a delayed sweetness and an aftertaste.
Monk Fruit Small, round fruit native to southern China; produced by removing the seeds and skin of the fruit, crushing the fruit, and collecting the juice	• Lakanto Monk Fruit Sweetener • Whole Earth Monk Fruit • Monk Fruit in the Raw	Zero calories	150 to 200 times sweeter	It can be used as a one-to-one sugar substitute. For example, 1 cup Monk Fruit in the Raw in place of 1 cup sugar.	Monk fruit sweeteners are stable at high temperatures and contain a bulking agent (usually erythritol) to help provide some of the functions of sugar.

BOX CONTINUES >

Sweetener and description	Brand name examples	Calories	Sweetness compared to table sugar	How to use	Good to know
Aspartame A low-calorie sweetener made from a combination of two amino acids—aspartic acid and phenylalanine	• NutraSweet • Equal	4 calories per gram	160 to 200 times sweeter	Use as a tabletop sweetener. Use in cold recipes or drinks or *after* a food is heated, such as in a custard. It is not recommended for baking.	Aspartame loses its sweetening capability when heated. Foods made with aspartame should not be consumed by people with a rare genetic disease called phenylketonuria (PKU).
Saccharin Synthetic sweetener, discovered in 1879; slowly absorbed, not metabolized by humans, excreted by the kidneys unchanged	• Sweet'N Low • Sugar Twin • Sweet Twin	Zero calories	200 to 700 times sweeter	Use as a tabletop sweetener. Use 2 teaspoons granulated or 1½ teaspoons liquid saccharin in place of ¼ cup sugar. When substituting saccharin, only replace part of the total amount of sugar; a quarter of the total is a good place to start.	Use saccharin in combination with sugar to replace the functions of volume and moisture that regular sugar provides. In high concentrations, saccharin has a bitter metallic aftertaste.
Erythritol A sugar alcohol and food additive produced by fermentation of cornstarch	Available as pure erythritol, or as erythritol combined with other sweeteners, such as oligosaccharides (sweet nondigestible carbohydrates), e.g., Swerve	Zero calories	70% as sweet	Use in a one-to-one ratio in place of sugar.	Erythritol is an ingredient in some sugar-substitute baking products (e.g., Truvia). Refer to manufacturer's website for tips on reducing the "cooling effect" (minty gum-like taste sensation) when baking with it.

Shopping List

- grapeseed oil
- brown rice flour
- canned pumpkin
- cocoa powder
- chia seeds
- chocolate chips
- salted pistachios
- almond extract

Chapter 5

Developing Recipes for Food Allergies and Intolerances

IN THIS CHAPTER, LEARN ABOUT:

- The differences between a food allergy, food intolerance, and food sensitivity

- Food allergen labeling laws and how to identify allergy ingredients on a food label

- How to use ingredient substitutions when developing or modifying recipes for each of the major food allergens

- Developing recipes for lactose intolerance and sulfite sensitivity

To create safe and successful recipes for people with food allergies and intolerances, a recipe developer must avoid or replace trigger food(s) or ingredient(s). This may sound straightforward, but it demands a great deal of ingredient knowledge, investigative skills, and culinary expertise. It also requires an understanding of the function of the ingredient being eliminated so appropriate substitutions and modifications can be made.

Precautions for preventing cross-contamination should be provided in the instructions for recipes developed for people with allergies and intolerances. And, of course, testing the recipe is key to ensuring it is successful and tastes delicious (see Chapter 8 for more on recipe testing).

Food Allergies versus Food Intolerances versus Food Sensitivities

According to Food Allergy Research and Education (FARE), approximately 32 million people in the United States have one or more food allergies, and—for unclear reasons—food allergies are on the rise. True food allergies involve an immune system response and come in various forms. An allergic reaction occurs when the body mistakes an ingredient in food, usually a protein, for a harmful substance and creates a defense system to fight it. As the body's immune system battles the "invading" food, a variety of symptoms may occur. Some exposures to food allergens set off a life-threatening allergic reaction known as anaphylaxis, a serious and possibly deadly reaction that impairs breathing, causes a sudden drop in blood pressure, and can send the body into shock. Other symptoms range from mild to severe, including rashes, hives, nausea, vomiting, diarrhea, breathing difficulties, and swelling around the mouth.

Food intolerances are often confused with food allergies, but food intolerances involve the digestive system rather than the immune system. An intolerance is a response that occurs when something in a food irritates the digestive system or when the food cannot be properly digested or broken down. This can lead to symptoms such as intestinal gas, abdominal pain, or diarrhea. Other symptoms of food intolerances can involve the skin and respiratory system. Generally speaking, reactions to food intolerances are usually less severe than those of food allergies, since they do not trigger the immune system. With food allergies even the smallest amount of an offending food has the potential to lead to anaphylaxis.

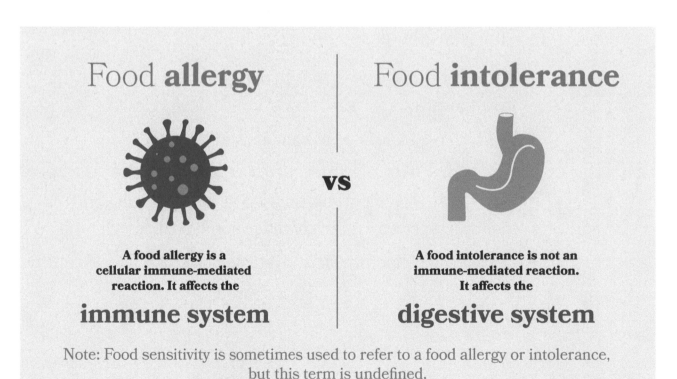

Food **allergy** | Food **intolerance**

vs

A food allergy is a cellular immune-mediated reaction. It affects the

immune system

A food intolerance is not an immune-mediated reaction. It affects the

digestive system

Note: Food sensitivity is sometimes used to refer to a food allergy or intolerance, but this term is undefined.

Food sensitivity, on the other hand, is often used as a catchphrase term for either a food allergy or intolerance. It can be used to describe a food or ingredient that triggers an allergic reaction or an intolerance, such as a sulfite sensitivity. There is no standard medical definition for a food sensitivity.

The guidance for recipe development in this chapter is primarily focused on food allergies, but the goal of developing recipes for food allergies, intolerances, and sensitivities is the same: to avoid the offending food or ingredient.

Food Allergen Labeling Laws

Food allergy labeling laws help make it easier for recipe developers and consumers to identify whether an allergen is present in a food product. These laws, regulated by the US Food and Drug Administration (FDA) under the Food Allergen Labeling and Consumer Protection Act of 2004 (FALCPA) and the Food Allergy Safety, Treatment, Education, and Research Act of 2021 (FASTER), mandate the nine major food allergens—milk, eggs, peanuts, tree nuts, soy, wheat, fish, crustacean shellfish, and sesame (as well as any ingredient containing protein derived from any one of these allergens)—to be listed on a packaged food label. This includes domestic food products and those imported from other countries that are regulated by the FDA.

The FDA also requires food manufacturers and processors to disclose the presence of sulfiting agents on food labels if the product has a concentration of 10 or more parts per million (ppm), regardless of whether the sulfites are components of an ingredient in the food or are used during processing. (See page 148 for more information on sulfite sensitivity.)

Voluntary Advisory Statements

Advisory statements for allergens can be confusing since there is no regulatory guidance on this type of precautionary labeling. Food label allergen regulations apply to ingredients only and do not include manufacturing practices that may result in unintentional cross-contamination with allergens during processing. While federal regulations do not require it, manufacturers can voluntarily include:

9 major proteins that trigger allergic reaction

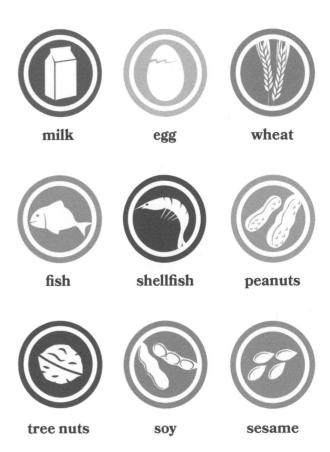

milk   egg   wheat

fish   shellfish   peanuts

tree nuts   soy   sesame

- **Allergen advisory statements**, which can include: "may contain," "processed in a facility that also processes," or "made on equipment that processes." These statement typically appear near the list of ingredients.

- **Allergen advisory phrases**, such as "peanut-free" and "egg-free," are not legally regulated. These phrases can be placed on a packaged food label but the food product may be manufactured in a facility where allergens are present. If unsure, contact the manufacturer directly for information about allergens, and keep in mind that a product's ingredients can be changed without warning, so it's best to read ingredient statements every time a product is used in a recipe.

Reading a Food Label for Allergens

Reading the package's ingredient list and "contains" statement is critical when developing recipes for people with food allergies, as ingredients and manufacturing processes change often. The law requires food labels to identify the food source of the nine major food allergens in **one of the following simple-to-understand ways**:

- **List the common name of the food allergen in the ingredient list**. The food allergen must be clearly identified (e.g., wheat flour, buttermilk, egg yolk).

> **INGREDIENTS:** CHOCOLATE COOKIES (BITTERSWEET CHOCOLATE, **SOY** LECITHIN, VANILLA FLAVOR), **EGGS**, SUGAR, ENRICHED **WHEAT** FLOUR, SEA SALT.

- **List the common name of the allergen in parentheses if it does not appear elsewhere in the ingredient list**. Food manufacturers choosing this option must list the allergen's common name in parentheses following the less common form of the name of the ingredient (e.g., lecithin [soy], whey [milk]). This includes listing the specific type of tree nut (e.g., almonds, pecans, walnuts), the specific type of fish (e.g., tuna, flounder, cod), and the specific type of crustacean shellfish (e.g., crab, lobster, shrimp).

> **INGREDIENTS:** WHEY PROTEIN (MILK), LECITHIN (SOY), SUGAR, NATURAL FLAVORS (ALMOND), SALT.

- **List the allergen name after or near the ingredients in a "contains" warning statement.** A "contains" warning is not required on a label if the allergen is already listed in the ingredient list. If a label doesn't include a "contains" statement, always read the ingredient list carefully to search for potential allergens. Only the nine major allergens are required to be listed in a "contains" statement.

> **INGREDIENTS:** WHEY PROTEIN, LECITHIN, SUGAR, NATURAL FLAVORS, SALT.
> **Contains: milk, soy, and tree nuts (almonds).**

FOOD ALLERGEN LABELING BY OTHER FEDERAL AGENCIES

The FDA regulates food allergen labeling on most packaged foods and drinks, under FALCPA and FASTER, except on meat products, poultry products, certain egg products, and some alcoholic beverages. Other federal agencies regulate these foods and beverages:

The US Department of Agriculture (USDA) regulates meat, poultry, and egg products and is not subject to FALCPA because these categories of foods are regulated by the Food Safety and Inspection service of the USDA. For these foods, allergen statements are voluntary.

Alcohol and Tobacco Tax and Trade Bureau (TTB) regulates alcoholic drinks, spirits, and beer and is not subject to FALCPA. TTB does permit voluntary labeling of major food allergens on the labels of wines, distilled spirits, and malt beverages. Note that alcohol labeling can be confusing since FDA has jurisdiction over certain alcoholic products (e.g., wine or hard cider under 7% alcohol by volume; beer made without malted barley and/or hops [e.g., gluten-free beer]; hard seltzers made from fermented sugar).

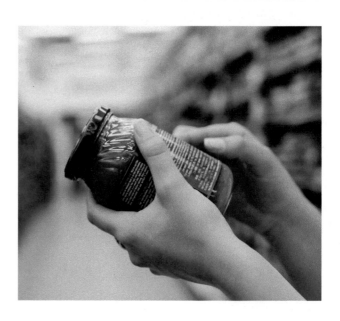

Peanut Allergy

A peanut allergy occurs when a person's immune system mistakenly identifies the proteins present in peanuts as harmful. Peanuts are one of the food allergens most commonly associated with anaphylaxis, a sudden life-threatening condition that requires immediate attention and treatment. A peanut allergy is different from an allergy to tree nuts (e.g., almonds, cashews, pistachios, walnuts, pecans). Peanuts are not actually true nuts; they are a legume (same family as beans, peas, and lentils).

It is safest to develop peanut-free recipes using alternate plant-based oils. Highly refined peanut oil is not required to be labeled as an allergen since the refining process separates the protein from the oil, resulting in an oil that contains negligible residual protein. It is therefore generally considered safe for those with a peanut allergy. However, in contrast, "crude," "extruded," "cold-pressed," and "gourmet" oils are not refined. These unrefined oils contain enough peanut protein to trigger an allergic reaction and must be listed on food labels as an allergen.

Developing Recipes for People with a Peanut Allergy

Do not use peanuts and products that contain peanut ingredients, which include:

- arachis oil (another name for peanut oil)
- artificial nuts (peanuts that have been deflavored and then reflavored with a nut such as pecan or walnut)
- beer nuts
- ground nuts
- mixed nuts
- lupin (or lupine or lupini, a common flour substitute in gluten-free foods—studies show a cross-reaction to this legume)
- mandelonas (peanuts soaked in almond flavoring)
- nut meat
- nut pieces
- peanuts
- peanut butter
- peanut flour
- peanut oil (cold-pressed, expelled, or extruded peanut oil)
- peanut protein hydrolysate

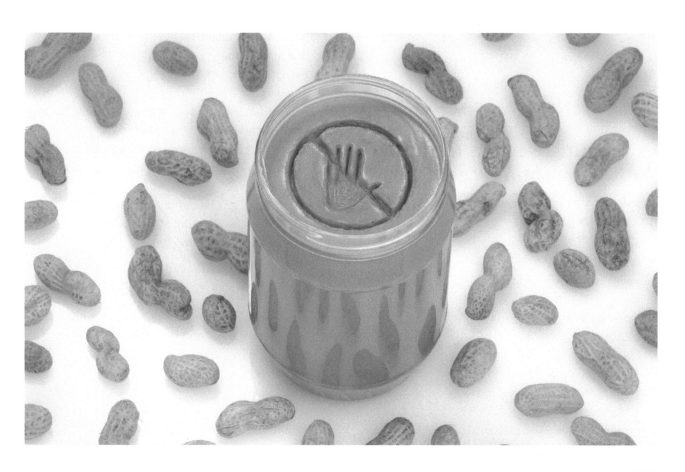

Tree Nut Allergy

As their name implies, tree nuts grow on trees. Peanuts, which grow underground, are considered legumes. A tree nut allergy occurs when a person's immune system mistakenly identifies the proteins present in tree nuts as harmful. Tree nut allergies can be life threatening, causing an anaphylactic reaction in some. Common tree nuts associated with allergies include walnuts, almonds, hazelnuts, pecans, cashews, pistachios, and pine nuts. While people with an allergy to one tree nut do not necessarily have an allergy to other tree nuts, it is best to avoid all types of tree nuts when developing tree nut–free recipes.

Also watch out for tree nuts in food products where they might seem unexpected, such as in cereals, crackers, cookies, candy, chocolates, energy bars, flavored coffee, frozen desserts, marinades, barbecue sauces, and some cold cuts (e.g., mortadella sometimes contains pistachios). Always read the ingredient list to verify.

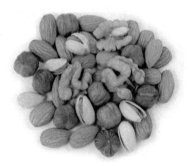

Developing Recipes for People With Tree Nut Allergies

Do not use tree nuts and products that contain tree nuts, which include:

- almonds
- artificial nuts
- beechnuts
- Brazil nuts
- butternuts
- cashews
- chestnuts
- chinquapin nuts
- gianduja (a chocolate-nut mixture)
- ginkgo nuts
- hazelnuts (filberts), hazelnut spread

Instead of	Use
Tree nuts	Seeds, including sunflower or roasted pumpkin seeds (pepitas), are a good replacement for tree nuts in granola, breads, and seed "butters"
	Roasted peas or chickpeas for added crunch in a salad
	Crushed pretzels for tree nut pie crusts or tree nut protein coating/breading
Tree nut oils	Tree nut–free oils like vegetable, canola, sunflower, soy, and coconut*

TREE NUT SUBSTITUTIONS

* Coconut, the seed of a drupaceous fruit, is typically not restricted in the diets of people with tree nut allergies since true coconut allergies are considered rare. Despite this, the US Food and Drug Administration identifies coconut as a tree nut and thus an allergen declaration is required.

- hickory nuts
- litchi/lichee/lychee nuts
- macadamia nuts
- marzipan/almond paste
- nangai nuts
- natural nut extracts (e.g., almond, walnut), but artificial extracts are generally safe
- nut butters (e.g., cashew butter, almond butter)
- nut distillates/alcoholic extracts
- nut flour/meal
- nut milks (e.g., almond milk, cashew milk)
- nut oils (e.g., walnut oil, almond oil)
- nut pastes (e.g., almond paste)
- pecans
- pesto
- pili nuts
- pine nuts (also referred to as indian, pignoli, pignolia, pignon, piñon, and pinyon nut)
- pistachios
- pralines
- shea nuts
- walnuts
- walnut hull extract (a flavoring)

Soy Allergy

A soy allergy occurs when a person's immune system mistakenly identifies certain soy proteins as harmful. For those with soy allergies, eating soy can cause mild symptoms such as hives and itching, but rarely will it cause a life-threatening anaphylactic reaction.

Soy, a product of soybeans, is part of the legume family, which also includes beans, peas, lentils, and peanuts. People with soy allergies are not necessarily allergic to other legumes.

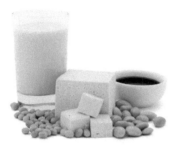

Developing Recipes for People With a Soy Allergy

Do not use soy and products that contain soy, which include:

- edamame
- miso
- natto
- shoyu
- soy (e.g., soy albumin, soy cheese, soy fiber, soy flour, soy grits, soy ice cream, soymilk, soy nuts, soy sprouts, soy yogurt, soy-based hamburgers)
- soy oil, cold-pressed, expelled, or extruded (note that highly refined soy oil is not required to be labeled as an allergen)
- soybean curds
- soybean granules
- soy sauce
- tamari
- tempeh (most commonly made with soybeans)
- teriyaki sauce
- tofu
- tofu "meats," such as hot dogs

Do not use products that contain the following ingredients:

- glycine max
- hydrolyzed vegetable protein (hvp)
- hydrolyzed plant protein
- textured vegetable protein (tvp)
- monoglycerides and diglycerides
- soya
- soy protein (concentrate, hydrolyzed, isolate)

Other ingredients that may contain soy include vegetable gums, vegetable starches, vegetable broth, artificial flavoring, and natural flavoring. Soy can also be found in some unexpected products, such as processed meats, canned tuna and meats, low-fat peanut butter, jarred sauces, breakfast cereals, and chocolate. Read the ingredient list on the food label.

SOY SUBSTITUTIONS

Instead of	Use
Tofu	Seitan or other types of beans
Miso	Vegetable or chicken broth/ stock
	Tahini
Soy sauce, tamari	A little extra salt
	Coconut aminos (made from the sap of the coconut palm)
	Fish sauce
	Worcestershire sauce
	Maggi seasoning (made from fermented wheat protein and contains umami-rich glutamate)
Cold pressed, expelled, or extruded soy oil	Alternate oils, such as corn, olive, canola, or avocado
Vegetable oil derived from soy	Vegetable and plant-based oils made without soybeans

Note: Highly refined soy oil is not required by the FDA to be labeled as an allergen. According to FARE, most people with soy allergies can safely eat highly refined soy oil and soy lecithin (made from highly refined soy oil).

Fish Allergy

A fish allergy occurs when a person's immune system mistakenly identifies fish protein or fish gelatin (which includes skin and bones) as harmful. For those with fish allergies, eating fish can cause mild to severe symptoms, such as swelling of the lips and tightening of the throat. A life-threatening anaphylactic reaction is less common.

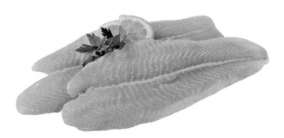

Developing Recipes for People With a Fish Allergy

Do not use finfish, which includes:

- anchovies
- bass
- catfish
- cod
- flounder
- grouper
- haddock
- hake
- halibut
- herring
- mahi-mahi
- perch
- pike
- pollock
- salmon
- scrod
- sole
- snapper
- swordfish
- sardines
- tilapia
- trout
- tuna

Do not use products that contain the following ingredients:

- Asian sauces and pastes containing fish-based stock, bonito flakes, or fish sauce
- barbecue sauce containing Worcestershire sauce
- bonita flakes (dried and fermented tuna)
- bouillabaisse
- Caesar salad dressing
- caviar/fish roe
- caponata (a Sicilian eggplant relish)
- fish gelatin (made from the skin and bones of fish)
- fish oil
- fish sauce
- fish stock
- imitation or artificial fish or shellfish made mainly from Alaskan pollock (e.g., surimi)
- Worcestershire sauce

FISH SUBSTITUTIONS

Instead of	Use
Products that contain fish	Read food labels and avoid products that contain fish ingredients; remove the ingredient or make substitutions based on the recipe you are developing
Worcestershire sauce	Soy sauce
	1 part soy sauce mixed with 1 part ketchup or apple cider vinegar
	Equal parts soy sauce, tamarind paste, and distilled white vinegar, mixed with a pinch of ground cloves and hot sauce
	1 part miso paste mixed with 1 part water
	Sherry or balsamic vinegar mixed with a pinch of onion powder and garlic powder
	Shaoxing wine
	Maggi seasoning sauce or Marmite
	Coconut aminos
Fish sauce	Bottled vegan fish sauce
	1 part soy sauce and 1 part rice vinegar plus pinch salt
	1 part soy sauce and 1 part freshly squeezed lime juice
	Coconut aminos and pinch salt
	Combine 3 cups water, ¼ ounces dried sliced shiitake mushrooms, 3 tablespoons salt, and 2 tablespoons soy sauce in a small pot over medium-low heat and simmer until reduced by half; strain

Crustacean Shellfish Allergy

A shellfish allergy occurs when a person's immune system mistakenly identifies certain proteins in shellfish as harmful. For those with shellfish allergies, eating shellfish can cause mild to life-threatening anaphylactic reactions.

Shellfish are organized into two subgroups: crustaceans (shrimp, crab, and lobster) and mollusks (clams, mussels, oysters, scallops, and octopus). Crustacean shellfish allergy is more common than mollusk shellfish allergy, but people who are allergic to crustacean shellfish may be advised to avoid mollusks as well. It's important to note that only crustacean shellfish, not mollusk shellfish, are required to be listed on food labels per FDA allergen labeling laws. Finfish allergies are separate from shellfish allergies. The protein in shellfish is different from finfish.

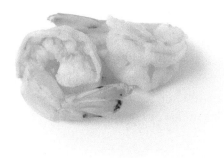

Developing Recipes for People With a Shellfish Allergy

Do not use shellfish and products that contain shellfish, which include:

- barnacles
- crab
- crawfish (also known as crawdads, crayfish, or ecrevisse)
- krill
- lobster (langouste, langoustine, moreton bay bugs, scampi, tomalley)
- prawns
- shrimp (crevette, scampi)

Although some people who are allergic to shellfish can eat mollusk shellfish safely, it's best to avoid using mollusks when developing recipes for people with shellfish allergies. Mollusk shellfish include:

- abalone
- clams (cherrystone, geoduck, littleneck, pismo, quahog)
- cockles
- cuttlefish
- limpets (lapas, opihi)
- mussels
- octopus
- oysters
- periwinkle
- sea cucumbers
- sea urchins
- scallops
- snails (escargot)
- squid (calamari)
- whelk (turban shell)

Do not use products that contain the following ingredients:

- bouillabaisse
- cricket flour (since crickets are arthropods, just like shrimp, crabs, and lobsters, they contain some of the same protein)
- cuttlefish ink
- glucosamine
- fish stock
- seafood flavoring (e.g., crab or clam extract)
- surimi (sometimes contains shellfish)

Sesame Allergy

A sesame allergy occurs when a person's immune system mistakenly identifies sesame seed proteins as harmful and triggers an immune response. For those with sesame allergies, eating sesame can cause symptoms ranging from mild (e.g., hives) to life-threatening (e.g. anaphylactic shock).

A product's ingredient list may include sesame or sesame (seed), or it may be listed under less familiar terms, such as benne, teel, or tahini. Sesame also may be hidden in an ingredient list under the terms "natural flavorings," "seasoning," or "spices." If an ingredient list is unclear, contact the product's manufacturer to determine whether sesame was used as an ingredient.

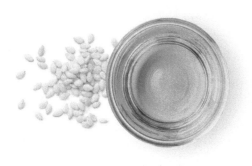

Developing Recipes for People With a Sesame Allergy

Do not use products that contain the following ingredients:

- benne, benne seed, benniseed
- gingelly and gingelly oil
- gomasio (sesame salt)
- halvah
- sesame flour
- sesame oil
- sesame paste
- sesame salt
- sesame seed
- sesamol
- sesamum indicum
- sesemolina
- sim sim
- tahini, tahina, or tehina
- til

Wheat Allergy

A wheat allergy occurs when a person's immune system mistakenly identifies wheat protein as harmful and triggers an immune response. It should not be confused with celiac disease, an autoimmune disorder. While wheat allergy and celiac disease are both adverse food reactions, the underlying causes are different.

A wheat allergy is an immune reaction to any of the proteins in wheat resulting in allergy symptoms involving the skin, gastrointestinal tract, respiratory system, and in some people, life-threatening anaphylaxis. In celiac disease, gluten, a protein found not only in wheat, but also in barley and rye, triggers an autoimmune response that attacks the small intestine. Symptoms can also involve the gastrointestinal tract (e.g., diarrhea and abdominal pain), but it's the inflammation and damage to the lining of the small intestine that makes this different from a wheat allergy.

Gaining an understanding of how wheat-based products—especially a product like all-purpose wheat flour—function in recipes will help you determine how to modify recipes and make substitutions. Look for products with a gluten-free label, since these are wheat-free. See Functional Role of Ingredients in Recipes on page 46 and Chapter 6 for more information on gluten-free food labeling, and wheat-free and gluten-free recipe development.

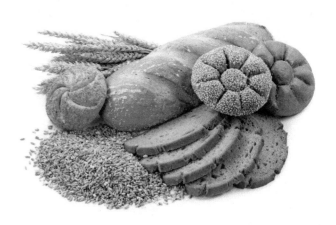

Developing Recipes for People With a Wheat Allergy

Do not use wheat and products that contain wheat, which include:

- ales/beers (sometimes made with wheat)
- bulgur (most often made from durum wheat)
- couscous (made from semolina)
- farina (made with milled wheat)
- farro (an ancient wheat grain)
- freekeh (derived from durum wheat)
- Kamut (an ancient wheat grain)
- matzo meal (made with wheat flour)
- Maggi seasoning (made from fermented wheat protein)
- noodles, pasta (made with wheat flour)
- udon noodles (made with wheat flour)
- panko breadcrumbs or cracker meal (made with wheat flour)
- seitan (wheat protein—used as a meat substitute)
- soy sauce (made from soybeans, wheat, salt, and water)
- spelt (an ancient wheat grain)
- surimi (imitation crab, most contain wheat)
- wheat berries (whole wheat kernel)
- wheat germ
- wheat flour: all-purpose, bread, cake, durum, unbleached, bleached, graham, 00 flour, pastry, self-rising, and whole wheat

Do not use products that contain the following ingredients:

- any variety of wheat: common wheat (also known as bread wheat, makes up most of the worldwide production), durum wheat (usually ground into semolina flour for pasta), club wheat (soft white wheat primarily used in pastries), and other types including einkorn, emmer, Kamut, and spelt
- any type of wheat flour
- wheat bran, wheat germ, wheat germ oil, wheat sprouts, sprouted wheat, wheat bran hydrolysate, and wheat protein isolate
- triticale wheat (bran, durum, germ, gluten, malt, sprouts, starch)
- gluten, wheat gluten, vital gluten, vital wheat gluten, fu (Japanese solidified wheat gluten)
- hydrolyzed wheat protein
- cereal extract—made from wheat
- soy sauce

WHEAT FLOUR SUBSTITUTIONS

Experiment with different nonwheat or wheat-free flour blends to find one that provides the functionality and texture needed. These include:

- amaranth flour
- barley and rye flours (these flours are acceptable for individuals allergic to wheat but not for individuals with celiac disease or non-celiac gluten sensitivity; see pages 160 and 165 for additional wheat-free ingredient substitution tips)
- buckwheat flour (despite the name, unrelated to wheat and safe to eat)
- chickpea flour
- corn flour
- gluten-free flour blends (homemade or packaged)
- oat flour
- quinoa flour
- rice flour
- tapioca flour

Egg Allergy

An egg allergy occurs when a person's immune system reacts negatively to the proteins present in eggs. Egg-free recipes are also appropriate for vegetarians who do not consume eggs and for those who follow a vegan diet.

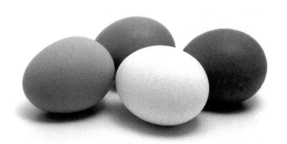

Do not use products that contain the following ingredients:

- albumin
- egg
- mayonnaise
- meringue powder
- globulin
- livetin
- lysozyme
- vitellin
- words starting with "ovo" or "ova" (e.g., ovalbumin)

Developing Recipes for People With an Egg Allergy

Do not use eggs and products that contain eggs, which include:

- all bird eggs, including those from chickens, ducks, quail, and geese
- egg substitutes
- dried powdered eggs
- eggnog
- meringue powder
- surimi (imitation crab)
- nougat
- marshmallow fluff
- fresh pasta (dry pastas are typically egg free)
- egg noodles
- mayonnaise
- ice cream and gelato

Eliminating Eggs From Recipes

Understanding the function of eggs in a recipe is essential (see Functional Role of Ingredients in Recipes on page 46). Recipes with relatively little egg content are easier to modify than recipes that rely on eggs (e.g., angel food cake, sponge cakes, popovers). When eliminating eggs from recipes, keep in mind that in addition to acting as a binding agent and providing moisture, eggs also help add to a dish's structure and stability, rise and lift, emulsification, and browning. Egg substitutes work best in recipes that require few eggs (e.g., cookies and muffins).

EGG SUBSTITUTIONS

Instead of 1 large egg, experiment with:

Homemade egg replacement
Mix together 1½ tablespoons tapioca starch or arrowroot powder, 3 tablespoons full-fat, plant-based dairy-free milk (e.g., coconut), and ¼ teaspoon baking powder.
OR
Mix 2 tablespoons arrowroot powder with 3 tablespoons water. (This is best in muffins and cakes.)*

Egg-replacement product
Mix 1½ teaspoons Ener-G Egg Replacer (a combination of a leavening agent and potato and tapioca starches) with 2 tablespoons warm water for a good egg substitute in cookies and cakes.
Other egg-replacement products include Follow Your Heart VeganEgg, JUST Egg, and Bob's Red Mill Egg Replacer.

BOX CONTINUES >

Soy lecithin
Use 1 tablespoon soy lecithin (provides binding properties and good for replacing yolks).*

Mashed fruit
Use ¼ cup mashed bananas, applesauce, or pumpkin puree; applesauce is a good binding agent for veggie burgers.

Flax "eggs"
Ground flaxseed is a good option for pancakes, quick breads, muffins, brownies, and cookies.
Whisk 1 tablespoon ground flaxseed (also known as ground flaxseed meal) into 3 tablespoons warm water and set aside for 10 minutes, or until the mixture thickens; flax "eggs" don't provide leavening, so also add ¼ to ½ teaspoon baking soda or baking powder to provide leavening if needed.

Chia "eggs"
Chia eggs are a good option for pancakes, quick breads, and muffins.
Whisk 1 tablespoon chia seeds into 3 tablespoons warm water and set aside for 10 minutes or until the mixture thickens; chia "eggs" don't provide leavening, so also add ¼ to ½ teaspoon baking soda or baking powder to provide leavening if needed.

Gelatin "egg"
Dissolve 1 packet (2½ teaspoons) unflavored gelatin in 2 tablespoons warm water OR dissolve 1 tablespoon unflavored gelatin in 3 tablespoons warm water; use immediately.

Aquafaba
Aquafaba, the liquid surrounding canned chickpeas or other canned beans or the liquid from cooking dried beans, makes a good egg substitute if it is the same consistency as egg white. If too watery, cook it until it reduces by about 25% (thicker is generally better).
- 3 tablespoons aquafaba = 1 whole egg
- 2 tablespoons aquafaba = 1 egg white

For an egg white substitute, whip aquafaba with a bit of cream of tartar or sugar until foamy.
Aquafaba works well in bars, cookies, and cakes, and as an emulsifier (e.g., good in mayonnaise and sauces).

Oat milk
Using an immersion or regular blender, blend 1½ ounces old-fashioned (not instant) rolled oats and 2 ounces water; push the oat milk through a fine mesh strainer and discard the solids; use immediately.

Tofu
Puree 3 to 4 tablespoons of silken tofu (good for cakes, quick breads, and cookies).

Baking powder or baking soda
Either of these substitutes works well in pancakes, cakes, and quick breads, as they provide leavening.
- Whisk together 1½ tablespoons water, 1½ tablespoons vegetable oil, and 1 teaspoon baking powder.
- Use 1 teaspoon baking soda and 1 tablespoon apple cider vinegar or distilled white vinegar.*

Yeast
Dissolve 1 teaspoon of yeast in ¼ cup warm water.

Instead of	Experiment with
Egg wash on breads or other baked goods	Milk or cream whisked with a little honey, maple syrup, or coconut nectar.
	For vegan recipes, use rice milk, soy milk, almond milk, or vegetable oil.
Coating a protein in egg before the breading stage	Dip or marinate the protein in buttermilk, unsweetened plant milk (e.g., rice milk), or water.
	Coat with thin layer of mustard, tahini, or hummus.

* Suggestions by Cynthia S. Ferron, MEd, CEPC, associate professor, Johnson & Wales University, College of Food Innovation & Technology

Milk Allergy

A cow's milk allergy is a reaction by the immune system to ingestion of either casein or whey, the two main proteins found in milk. Recipes developed for a milk-free diet are also appropriate for those who follow a vegetarian, dairy-free, or lactose-free diet. An important difference is that someone with lactose intolerance can tolerate some milk products (e.g., kefir, hard cheese), whereas a person with a milk allergy cannot tolerate any milk or dairy products. See page 146 for more on lactose intolerance.

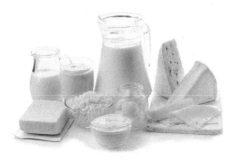

Developing Recipes for People With a Milk Allergy

Do not use milk or dairy products (all dairy products contain milk), which include:

- milk in all forms (e.g., nonfat milk, low-fat milk, whole milk, buttermilk, powdered milk, condensed milk, evaporated milk, goat milk, milks from other animals, malted milk)
- heavy whipping cream, half-and-half, nondairy creamers, heavy cream powder
- sour cream
- butter or ghee
- yogurt
- pudding
- ice cream or gelato
- cheese, including ricotta and cottage; all food products with artificial cheese flavors
- whey and casein protein powders

Be cautious about using ingredients that **may** contain milk, such as:

- nondairy products (some may contain casein, whey, or other derivatives)
- tuna products containing the milk protein casein

- lunch meats, hot dogs, and sausages (some use casein as a binder)
- plant-based foods
- shellfish, which is sometimes dipped in milk to reduce the fishy odor (ask the vendor or fishmonger)
- commercially prepared bread, rolls, and cereals (some use milk solids or casein)
- margarine, a type of artificial butter that may include milk or added ingredients like whey or casein
- lactic acid starter culture and other bacterial cultures
- chocolate (some types are milk free; see Does All Chocolate Contain Milk? on page 143)
- nougat
- caramel candy and sauce

Read the ingredient list on the food label to verify that it does not contain the following ingredients:

- artificial cheese or butter flavors
- butter
- casein
- casein hydrolysates
- caseinates (in all forms)
- curds
- diacetyl
- ghee
- lactalbumin
- lactalbumin phosphate
- lactoferrin
- lactose
- lactulose
- margarine
- milk in all forms
- milk protein hydrolysate
- recaldent
- rennet casein
- tagatose
- whey in all forms, including whey protein hydrolysates

Eliminating Milk From Recipes

There are numerous options for eliminating milk and milk products during recipe development because milk has varying functions in recipes, including:

- adds nutrients
- helps darken crust (due to the lactose [milk sugar] and proteins present in milk)
- softens crust texture
- adds moisture to doughs
- helps give breads a longer shelf life (partly due to milk fat)
- improves flavor (helps blend flavors and reduces the raw flour taste)

Plant-Based Milk Substitutes for Dairy Milk

Experiment with different plant-based milks when developing milk-free recipes. When testing variations, keep in mind how the flavors of plant-based milks may affect the final product. Some products may be available in sweetened or unsweetened varieties; select appropriately based on the type of recipe being developed. See page 74 for more on plant-based milks.

Soy milk Soy milk is an all-purpose plant milk option, as it works well in baking and cooking. Its higher protein content can help contribute to the structure of doughs and batters, but some may not care for the flavor soy adds to baked goods.

Pea milk This milk is similar to soy milk in terms of protein content; it also fares well in baking and cooking.

Oat milk While it is not as high in protein as soy and pea milks, oat milk has a mild, sweet taste and similar thickness to cow's milk, making it a good substitute in baked goods and smoothies.

Nut milks Milks made from nuts (e.g., almond and cashew) are good for sauces and smoothies; cashew milk often works well in baked goods.

Coconut milk Since it typically has a higher fat content, coconut milk adds richness to beverages, rice puddings, and creamy soups.

Milk-Free Substitutes for Butter

Butter, a dairy product made by churning fresh cream or milk, provides moisture and flavor in baking and flakiness in croissants and pastries. The minimum amount of butterfat required for butter sold in the United States is 80%, and another 16% to 18% of butter is water. The rest of the content is devoted to milk solids, such as proteins, lactose, and minerals, and, in the case of salted butter, salt. The higher the butterfat content is, the creamier the mouthfeel will be and the firmer and slower the butter will melt. The water in the butter helps hydrate flour and starches in recipes, and the fat adds tenderness and flavor.

Quick Tip

"Coconut oil is a good replacement for butter. Consider refined coconut oil when developing plant-based or vegan recipes for pie crusts, biscuits, and scones (or any recipe where you want cold bits of fat dispersed in the flour). It has a melting point of 78° F, which is close to butter's melting point of 90° F and has a mouthfeel that is similar to butter. Simply melt the coconut oil, measure it for the recipe, then chill until solid. Run warm water over the cup or container to allow easy removal of the solid oil, then either cut it in or shred it into the flour mixture. Melted, it also makes a good substitute for butter in phyllo pastries, which come out crisp and stay crisp longer than they would if made with liquid oils."

—Robin Asbell, plant-based chef and cookbook author of *Big Vegan*

While no substitute perfectly captures butter's flavor and texture, plant-based butter alternatives mimic some of butter's qualities. The percentage of fat and water varies among different plant-based products; as a result, the texture and flavor of baked goods made with them varies as well. Plant-based butter alternatives are usually made from a mixture of vegetable oils (e.g., coconut, sunflower), water, emulsifiers (e.g., sunflower lecithin, xanthan gum, psyllium husk), and protein (e.g., soy, nuts, cashews).

When substituting for butter in baking, choose solid plant-based butter alternatives or solid coconut oil. If a recipe calls for melted butter, substitute melted coconut oil or vegetable oil instead.

MILK SUBSTITUTIONS

Experiment with these options for replacing milk and dairy products in milk-free, dairy-free, and vegan recipes. The substitution you choose will depend on the type of savory or baking recipe being developed.

Instead of	Experiment with
Milk	One of the following in a 1:1 ratio in place of milk: • plain water (in flavorful baked goods) • plant-based milk: unsweetened, fortified soy milk (most like cow's milk in terms of protein content and overall nutritional profile; good choice for baking). Try other unsweetened plant-based milks, such as oat, coconut, almond, rice, hemp, quinoa, flax, pea, and potato. *Note: Goat milk is not considered a safe alternative for milk allergies.*
Powdered milk	Plant-based milk powders, such as soy, rice, potato, and cashew Raw cashews ground into a powder
Evaporated milk	Soy or other plant-based coffee creamer or plant-based plain yogurt Plant-based evaporated milk substitute (such as Carnation Almond Cooking Milk)
Buttermilk	Distilled white vinegar, apple cider vinegar, or lemon juice: Add 1 tablespoon to 1 cup unsweetened plant-based milk; this substitute will provide the acidity of buttermilk but not the flavor. Plant-based sour cream or plain yogurt. Whisk in enough water or plant-based milk to obtain a buttermilk consistency. Cream of tartar: Mix 1½ teaspoons cream of tartar to dry recipe ingredients. Then add a plant-based milk. (Cream of tartar tends to clump when mixed directly into liquid.)
Sweetened condensed milk	Coconut milk: Mix 1 can of full-fat coconut milk (about 13.5 ounces) with ⅓ cup granulated sugar in a pot. Heat to a boil. Simmer about 45 minutes, whisking about every 5 minutes. Canned cream of coconut, which contains added sugar (*do not use canned coconut cream*). Potato milk: Mix ½ cup potato flour (powder) with 1 cup hot water; heat over medium heat and whisk in 1½ cups sugar until fully dissolved. Plant-based sweetened condensed milk substitute (such as Nature's Charm Sweetened Condensed Coconut Milk)
Half-and-half or heavy cream	Silken tofu, pureed. Thin with unsweetened soy milk to obtain the desired consistency. Coconut milk cream (from a can of unsweetened, full-fat coconut milk): Refrigerate overnight 1 can of unsweetened full-fat coconut milk (ingredients should only be coconut and water); remove the solid coconut cream that floats to the top. For heavy cream, use coconut cream by itself; for half-and-half, blend the coconut cream with an equal amount of unsweetened plant-based milk. Plant-based milk and neutral oil: Use a 2:1 ratio mixture of unsweetened plant-based milk (⅔ cup) and melted plant-based butter or vegetable oil (⅓ cup). If needed, thicken with tapioca flour or cornstarch. Cashew cream for heavy cream: Soak 1 cup cashews in water overnight. Discard soaking liquid. Using a high-speed blender, blend cashews with ¾ cup water into a smooth cream. Plant-based half-and-half substitute (brands include Califia, Silk); plant-based heavy cream substitute (such as Silk Heavy Whipping Cream Alternative).

BOX CONTINUES >

Whipped cream	Coconut milk cream (from a can of unsweetened, full-fat coconut milk): Refrigerate overnight 1 can of full-fat coconut milk (ingredients should only be coconut and water); remove the solid coconut cream that floats to the top. Whip with confectioners' sugar.
Butter	Vegetable oil: In cooking, use a 1:1 ratio. In baking, generally less oil than butter is used; keeping a 1:1 ratio can make the recipe taste somewhat greasy. Start with ¾ cup oil for 1 cup butter or ⅓ cup oil for ½ cup butter.
	Refined coconut oil (melted). This has a similar mouthfeel and melting point to butter with less coconut flavor.
	Lard, all-vegetable shortening, or a blend of plant-based butter and vegetable shortening (consider these options if flakiness is desired, e.g., for pie crust or shortbread). Lard is not vegan, but it is milk free.
	Pureed fruits or vegetables (e.g., avocado, apples, prunes, sweet potatoes, pumpkin, carrots, zucchini). Use half the amount of puree than the butter needed in a recipe, alone or in combination with vegetable oil (e.g., for 1 cup butter, start with ½ cup puree and 2 tablespoons vegetable oil; experiment by adding more oil as needed, up to ½ cup puree and ½ cup oil).
	Plant-based butter substitute. Use in stick form as these usually contain less water (such as Earth Balance Vegan Buttery Sticks and Miyoko's Creamery).
Cheese	Plant-based cheese (brands include Daiya, Follow Your Heart, Violife)
Cream cheese	Raw cashews soaked in water until softened; pureed with a little freshly squeezed lemon juice and salt.
	Soft tree-nut cheeses (such as Treeline Soft French-Style Nut Cheese)
	Plant-based cream cheese substitute (such as Miyoko's Creamery Vegan Plainly Classic Cream Cheese or Tofutti)
Sour cream	Firm silken tofu, pureed. Use alone or make a dairy-free sour cream. For example, puree 1 (12-ounce) package extra-firm or firm silken tofu, 1 tablespoon apple cider vinegar, 1 tablespoon freshly squeezed lemon juice, and 1 pinch salt.
	Plant-based unsweetened plain yogurt (e.g., made with soy, almond, or coconut milk).
	Plant-based sour cream substitute (brands include Kite Hill, Forager, Tofutti)
Yogurt	Plant-based yogurt
Whey and casein protein powders	Plant-based protein powder
Chocolate (milk chocolate and white chocolate contain milk solids)	Cocoa nibs
	Dutch process cocoa powder
	Milk-free chocolates (brands include Hu, Enjoy Life)
	Note: Many brands of semisweet or bittersweet dark chocolate are naturally free of milk ingredients; read the ingredient list carefully to ensure the product does not contain milkfat, milk solids, lactose, cream, whey, or caseinates. See Does All Chocolate Contain Milk? on page 143 for more information.

USING DAIRY-FREE LABEL CLAIMS AND KOSHER SYMBOLS TO HELP IDENTIFY MILK-FREE PRODUCTS

Dairy-free and nondairy label claims and kosher symbols can be helpful tools for quickly finding milk-free products to use in recipe development, but it's important to understand what they mean and their limitations.

Dairy free and nondairy label claims

Do not rely solely on a product's label descriptor *dairy free* or *nondairy* when developing recipes for people with milk allergies (or vegan diets). Instead, carefully read the ingredient list on the food label for evidence of any milk proteins.

Dairy free: This claim *should* indicate that a product is made without any dairy (milk-based) ingredients. However, since the US Food and Drug Administration has no rules for using a dairy-free label claim—be careful. A product bearing this unregulated term may possibly contain milk proteins (casein, sodium caseinate, or whey).

Nondairy: Use of the term nondairy is regulated, but even that doesn't guarantee that the product is milk free. Caseinates, which are milk-derived ingredients, can be used in nondairy products as long as the ingredient statement includes the word "milk" or "milk derivative" after the caseinate ingredient in parentheses. For example, a creamer labeled as being nondairy meets the requirement by listing "sodium caseinate (milk derivative)" in the ingredient list.

Kosher symbols

A quick scan of a food label for kosher symbols is a good starting point to find out whether the product contains dairy or if it is dairy-free (pareve). However, these symbols are intended for those who comply with Jewish dietary laws, so they do not necessarily meet requirements for allergy disclosures. Read the ingredient list and contact the manufacturer to confirm. (See page 54 for examples of kosher symbols.)

Kosher dairy: The word dairy or the letter D following the kosher symbol (e.g., Ⓤ) on a product label means the product contains milk or a milk derivative.

Pareve: The term that refers to foods that contain neither milk nor meat. In other words, they are dairy free and meat free. Food products that are dairy free will have a kosher symbol (e.g., Ⓤ) followed by the word pareve. However, it's possible that a pareve-labeled product contains a small amount of milk protein from airborne particles. Check with the manufacturer to ensure it's 100% milk free.

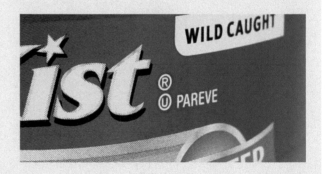

DOES ALL CHOCOLATE CONTAIN MILK?

Pure chocolate is made from the cacao bean of the cacao tree and is naturally free of milk. However, milk is an ingredient in many chocolate products, which makes them off-limits for people with milk allergies.

Milk-free chocolate products

Chocolate liquor is the purest form of chocolate. It is made by finely grinding cocoa nibs through rollers; the term "liquor" (or "cocoa mass") refers to the liquid state the substance takes on when it's warm. It contains no alcohol.

Cocoa solids includes all of the solid substances from cacao beans except cocoa butter.

Cocoa butter is the vegetable fat naturally present in cacao beans. It's referred to as a "butter" because of its creamy texture.

Cocoa nibs are small bits of roasted cacao beans.

Cocoa powder and Dutch process cocoa powder is the dried solid material left over once the cocoa butter (fat) is removed from chocolate liquor. Dutch processing is the term for treating a chocolate product with alkali, creating a darker brown cocoa powder with a more mellow flavor.

Baking chocolate is traditionally pure, unsweetened chocolate liquor pressed from cacao beans. Note that bittersweet and semisweet baking chocolate are not the same as baking chocolate, and they may contain milk.

Soy lecithin and flavorings (e.g., vanilla extract), which are common ingredients in chocolate products, are milk free.

Chocolate products that contain milk*

Milk chocolate contains a minimum of 10% chocolate liquor, a minimum of 12% milk solids, and a minimum of 3.39% milkfat.

White chocolate contains at least 20% cocoa butter, 14% milk solids, and 3.5% milkfat.

Instant hot cocoa mix product contains cocoa, sugar, dehydrated milk, and other ingredients.

Chocolate products that may contain milk*

Semisweet chocolate (usually in the 60% cacao range) contains a minimum of 35% chocolate liquor and may or may not contain milk solids.

Bittersweet chocolate (usually in 70% cacao range) contains a minimum of 35% chocolate liquor and may or may not contain milk solids.

Dark chocolate, a term that is not regulated by the US Food and Drug Administration, is often used interchangeably to describe bittersweet and semisweet chocolate. Milk may be present in dark, bittersweet, and semisweet chocolate.

A "lactose free" labeled chocolate product is not necessarily milk free. Even if the milk sugar lactose is removed from a chocolate product, milk proteins are still present.

* Ingredients that indicate the presence of milk in a chocolate product: milkfat, milk solids, lactose, cream, whey, or sodium caseinates.

This classic pumpkin bread is made milk-free and egg-free by using a seed-based oil instead of butter, and chia seed gel instead of eggs. These ingredient substitutions work well for any quick bread recipe. The quick bread is moist and delicious and perfect for those following a dairy-free or vegan diet. It also offers:

- a healthier fat profile by using sunflower (or grapeseed oil) instead of butter
- added fiber and a "nuttier" whole grain goodness by using whole wheat pastry flour instead of all-purpose flour
- beneficial cocoa polyphenols from the dark chocolate
- extra texture and wholesome plant-based nutrition—unsaturated fatty acids, potassium, and fiber—from the pistachios

Dark Chocolate Pumpkin Bread

By Jackie Newgent, RDN, CDN

Preparation time: 20 minutes
Cooking time: 55 minutes
Yield: 9 servings (one 9- by 5-inch loaf)

¼ cup plus 1 teaspoon sunflower or grapeseed oil, divided use
1¼ cups plus 1 tablespoon whole wheat pastry flour, divided use
¾ cup plus 1 tablespoon turbinado or granulated sugar, divided use
1 (15-ounce) can no-salt-added pumpkin puree
3 tablespoons cold water
1 tablespoon chia seeds
1½ teaspoons vanilla extract
¼ teaspoon almond or chocolate extract
⅓ cup plus 1 teaspoon unsweetened cocoa powder, divided use
½ teaspoon baking powder
½ teaspoon baking soda
½ teaspoon ground cinnamon
½ teaspoon sea salt or table salt
⅔ cup bittersweet chocolate chips or chunks (preferably 70% cacao)
⅓ cup salted roasted shelled pistachios, chopped

1. Heat the oven to 350° F. Lightly brush a 9- by 5-inch loaf pan with 1 teaspoon of the oil and dust with 1 tablespoon of the flour.

2. In a large bowl, stir the remaining ¼ cup oil with ¾ cup of the sugar until combined. Add the pumpkin, water, chia seeds, vanilla extract, and almond extract; stir until well combined.

3. In a medium bowl, whisk together the remaining 1¼ cups flour, ⅓ cup of the cocoa powder, the baking powder, baking soda, cinnamon, and salt until evenly mixed. Add the flour mixture to the pumpkin mixture and stir until just combined. Stir in the chocolate chips and pistachios.

4. Transfer the batter to the loaf pan and smooth the top. Dust the top with the remaining 1 teaspoon cocoa powder and sprinkle with the remaining 1 tablespoon sugar. Bake until springy to the touch, about 55 minutes. Cool in the pan on a wire rack for 15 minutes.

5. Remove the bread from the pan and completely cool before slicing. Cut into 9 slices and serve.

Nutrition per serving: 300 calories, 14 grams total fat, 3 grams saturated fat, 250 milligrams sodium, 46 grams carbohydrate, 6 grams fiber, 28 grams total sugar, 4 grams protein

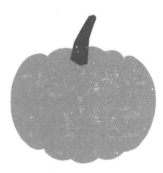

This satisfying milk-free soup has a secret ingredient full of plant-based protein: silken tofu. Standing in for the typical heavy cream or half-and-half often used in a pureed soup, silken tofu provides dairy-free creaminess and richness. The tomatoes are chock-full of the antioxidant lycopene, which supports a healthy heart and bone health. And consuming lycopene-containing foods with a fat source, such as olive oil, helps the absorption of lycopene.

Creamy Tomato Soup
By Abbie Gellman, MS, RD, CDN

Preparation time: 20 minutes
Cooking time: 15 minutes
Yield: 4 servings (1¾ cups per serving)

1 tablespoon extra-virgin olive oil
1 onion, diced
2 cloves garlic, sliced
1 tablespoon no-salt-added tomato paste
2 pounds tomatoes, chopped
½ cup no-salt-added vegetable stock or broth
1 teaspoon kosher salt
¼ teaspoon ground black pepper
¾ cup fresh basil, chopped, divided use
½ (16-ounce) package silken tofu, drained
1 cup cherry tomatoes, quartered

1. Heat the oil in a large saucepan over medium-high heat. Add the onion and sauté until light golden, 5 to 6 minutes. Add the garlic and sauté for 30 seconds. Add the tomato paste and sauté for 30 seconds. Add the tomatoes and cook down a bit, 5 to 10 minutes. Add the stock, salt, pepper, and about ⅔ of the basil.

2. Carefully transfer half the mixture to a high-powered blender (such as a Vitamix), add half the tofu, and puree. Transfer to a bowl and repeat with the remaining soup and tofu. Return all the soup to the saucepan and simmer for about 5 minutes, until heated through.

3. Divide the cherry tomatoes among four bowls. Add soup to each and garnish with the remaining basil.

Note: *To make part of the soup ahead, complete step 1 and refrigerate for up to 5 days or freeze for up to 3 months. Just before serving, complete steps 2 and 3. This is a great way to save some of summer's bounty of tomatoes.*

Nutrition per serving: 130 calories, 6 grams fat, 1 gram saturated fat, 325 milligrams sodium, 17 grams carbohydrate, 4 grams fiber, 10 grams total sugar, 6 grams protein

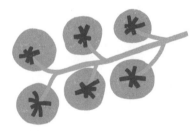

Lactose Intolerance

Lactose intolerance occurs when the body is unable to fully digest the sugar (lactose) in milk. As a result, unpleasant symptoms like abdominal bloating, gas, cramps, and diarrhea may occur after those with lactose intolerance consume dairy products. The intolerance is caused by a shortage of the enzyme lactase, which breaks down the lactose in milk and other dairy products made from milk, including yogurt, ice cream, soft cheeses, and butter.

While lactose intolerance can cause significant discomfort, it is not life-threatening or considered an allergy. The condition has been linked to different causes, including a general decline in levels of lactase enzyme as a person ages and lactase deficiency, which can occur as a result of diseases that affect the lining of the intestines, such as celiac disease, or chemotherapy treatments.

People with lactose intolerance can sometimes tolerate small amounts of lactose in their diet; specifically, many people can consume aged cheeses and yogurt products, which tend to have lower levels of lactose than milk, but this may vary. Kefir and yogurt contain bacteria cultures that ferment, or break down, the lactose naturally present in dairy to produce lactic acid. As a result, kefir and yogurt contain relatively little lactose, so these products are generally well tolerated by people with lactose intolerance.

SUBSTITUTIONS TO REDUCE OR ELIMINATE LACTOSE

Foods with lactose	Use
Milk products including milk, buttermilk, heavy cream, half-and-half, sour cream, evaporated and condensed milk, dry milk powder, whey powder	Lactose-free milk
	Plant-based milks, including soy, almond, rice, hemp, and oat milk
	Nondairy or soy milk creamer
	Plant-based sour cream
	Plant-based protein powder
	Pureed silken tofu
	Plant-based yogurt
	Yogurt (usually well-tolerated)
	Kefir
Fats	Butter and margarine are usually tolerated since they contain no or trace amounts of lactose; if unsure of sensitivity, use:
	• ghee instead of butter (contains no lactose)
	• vegetable oil or plant-based butter (vegan or nondairy butter)
Fresh, soft cheeses (which contain higher levels of lactose): ricotta, cottage, mozzarella, and burrata cheese	Aged cheeses, including Parmesan, Grana Padano, Manchego, and aged cheddar
	Lactose-free cottage cheese
Ice cream	Lactose-free ice cream
Sherbet	Sorbet
Packaged food products that likely contain milk ingredients, including pancake and waffle mixes; hot chocolate mixes; and prepared mashed potatoes	Homemade versions of each made with lactose-free or plant-based milk

Developing Recipes for People With Lactose Intolerance

The FDA does not provide a definition for "lactose free" or "lactose reduced" on food labels, but manufacturers must provide truthful information on their labels regarding the presence of lactose or if it has been reduced. Sources of lactose can be found on ingredient labels by searching for any milk ingredients.

Read labels carefully and avoid milk and products that contain milk, which include:

- buttermilk
- cream
- milk
- milk solids
- milk powder
- malted milk
- nonfat dry milk
- lactose or lactose monohydrate
- whey
- whey solids (and curds)

The following ingredients **do not** contain lactose:

- casein
- lactilol (a sugar substitute)
- lactate (lactic acid)
- lactic acid
- milk protein

LACTOSE CONTENT OF COMMON FOODS

Food	Serving size	Lactose (grams)
Milk (nonfat, 1%, 2%, whole)	1 cup	11–13
Chocolate milk	1 cup	11
Goat milk	1 cup	10–12
Buttermilk	1 cup	9
Cream, light	½ cup	4
Half-and-half	½ cup	5
Evaporated milk	½ cup	25
Condensed milk (sweetened)	½ cup	15
Kefir	1 cup	No conclusive amount. The longer the fermentation process lasts, the less lactose remains.
Ice cream	½ cup	6
Sherbet	1 cup	4–6
Yogurt	6 ounces	5–10*
Greek yogurt	6 ounces	4
Sour cream	¼ cup	2
Cream cheese	1½ ounces	1.5
Cottage cheese (2%)	½ cup	3
Cheese, hard	1 ounce	0–2
Mozzarella cheese	1 ounce	Less than 1
Parmesan cheese	1½ ounces	0
Whipped cream topping	2 tablespoons	Less than 0.5
Butter or margarine	1 teaspoon	Trace

* Live and active cultures in yogurt help break down lactose. Greek yogurt contains less lactose than regular yogurt since the watery part of the yogurt (the whey) has been strained out in processing, thus removing much of the lactose.

Adapted from *Health Professional's Guide to Food Allergies and Intolerances* by Janice M. Vickerstaff Joneja. 2013. Academy of Nutrition and Dietetics.

Sulfite Sensitivity

Sulfite additives are used widely in the food industry as preservatives. They help prevent spoilage, browning, and discoloration in foods and beverages during preparation, storage, and distribution. People who are sensitive to sulfite additives may experience a range of symptoms after exposure; respiratory symptoms are the most common type. In fact, sulfites can trigger an asthma attack in people who have both a sulfite sensitivity and asthma.

Most people with sulfite sensitivity only experience reactions when they consume foods and drinks to which sulfites have been added, but some highly sensitive individuals may also react to the sulfites that naturally occur in such foods as eggs, fermented foods, asparagus, arugula, salmon, dried cod, onions, garlic, cornstarch, and maple syrup.

Developing Recipes for People With a Sulfite Sensitivity

Check the ingredient list carefully to avoid using products that contain the following sulfiting agents: sulfur dioxide, potassium bisulfite, potassium metabisulfite, sodium bisulfite, sodium metabisulfite, and sodium sulfite. Other tips include the following:

- Look for a "contains sulfites" statement on food and beverage labels. The FDA requires food manufacturers and processors to disclose the presence of sulfiting agents if the product has a concentration of 10 or more parts per million (ppm), regardless of whether the sulfites are components of an ingredient in the food or are used during processing. This typically occurs when sulfites are added, and the specific name of the sulfite must be declared.

- Be aware that sulfites may be added to products that you might not expect (e.g., dried fruits, dried soup mixes, bottled lemon juice, bottled lime juice, maraschino cherries, canned coconut milk, sriracha sauce, chili paste).

- Fermented products like pickles, relishes, sauerkraut, pickled cocktail onions, and malt, cider, and wine vinegars often contain sulfites and may be labeled as such. Sulfites are a natural by-product of the fermentation process of yeast in these foods. Foods that naturally contain sulfites at levels below 10 ppm are not required to be labeled as containing sulfites.

- In wine, sulfites develop naturally during the fermentation process (in very small amounts); more sulfites are sometimes added to preserve and stabilize the wine. Wines that contain 10 ppm or more of sulfite must be labeled with a "contains sulfites" warning.

- US Department of Agriculture (USDA) Certified Organic varieties of foods never contain added sulfites. Many light-colored dried fruits that are conventionally grown, including golden raisins, dried apricots, dried apples, and dried pears, are treated with sulfites to maintain their light color and prevent darkening. If you choose organic versions of these light-colored fruits, they will not contain sulfites. However, be aware that some foods and beverages, including some wines and vinegars, may still contain naturally occurring sulfites.

ADDITIONAL TRIGGERING FOODS OR INGREDIENTS THAT MAY CAUSE ADVERSE REACTIONS

Fresh fruits and **vegetables** (e.g., apples, carrots, peaches, plums, tomatoes, bananas) have been known to cause allergic reactions in some individuals who are allergic to pollen. This cross-reaction that mainly occurs in the oral cavity (lips and mouth) after consuming trigger foods in their raw form is known as oral allergy syndrome (OAS).

Seeds including sunflower and poppy seeds and **spices** like mustard, coriander, and garlic have been known to cause allergic reactions.

Recipe Development Resources for Food Allergies and Intolerances

In addition to the Recipe Development Resources listed in Chapters 1 to 3, consult these websites when developing recipes for people with food allergies, intolerances, and sensitivities.

Allergic Living:
allergicliving.com

American Academy of Allergy, Asthma & Immunology:
aaaai.org/Conditions-Treatments/Allergies

American College of Allergy, Asthma and Immunology:
acaai.org/allergies/types/food-allergies/types-food-allergy

Food Allergy Research & Education (FARE):
foodallergy.org

Kids with Food Allergies (Asthma and Allergy Foundation of America):
kidswithfoodallergies.org

Bibliography

Draft guidance for industry: voluntary disclosure of sesame as an allergen. US Food & Drug Administration website. November 2020. Accessed June 30, 2021. fda.gov/regulatory -information/search-fda-guidance-documents/draft-guidance-industry-voluntary-disclosure -sesame-allergen

Food allergy essentials: common allergens. Food Allergy Research and Education website. Accessed June 30, 2021. foodallergy.org/living-food-allergies/food-allergy-essentials /common-allergens

Food Safety & Inspection Service. Allergens—voluntary labeling statements. US Department of Agriculture website. Accessed June 30, 2021. fsis.usda.gov/guidelines/2013-0010

Food Safety & Inspection Service. Food allergies. USDA website. Accessed June 30, 2021. fsis.usda.gov/food-safety/safe-food-handling-and-preparation/food-safety-basics/food -allergies#11

Sadowski L. Egg replacers: when and how to use. Allergic Living website. Accessed June 30, 2021. allergicliving.com/2016/09/20/egg-replacers-when-and-how-to-use

Sicherer SH. *Food Allergies: A Complete Guide for Eating When Your Life Depends on It.* Baltimore: Johns Hopkins University Press; 2017.

Sulfite sensitivity. The Asthma & Allergy Center website. Accessed June 30, 2021. asthmaandallergycenter.com/article/sulfite-sensitivity

Types of food allergies. American College of Asthma, Allergy, and Immunology website. Accessed June 30, 2021. acaai.org/allergies/types/food-allergies/types-food-allergy

US Food & Drug Administration Food allergies. FDA website. Accessed June 24, 2021. fda.gov/food/food-labeling-nutrition/food-allergies

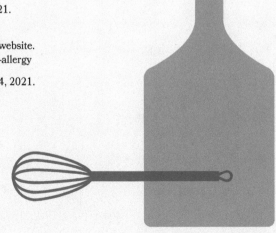

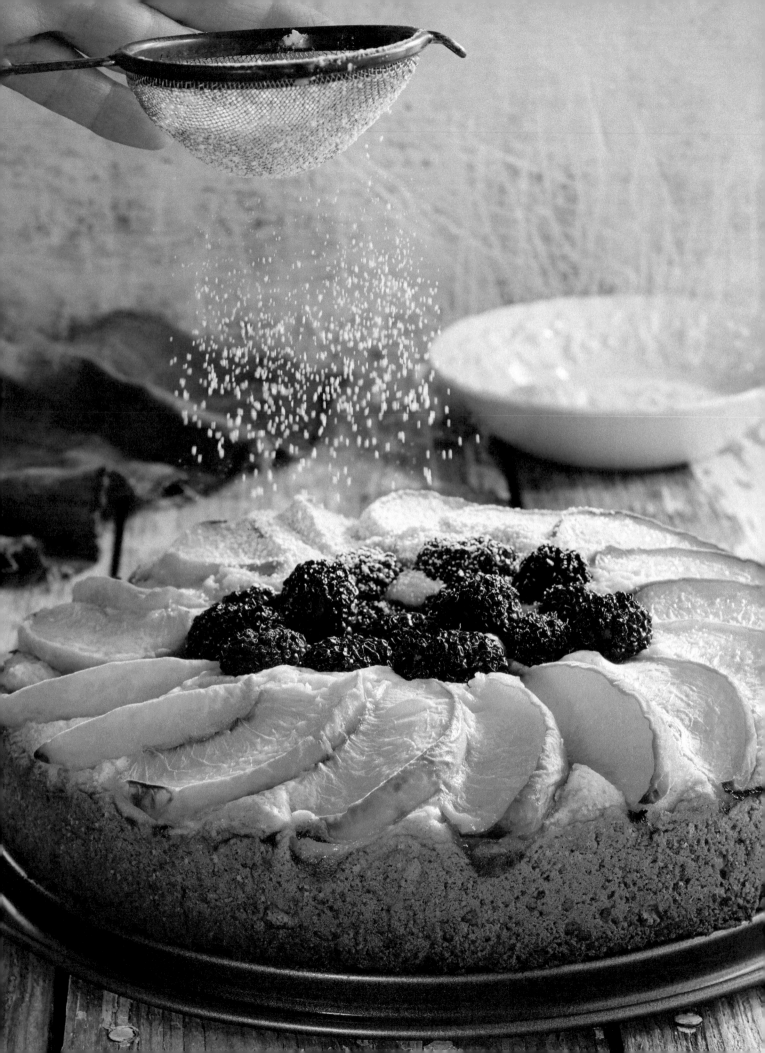

Chapter 6

Developing Gluten-Free and Low FODMAP Recipes

In this chapter, learn about:

- Gluten-free label regulations and how to identify foods and ingredients that contain gluten

- How to choose and use a gluten-free flour to replace all-purpose and other wheat flours in baking and cooking

- The purpose of a low FODMAP diet and how foods are categorized

- Developing recipes for the low FODMAP diet

Recipe development for people with certain medical conditions requires nutrition knowledge, an understanding of the culinary function of the ingredient being modified or eliminated, and kitchen creativity to develop delicious and foolproof recipes that align with the nutrition care guidelines. This chapter focuses on developing recipes for two therapeutic diets that fall in this category: a gluten-free diet for people with celiac disease and non-celiac gluten sensitivity and a low FODMAP diet (low in fermentable oligosaccharides, disaccharides, monosaccharides, and polyols) for people with irritable bowel syndrome or other gastrointestinal symptoms.

Developing Recipes for People With Celiac Disease and Non-Celiac Gluten Sensitivity

There are varying reasons why people might follow a gluten-free diet. But for those with celiac disease or non-celiac gluten-sensitivity, following a gluten-free diet is essential.

Celiac is classified as an autoimmune digestive disease that causes inflammation and severe damage to the small intestine. Non-celiac gluten sensitivity, on the other hand, is classified as a digestive condition or disorder. People with non-celiac gluten sensitivity present with symptoms triggered by gluten consumption, but they do not have celiac-specific antibodies or damage to the lining of small intestine, and they do not have immunoglobulin E (IgE) antibodies to wheat, which is a sign of a wheat allergy.

People with celiac disease and non-celiac gluten sensitivity can experience a range of symptoms after consuming gluten (a protein found in wheat, rye, barley, and sometimes oats)—everything from abdominal bloating and pain to chronic diarrhea. Other non-gastrointestinal symptoms can include skin rashes, mouth ulcers, fatigue, joint pain, and tingling and numbness in the legs. If left untreated, celiac disease can result in serious complications, including vitamin and mineral deficiencies, intestinal damage, cancer, and coronary artery disease. **The primary treatment for both celiac disease and non-celiac gluten sensitivity is to follow a gluten-free diet that eliminates all sources of gluten.**

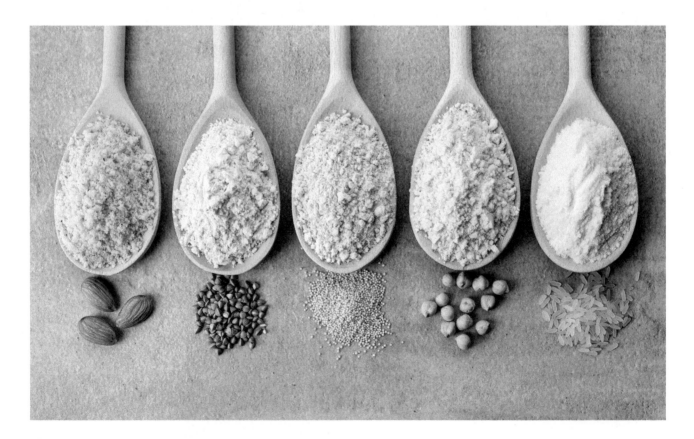

WHERE IS GLUTEN FOUND?

Gluten is a protein found in all forms of wheat, barley, and rye. Below are various forms of wheat, barley, and rye and some common ingredients made from these grains. Do not use any of these products when developing gluten-free recipes. Oats are naturally gluten-free; however, oats grown, harvested, milled, and transported near gluten-containing grains may lead to cross contamination of the oats. Look for oats labeled gluten-free.

Wheat

- Any variety of wheat: common wheat, durum wheat, club wheat; other types include einkorn and emmer
- Wheat flour: all-purpose, bread, cake, durum, unbleached, bleached, graham, 00 flour, pastry, self-rising, and whole wheat
- Wheat germ, wheat germ oil, wheat bran
- Triticale wheat (bran, durum, germ, gluten, malt, sprouts, starch)
- Wheat berries (whole wheat kernel)
- Wheat sprouts, sprouted wheat

Common wheat-containing foods and condiments:

- Bulgur (cracked whole grain wheat berries)
- Couscous (rolled durum wheat semolina)
- Farina (a form of milled wheat)
- Farro (an ancient wheat grain from the plants spelt, emmer, and einkorn)
- Freekeh (durum wheat that is roasted and crushed)
- Kamut (from Khorasan wheat)
- Maggi seasoning (made from fermented wheat protein)
- Matzo, matzo meal (made with wheat flour)
- Noodles, pasta (made with wheat flour)
- Panko breadcrumbs or cracker meal (made with wheat flour)
- Seitan (wheat protein—used as a meat substitute)
- Soy sauce (made from soybeans, wheat, salt, and water)
- Spelt (species of wheat)
- Surimi (imitation crab, most contain wheat)
- Udon noodles (made with wheat flour)

Common wheat-containing ingredients:

- Cereal extract—made from wheat
- Gluten, wheat gluten, vital gluten, vital wheat gluten, fu (Japanese solidified wheat gluten)
- Hydrolyzed wheat protein
- Wheat bran hydrolysate
- Wheat protein isolate

Barley

- Whole grain or pearled barley
- Barley flour or malted barley flour

Common barley-containing beverages, foods, and condiments:

- Beer, ale, porter, stout (made with barley; some contain wheat)
- Brewer's yeast (made from barley)
- Marmite, Vegemite (paste made from brewer's yeast extract)
- Malt vinegar (made from barley)

Common barley-containing ingredients:

- Autolyzed yeast extract
- Cereal extract—made from barley
- Hydrolyzed barley protein
- Malt, malt flavoring, malt syrup, malt extract
- Yeast extract

Rye

- Rye berries, including cracked rye and rye flakes
- Rye flour (all types of rye flours, rye meal, pumpernickel)
- Triticale (a cross between wheat and rye)

Understanding Gluten-Free Labeling

When developing gluten-free recipes, choose products that are labeled gluten-free or that have third-party gluten-free certification logos on their labels. These identifications are voluntary, so if a product does not have a claim or certification on its label, it may still be gluten-free. Always read the ingredient list to verify. See Do These Ingredients Contain Gluten? on page 156 for the gluten status of common ingredients.

Because wheat is considered an allergen under the Food Allergen Labeling and Consumer Protection Act (FALCPA), food products regulated by the FDA that contain wheat must carry a "contains wheat" warning statement or must include the word "wheat" in the ingredient list. However, a food that is labeled "wheat-free" may not be gluten-free because the product may contain barley or rye. There is no FDA "Contains" statement for barley, rye, or gluten, so carefully check the ingredient list for these three ingredients and other ingredients derived from these grains.

Regulation of Gluten-Free Label Claims

There are two FDA rules that help ensure products labeled "gluten-free" are truly free of gluten: the Gluten-Free Labeling of Foods rule of 2013 and the Gluten-Free Labeling of Fermented and Hydrolyzed Foods rule of 2020.

The Gluten-Free Labeling of Foods rule states that if a manufacturer labels their product "gluten-free" it must contain fewer than 20 parts per million (ppm) of gluten in the final product. Whether a food is manufactured to be free of gluten or by nature is free of gluten, it may bear a gluten-free labeling claim, giving the consumer the expectation that if any gluten is present, it is present at less than 20 ppm in the final product.

The rule on Gluten-Free Labeling of Fermented and Hydrolyzed Foods establishes additional compliance requirements to limit consumer confusion when reading an ingredient list on a food product labeled "gluten-free" for fermented and hydrolyzed foods or foods that contain fermented or hydrolyzed ingredients. Beer is an example of a fermented food and hydrolyzed wheat protein is an example of a hydrolyzed ingredient. Hydrolysis refers to the way a protein is broken down. Hydrolyzed proteins, including wheat and barley, are used to improve flavor or texture in processed foods such as soups, sauces, and seasonings.

Under this rule, any manufacturer can use the "gluten-free" claim on a product if their records document the product is gluten-free in compliance with the 2013 labeling rule and is free of wheat and barley fermented or hydrolyzed ingredients. The FDA added this safeguard since there is no scientifically valid testing method effective in detecting and quantifying the equivalent of 20 ppm intact gluten for foods containing fermented or hydrolyzed ingredients.

FOOD PRODUCTS THAT MAY CONTAIN "HIDDEN" GLUTEN

Closely read the ingredient labels on the following products when using them in recipe development:

- Cereals like cornflakes and rice puffs (often contain malt extract/flavoring)
- Soups and premade sauces
- Foods with added sauces, marinades, seasonings, and flavorings
- Seasoning mixes, spice mixes, and flavoring enhancers (e.g., Maggi seasoning, bouillon containing autolyzed yeast protein [barley])
- Condiments, such as salad dressings and BBQ sauce
- Processed lunch meat and self-basting turkey (seasonings and binders may contain gluten)
- Meat substitutes (many contain not only wheat but other allergens such as soy and tree nuts)
- Surimi (imitation crab): most contain wheat
- Candies, such as licorice (made using wheat flour) and certain candy bars; check the brand's website or product labels

When using imported food products in recipes, read the ingredient label carefully for possible gluten-containing ingredients or look for the gluten-free label claim. According to the FDA, products imported from other countries into the United States must meet the same FDA "gluten-free" labeling requirements as domestically produced products.

Gluten-Free Label Certifications

Some manufacturers may choose to pursue an independent third-party certification for their gluten-free food products so consumers can more quickly and easily identify the product as safe. Certification includes submission of a full ingredient list and list of suppliers to ensure no cross-contamination prior to the ingredients arriving at the facility and confirm manufacturing practices meet certification requirements too. The largest third-party certifications include:

- Gluten-Free Certification Organization (GFCO)

- Gluten-Free Certification Program (GFCP) endorsed by Beyond Celiac organization

- Gluten-Free Food Program (GF) endorsed by the National Celiac Association and Canadian Celiac Association

- National Sanitation Foundation International (NSF)

The certification testing process ensures that the product contains less than the FDA's gluten-free label claim requirement of 20 parts per million (ppm) of gluten. Some certifications follow more strict gluten standards, limiting the presence of gluten to less than 10 ppm (GFCO) or 5 ppm (GF).

Quick Tip

"The FDA's gluten-free labeling rule does not cover foods regulated by the USDA [US Department of Agriculture]. But (and this is important), the USDA has shared that while they are not planning to define gluten-free under USDA rules, a manufacturer under their jurisdiction who labels a food gluten-free must comply with FDA rules. In addition (and this is more than what is required by FDA), if a food regulated by the USDA includes a gluten-free claim, the label of that food must be preapproved by the USDA." —Tricia Thompson, founder, Gluten Free Watchdog, LLC

Quick Tip

"Many certified gluten-free products, particularly those made in Europe, contain the ingredient gluten-free wheat starch. Though it seems counterintuitive, there is no evidence showing that foods made with gluten-removed wheat starch are harmful to people with celiac disease. Gluten-free wheat starch improves the flavor and texture of gluten-free products. It is made by removing the endosperm from the wheat grain, dissolving the water-soluble starch in water, and then evaporating the water to create a fine, powdery starch. To make sure the wheat starch is truly gluten-free, it goes through multiple rounds of testing using the ELISA method (a validation testing method for presence of gluten). For example, Schär has been using this ingredient in certain products for nearly 20 years, and more than 90% of the wheat starch used has tested below 5 ppm." —Meghan Donnelly, MS, RDN, Nutrition Service Manager, Dr. Schär USA

DO THESE INGREDIENTS CONTAIN GLUTEN?

Many gluten-free food products do not carry a gluten-free label claim but actually may be gluten-free, so always read the ingredient list. The following are ingredients that can be confusing to determine if they are gluten-free or not.

Ingredient	Gluten status	Notes
Artificial flavors	Gluten-free	These chemical compounds or mixtures of compounds mimic natural flavors.
Natural flavors	Gluten-free (most likely)	Derived from many different sources of plants or animals, their function is to flavor foods. Double-check ingredient list and any "**contains**" warning statements to ensure no wheat, barley, rye, or malt is listed.
Caramel coloring and color additives	Gluten-free	Caramel coloring is most often made from cornstarch and blended with chemical compounds. Color additives are derived from chemicals and dyes.
Monosodium glutamate (MSG)	Gluten-free	Used as a flavor enhancer, MSG is the sodium salt of the amino acid, glutamic acid. Glutamic acid is produced through the fermentation of starch found in ingredients like sugar beets, sugar cane, cassava, or molasses.
Maltodextrin	Gluten-free	Maltodextrin is typically made from cornstarch, making it naturally gluten-free. If wheat or barley is listed as the source of maltodextrin, it is unlikely to contain 20 ppm (or more) gluten.
Modified food starch	Gluten-free	Modified food starch is most often made from cornstarch. If it is made from another starch, such as wheat, it must be described as such in the ingredient list, in a "contains" warning statement, or both.
Cornstarch	Gluten-free	Any ingredient labeled as *starch* in an US Food and Drug Administration (FDA)–regulated product is cornstarch, but anything labeled "starch" in a US Department of Agriculture (USDA)–regulated product could be cornstarch or wheat starch.
Wheat starch	Gluten-free	Wheat starch is permitted in foods labeled gluten-free because gluten is removed when wheat starch is processed; the final food product must contain no more than 20 ppm of gluten to comply with the FDA rule for gluten-free. If a product contains wheat starch, look for the gluten-free label claim for extra assurance.
Glucose syrup	Gluten-free	Glucose syrup is usually made from cornstarch, but it can also be made from potato or wheat starch. Regardless of the starting material, glucose syrup is considered gluten-free since it is highly processed to remove all proteins, including gluten.
Rice or brown rice syrup	Gluten-free	Rice and brown rice syrups are made by adding enzymes to rice to break down its starch into sugar. These enzymes may be derived from barley, but if they contain less than 5 ppm of gluten, as they normally do, they are considered gluten-free; look for a gluten-free label.
Wheat grass and barley grass	Gluten-free	Freshly sprouted young grasses of wheat and barley plants are gluten-free as long as they are 100% free of any cross contamination from the wheat and barley grains they produce at maturity. The FDA allows wheat or barley grass (or grass juice) to be labeled gluten-free if they contain less than 20 ppm of gluten; make sure any product used in recipe development is labeled as gluten-free.

BOX CONTINUES >

Ingredient	Gluten status	Notes
Malt	Contains gluten	This flavoring agent is usually made from barley and may be listed among ingredients as malt, malt flavoring, malt extract, malt vinegar, or malt syrup. The word "malt" in an ingredient list means "barley malt" unless another source is named. Malted milk powder is an evaporated powder made from malted barley, wheat flour, and whole milk.
Hydrolyzed protein ingredients		
Hydrolyzed soy protein and hydrolyzed milk protein	Gluten-free	These ingredients are used as flavor enhancers made from a plant source, such as soy, wheat, or barley, or from an animal source, such as milk. The FDA requires the source to be identified on the label (e.g., hydrolyzed soy protein).
Hydrolyzed wheat protein and hydrolyzed barley protein	May contain gluten	Products containing hydrolyzed wheat protein or hydrolyzed barley protein cannot be labeled gluten-free, regardless of the gluten level found during testing.
Yeast ingredients		
Nutritional yeast	Gluten-free	Made from *Saccharomyces cerevisiae* yeast, nutritional yeast is typically grown on molasses from sugar beets or cane.
Active dry yeast and instant yeast	Gluten-free	Active dry and instant yeasts are commonly used to bake breads.
Autolyzed yeast	Gluten-free	Also known as baker's yeast, this food additive is used to improve flavor and nutritional value of many food and bakery products.
Brewer's yeast	Most contain gluten	Brewer's yeast is the same yeast species as nutritional yeast, but most brewer's yeasts are not gluten-free as they are a by-product of beer production and therefore contain barley malt. Some brands produced with sugar beets are gluten-free, so check labels carefully.
Yeast extract and autolyzed yeast extract (not the same ingredient as autolyzed yeast)	May contain gluten	These extracts made from spent yeast (a by-product of the beer production process) or sugar beets are used as flavoring agents in a variety of food products.
		Avoid using products that contain yeast extract or autolyzed yeast extract unless labeled as gluten-free. If a food product, such as bouillon cubes, lists "yeast extract" or "autolyzed yeast extract" as an ingredient without listing its source—e.g., "autolyzed yeast extract (barley)"—contact the manufacturer to ask for the source or look for a product that is labeled gluten-free.
		Marmite and Vegemite are brands of yeast extract food products that contain gluten. They are used as a spread or ingredient in cooking to add a savory umami flavor. (Vegemite offers a gluten-free version made from baker's yeast grown on molasses).

Important: *Foods regulated by USDA, which include meat, poultry, and egg products, that carry a gluten-free label claim must follow FDA's gluten labeling guidelines. If a USDA-regulated product is not labeled gluten-free, always check for the ingredients dextrin and starch in the ingredient list, and call the manufacturer to determine the grain source since these may not be identified.*

Gluten in Alcoholic Beverages

The Alcohol and Tobacco Tax and Trade Bureau (TTB) governs voluntary gluten content statements on labels of wines, distilled spirits, fermented ciders, and many malt beverages (e.g., traditional beers made with both barley and hops). However, some wines containing less than 7% alcohol by volume, hard seltzers, and beers that do not meet the definition of a "malt beverage" are regulated by the FDA, which generally requires products to include Nutrition Facts labels and ingredient statements.

Alcoholic beverages that are gluten-free include:

- **unflavored hard liquor** (also referred to as distilled spirits) including brandy, gin, rum, tequila, vodka, and whiskey. Even if wheat, barley, or rye is used to make the distillate, all gluten is removed during the distillation process.

- **fortified wines** (e.g., Marsala, Madeira, vermouth, port, sherry). These grape-based wines have extra alcohol added in the form of a flavorless grape brandy.

- **red, white, and sparkling wines**. Wine is predominantly made from grapes, and the fermentation process does not include gluten.

- **hard ciders**. These beverages are made from naturally gluten-free fruits (typically apples).

- **gluten-free beers**. Only beers made with these ingredients are gluten-free: millet malt, buckwheat malt, malted rice, chestnuts, and lentils; hops (flowers of the hop plant are naturally gluten-free); gluten-free yeast grown in a gluten-free environment. Some gluten-free beers are produced in a dedicated gluten-free brewery for additional safety. Look for the terms "gluten-free" or "certified gluten-free" on the label.

Alcoholic beverages that may contain gluten include:

- **flavored hard liquor** that has flavoring ingredients added after distillation, as these may contain gluten. Look for the terms "gluten-free" or "certified gluten-free" on the label.

- **"gluten-reduced" or "gluten removed" beer**. These beers contain barley, wheat, or rye ingredients but undergo a process of enzymatic removal of gluten. They cannot be marketed as gluten-free because the FDA has ruled that there is no valid method for testing and evaluating the gluten content of beer or other fermented products.

Alcoholic beverages that contain gluten include:

- **regular beer made with barley, rye, or wheat** (gluten containing grains). When beer is brewed, no distillation takes place, so the gluten protein remains.

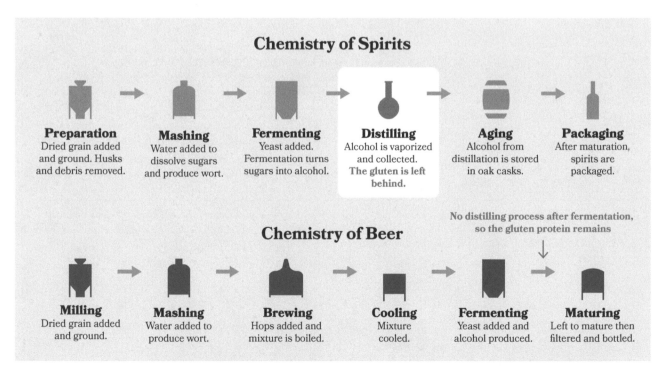

Chemistry of Spirits

Preparation
Dried grain added and ground. Husks and debris removed.

Mashing
Water added to dissolve sugars and produce wort.

Fermenting
Yeast added. Fermentation turns sugars into alcohol.

Distilling
Alcohol is vaporized and collected. **The gluten is left behind.**

Aging
Alcohol from distillation is stored in oak casks.

Packaging
After maturation, spirits are packaged.

Chemistry of Beer

No distilling process after fermentation, so the gluten protein remains

Milling
Dried grain added and ground.

Mashing
Water added to produce wort.

Brewing
Hops added and mixture is boiled.

Cooling
Mixture cooled.

Fermenting
Yeast added and alcohol produced.

Maturing
Left to mature then filtered and bottled.

Gluten-Free Recipe Development

Developing gluten-free recipes is more straightforward than it may seem—especially since there are many foods that are *naturally* gluten-free, and many gluten-free products are readily available at the grocery store. Recipe developers should follow these steps:

1. Use naturally gluten-free foods whenever possible (see Naturally Gluten-Free Foods, Gluten-Free Substitutions for Savory Recipes on page 160, and Gluten-Free Flours and Starches for Baking Recipes on page 165).

2. Use food products that are labeled gluten-free or have a gluten-free certification logo. Specify the brand if necessary.

3. On other products, always read the ingredient list to ensure that no wheat, barley, or rye or their derivatives (e.g., barley malt) are listed. Do not use products with label warnings that state "Contains wheat."

4. If unclear about any ingredients or if verification is needed, call the manufacturer, or visit their website.

Quick Tip

"While gluten-free grains do not inherently contain any gluten, some are grown, harvested, and processed in a facility that also manufactures wheat, increasing the risk for cross contact. It's safest to call for ingredients labeled or certified as gluten-free when writing gluten-free recipes." —Lori Welstead, MS, RDN, University of Chicago, Adult Outpatient GI Dietitian at University of Chicago, Nutrition Advisor for the Celiac Disease Center

NATURALLY GLUTEN-FREE FOODS

Fruits

Vegetables

Dairy products

Eggs

Fish and seafood

Meat and poultry

Tofu

Beans (e.g., black, kidney, navy, pinto, adzuki, fava, garbanzo beans/chickpeas, soybeans)

Lentils, black-eyed peas, and peas*

Nuts (e.g., peanuts, almonds, walnuts, pecans, pistachios)

Seeds (e.g., chia, sesame, flax)

All oils

Vinegars (e.g., apple cider, balsamic, red wine, sherry, rice)

Gluten-free grains and noodles
- Amaranth
- Buckwheat (kasha)
- Cornmeal and polenta
- Millet
- Oats and oat groats that are labeled gluten-free**
- Quinoa
- Rice: arborio, basmati, black, brown, jasmine, white, wild
- Rice noodles
- Soba noodles *(choose 100% buckwheat varieties; read the label carefully, as many contain added wheat)*
- Sorghum
- Teff

* When creating recipes that use legumes of any kind—especially lentils—include instructions to sort through and rinse them thoroughly. Sometimes, errant wheat and barley grains can end up in bags of lentils.

** Oats are inherently gluten-free but may be processed in facilities that also process wheat. This can lead to possible cross-contamination at manufacturing facilities.

GLUTEN-FREE SUBSTITUTIONS FOR SAVORY RECIPES

Understanding how wheat flour or other gluten-containing ingredients function in a recipe will help you decide how to modify and make substitutions.

Instead of	Use
Wheat flour (for thickening a pan sauce or making a gravy or stew)	Substitute in a 1:1 ratio: • sweet rice flour, also known as glutinous rice flour (used more like a starch, preferable when making a roux for gravy and sauces) • arrowroot • potato starch • tapioca starch • store-bought gluten-free flour blend Cornstarch (use half the amount of cornstarch as flour; 1 tablespoon cornstarch = 2 tablespoons flour). If thickening a hot liquid, first whisk the cornstarch with a little cold water until it becomes a smooth slurry and then stir the slurry into the hot liquid.
Wheat flour (for dusting with flour alone and in the process of breading)	Cornstarch Rice flour Sweet rice flour
Breadcrumbs	Store-bought gluten-free breadcrumbs Homemade gluten-free bread, dried in oven, ground to a crumb; alone or mixed with a little cornstarch Cornmeal Potato flakes Gluten-free oats (for meat loaf or meatballs) For a crunchy topping or breading, use: • chickpea crumbs • crushed cornflakes or puffed rice cereal (check to ensure there are no malt ingredients) • rice cakes processed to a fine or coarse crumb
Matzo	Gluten-free matzo
Wheat grains (bulgur, couscous, farina, freekeh, Kamut, spelt, and wheatberries)	Amaranth (whole grain) Buckwheat groats (whole grain) Cornmeal and polenta Millet (whole grain) Oat groats (whole grain) Quinoa (whole grain) Rice: wild, brown, black, and purple (whole grain); white, basmati, jasmine, arborio Sorghum (whole grain) Teff (whole grain) Note: It is safest to use oats labeled gluten-free since there can be contamination with gluten-containing grains during seeding, growing, harvest, storage, transport, and milling. Some companies follow a "purity protocol" to produce safe gluten-free oats.

BOX CONTINUES >

Instead of	Use
Pasta	Gluten-free pasta (note: only cook gluten-free pasta until al dente, as it gets mushy quickly if it's overcooked; toss immediately with a bit of oil or sauce to prevent pasta from sticking or rinse under cold water to stop the cooking process and then toss with sauce)
	Pulse-based pasta (made from peas, lentils, chickpeas)
Chow mein, lo mein, or udon noodles	Glass or cellophane noodles (made from mung beans)
	Rice noodles
	Soba noodles (choose 100% buckwheat varieties; read the label as many soba noodles have wheat added)
Asian ingredients/condiments, including: • hoisin sauce/sweet bean sauce • oyster sauce • soy (light, dark, and black) • teriyaki sauce • pot sticker and gyoza wrapper	Coconut aminos (made from the sap of the coconut palm) Coconut aminos teriyaki sauce Gluten-free hoisin sauce Gluten-free oyster sauce Gluten-free soy sauce Gluten-free teriyaki sauce Liquid aminos (made from soybeans) Tamari (a Japanese sauce primarily made from soybeans; check label) Other naturally gluten-free Asian ingredients, such as: • fish sauce (brands include Red Boat, Thai Kitchen) • gochujang, sriracha, sambal oelek, chili paste, chili garlic sauce • mirin or rice wine vinegar (naturally gluten-free when produced only with rice) • miso (read the ingredient label to ensure no barley is used) • monosodium glutamate (MSG) • rice paper or rice wrappers (for egg or spring rolls) • tamarind paste • Thai curry paste (red, green, yellow) Note: Always read the ingredient list to ensure the product contains no wheat or barley, especially with imported products. Do not use products that include "hydrolyzed vegetable protein (HVP)" or "hydrolyzed protein" in the ingredient list because the source of the protein is not identified and may be made from wheat. Some imported rice vinegars may contain a mix of rice and other grains, such as wheat or malt (barley).
Shaoxing wine (a type of wine from Shaoxing, China, made by fermenting rice, water, and a small amount of wheat)	Chinese rice wine (e.g., mijiu, michiu) Korean rice wine (e.g., Cheongju), for cooking Premium sake (a Japanese rice wine) clearly identified as premium on the label; types include junmai (meaning pure rice), honjozo, ginjo, daiginjo, tokubetsu junmai, tokubetsu honjozo, junmai ginjo, and junmai daiginjo (e.g., TYKU) Pale dry sherry Gluten-free stock: chicken, vegetable, or meat
Fermented black bean paste (often has wheat added)	Fermented black beans (black soybeans fermented with salt) can be used to make a gluten-free black bean paste or sauce (see recipe on page 163).
Dashi powder (contains hydrolyzed wheat protein)	Make homemade dashi with dried kombu (kelp) and bonito (dried bonito fish flakes).

BOX CONTINUES >

Instead of	Use
Packaged products, such as: • bouillon cubes (may contain hydrolyzed wheat or barley) • Marmite (barley) • Vegemite (wheat and barley) • Maggi seasoning • licorice (made with wheat flour) • Rice Krispies (contains malt syrup)	Homemade or canned broth (check label) Roasted chicken, beef, or veal stock or base (brands include: Gourmet Glace De Poulet Gold, More than Gourmet Roasted Chicken Demi-Glace, and Better Than Bouillon) Ketchup Mustard Mayonnaise Worcestershire sauce (Lea & Perrins brand is gluten-free; check labels of other brands) Tabasco, and most other hot sauces Harissa Gluten-free Vegemite Gravy Master, Kitchen Bouquet Gluten-free licorice and gummies (check the manufacturer's website) Gluten-free puffed rice (check label) For other gluten-free products: Look for a gluten-free claim on the label. Remember that many products are gluten-free but aren't labeled as such, but always read the ingredient list carefully to ensure it doesn't include wheat, barley, rye, malt, brewer's yeast, or yeast extract as an ingredient.
Malt vinegar (from malted barley) **Black vinegar** (often contains wheat bran)	Any other vinegar (e.g., distilled white, apple cider, white wine, red wine, balsamic, sherry wine, rice)

Quick Tip

"Rice flour is a versatile fine-textured, neutral flour used in gluten-free baking and cooking—whether for breading, for thickening sauces and gravies, or for gluten-free baked products. White rice flour is ground from long- or medium-grain rice. Sweet white rice flour is made from high-starch, short-grain glutinous rice, aka 'sticky rice.' It is not sweet, and it does not contain gluten, despite the 'glutinous' and 'sweet' descriptors. Due to its higher starch content, sweet rice flour is a more efficient thickener for sauces and gravies, and when used in baking, [it] has a more sticky and chewy texture." —Denise Herrera, VP Food & Beverage, Burtons Grill & Bar

WHAT IS MALT?

Malt is a name given to grains (typically barley) that go through a malting process in which they are dried, allowed to sprout, dried a second time, and then often ground into a powder.

Malt is added to a variety of foods and beverages to provide sweetness, flavor, and color in many different forms—everything from malt vinegar to malted milk powder. It's safe to assume that the single word "malt" in an ingredient list is intended to mean barley malt unless another source is named.

Recipe Example: Making a homemade gluten-free sauce

Black bean sauce is the "secret ingredient" in many of the best Chinese recipes, but unfortunately, store-bought versions of Asian fermented black bean sauce or paste usually contain wheat. This homemade version uses preserved black beans—an umami ingredient made of black beans and salt—along with gluten-free soy sauce and dry sherry (instead of the gluten-containing Shaoxing wine). If you prefer a smoother sauce or paste, puree with an immersion or regular blender.

Black Bean Sauce

By Cinde Little, gluten-free health educator and founder of everydayglutenfreegourmet.ca

Preparation time: 10 minutes
Cooking time: 5 minutes
Yield: about ¾ cup (1 tablespoon per serving)

¼ cup chicken stock
2 tablespoons dry sherry or sherry wine
1 tablespoon gluten-free soy sauce
1½ teaspoons cornstarch
1 teaspoon sugar
2 tablespoons vegetable oil
2 tablespoons preserved Chinese black beans, drained, rinsed, and chopped
4 cloves garlic, minced (about 2 tablespoons)

1. Whisk together the stock, sherry, soy sauce, cornstarch, and sugar in a liquid measuring cup.

2. Heat the oil in a saucepan over medium-high heat until hot. Add the black beans and garlic and cook, stirring, for about 30 seconds. Add the stock mixture and cook, stirring continuously, until the sauce thickens, 2 to 4 minutes. Remove from the heat and allow to cool.

3. Pour into jar and label it. Store in the refrigerator for 3 to 4 months. Make sure you use a clean utensil each time you dip into jar.

Nutrition per 1-tablespoon serving: 112 calories, 2.5 grams fat, 0 grams saturated fat, 92 milligrams sodium, 8 grams carbohydrate, 2.5 grams fiber, 0 grams total sugar, 1 gram protein

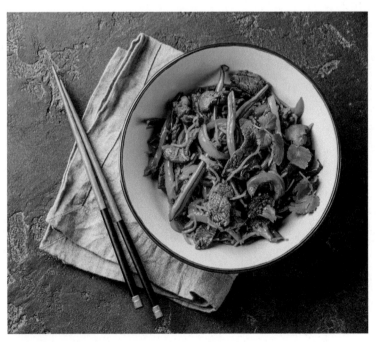

Beef with black bean sauce

Gluten-Free Baking

There are no straightforward rules in gluten-free baking, as the choices of ingredients and amounts used are dependent on the type of baked good recipe being developed. In gluten-free baking, many classic baking techniques are not relevant or necessary—for example, there is no need to instruct how to limit gluten development (in cakes, cookies, and muffins) or encourage gluten development (in breads and pastries).

Using gluten-free flour in baking requires rethinking ingredients completely, including usage and baking technique. Each gluten-free flour works differently in different types of recipes. The gluten-free baking process is based on trial and error—experiment, analyze your findings, and be a good observer. When developing gluten-free recipes, it's often best to start with a familiar and successful gluten-free recipe and make modifications to it.

Gluten-free baking can be challenging because all-purpose flour (made from a combination of hard and soft wheat) is the base ingredient of almost all baked goods, and it cannot be used in any gluten-free recipe. All-purpose flour contains the proteins glutenin and gliadin, which interact with each other when mixed with water to form gluten. Once it is heated, this elastic gluten framework stretches to allow baked goods the ability to hold a new, larger size and shape, trapping the leavening gases that expand during rising and baking.

Gluten-free flours do not contain gluten-forming proteins and contain less protein overall than wheat flours. As a result, gluten-free flours cannot create the structure and lift needed in baked goods. To compensate for this, in gluten-free baking, binders and leaveners are used to take on some of these functional properties. Binders (e.g., xanthan gum, psyllium husk) help bind together the protein and starch molecules, which give the baked goods the structure they need, and leaveners (e.g., baking powder, baking soda) help with the rise. This is why gluten-free flours need to be used in combination with starches and binders or leaveners.

Quick Tip

"When my students are developing recipes, I always ask them, 'What are you trying to accomplish with this recipe?' It's important to think about ingredient function and flavor when developing recipes. For example, with gluten-free baking, you might notice that using tapioca starch in the flour blend adds a chewy quality to gluten-free pizza doughs, but with gluten-free muffins, the result is less desirable. So, you might try another starch in your flour blend—like potato or corn starch—and discover this modification helps produce a softer and more tender crumb."

—Peter Reinhart, faculty member at Johnson & Wales University and author of many books on bread and baking

Quick Tip

"[For gluten-free baking recipe development,] start with a recipe that you like and that you know works because you've tried it, and then start to experiment from there, changing one ingredient or technique at a time. Starting with a reliable recipe is a great way to create something new and learn at the same time."

—Alice Medrich, pastry chef and James Beard–Award-winning cookbook author

Quick Tip

"There are no general rules or formulas that apply to all gluten-free flours. Don't assume that swapping one gluten-free flour for another will work in a recipe. Gluten-free recipe development involves a lot of experimentation and testing, since the variety of gluten-free flours work differently in different types of recipes." —Alice Medrich, pastry chef and James Beard–Award-winning cookbook author

GLUTEN-FREE FLOURS AND STARCHES FOR BAKING

Flours

A single-ingredient flour will work for some recipes, but a homemade blend made with a combination of gluten-free flours and starches is often more effective; these flours and starches include:

- almond flour
- buckwheat flour
- cassava flour
- chickpea flour
- coconut flour
- corn flour (dried masa)
- flaxseed meal
- millet flour
- nonfat milk powder (used in gluten-free flour blends)
- oat flour
- pea flour
- potato flour
- quinoa flour
- rice flour (white, brown, sweet/glutinous)
- sorghum flour
- soy flour
- teff flour

Or use a commercial gluten-free flour blend, such as:

- Authentic Foods Gluten-Free Classical Blend
- Better Batter
- Bob's Red Mill Gluten-Free All-Purpose Baking Flour
- Cup4Cup Gluten-Free Flour
- Judee's All-Purpose Gluten-Free Bread Flour Mix
- King Arthur Gluten-Free Multipurpose Flour
- Molino Piantoni La Senza Glutine

Starches

Gluten-free starches include:

- arrowroot
- cornstarch
- potato starch
- tapioca starch (made from cassava starch)
- white rice and sweet rice flour (can act as a starch)

Tips for using gluten-free flours

Measure accurately; weigh gluten-free flours instead of measuring them in cups.

Store gluten-free flours in airtight containers in a cool, dark place. Storing them in the refrigerator or freezer keeps them fresh longer.

A superfine grind of flour helps create a lighter and more delicate product.

Most gluten-free commercial flour blends do not work well in yeast breads; consider making your own flour blend.

Test the recipe with a specific gluten-free flour or commercial gluten-free flour blend. They are not all the same. Unlike all-purpose flour, which is entirely made of wheat, gluten-free commercial blends are made with varying amounts and types of flours and may or may not include gluten-free gums. (See Xanthan Gum and Guar Gum in Gluten-Free Baking on page 167).

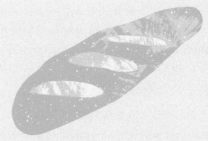

TIPS FOR USING GLUTEN-FREE BINDERS, LEAVENERS, AND FLAVORING EXTRACTS IN BAKING

Binders (eggs, nonfat milk powder, xanthan or guar gum, psyllium husk)

Use a binder to assist with structure and thickening, enhance texture, prevent crumbling, control spread of the batter/dough, and help lock in moisture. A little goes a long way.

Egg
Add an extra egg and whip the eggs into a foam to provide additional structure.

Replace 1 whole egg with 2 egg whites for a bit more added protein, which provides more structure.

Nonfat milk powder
Adding nonfat milk powder (contains lactose) can help with structure, tenderness, and browning.

Xanthan or guar gum
Adding ¼ teaspoon xanthan gum per 1 cup gluten-free flour can help with structure and prevent crumbling.

Do not use xanthan gum if you are using a commercial gluten-free flour blend that already contains xanthan gum; check the ingredient list carefully.

Some professionals suggest using xanthan gum in baked goods and guar gum in cold foods, such as ice cream and dressings.

Psyllium husk
Add 1 tablespoon psyllium husk per 1 cup gluten-free flour, but raise or lower the amount depending on the product; use less for cookies, for example, or more for sandwich breads (based on the outcome desired). Psyllium husk helps mimic the structure of gluten in flour.

Other binder suggestions
Ground chia seed or ground flaxseed; use an equal amount in place of xanthan gum.

Cream cheese helps as a binder since it contains gums.

Leaveners (baking soda, baking powder, baker's yeast, active dry yeast)

Add a little extra baking powder or baking soda to batters for gluten-free cakes, quick breads, and muffins to make them less dense.

Some chefs recommend using 25% more baking soda or baking powder when converting a recipe to gluten-free.

For cookies, it might be necessary to decrease the amount of baking soda to prevent excess spread.

Flavoring extracts (vanilla, almond, lemon, peppermint)

Infuse extra flavor into baked goods without worry. All flavoring extracts contain distilled alcohol, and distilled alcohol is gluten-free.

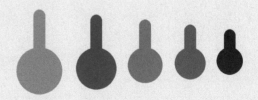

XANTHAN GUM AND GUAR GUM IN GLUTEN-FREE BAKING

Xanthan and guar gums are both powdery white substances that act as binders, stabilizers, thickeners, and emulsifiers. Xanthan gum is produced by taking a carbohydrate, such as glucose or sucrose, and fermenting it with the *Xanthamonas* bacteria, and then grinding it into a fine powder. Guar gum is produced by dehusking, milling, and then finely grinding the seed of the guar plant into a powder.

Why use xanthan and guar gum

These gums are often the secret ingredient in gluten-free baking. Since gluten-free flour and all-purpose wheat flour are not replaced in a 1:1 ratio in recipes, additional ingredients like xanthan gum or guar gum are often required to re-create some of the functions of gluten in wheat flour.

How to use xanthan and guar gum

If the gluten-free flour blend you are using does not contain xanthan gum or guar gum, consider adding some to help solve common problems associated with gluten-free baking, like a crumbly texture or a lack of structure. Not all gluten-free baking recipes require the addition of a gum, so when and if you decide to use one, start with the smallest amount first and increase as needed after testing and tasting each version. In general, 1 teaspoon guar gum = ½ teaspoon xanthan gum.

Type of recipe	For each 1 cup gluten-free flour, add either:	
	Xanthan gum	Guar gum
Cookies	¼ teaspoon	¼ to ½ teaspoon
Cakes	½ teaspoon	¾ teaspoon
Muffins and quick breads	¾ teaspoon	1 teaspoon
Pancakes and waffles	⅛ to ¼ teaspoon	¾ teaspoon
Breads	1 to 1½ teaspoons	1½ to 2 teaspoons
Pizza dough	2 teaspoons	1 tablespoon

Sources: A guide to xanthan gum: the gluten-free baker's secret weapon, by Alyssa Rimmer: kingarthurbaking.com/blog/2015/08/05/xanthan-gum | Guar gum vs. xanthan gum, by Cassidy Stockton: bobsredmill.com/blog/recipes/guar-gum-vs-xanthan-gum

Quick Tip

"Choosing to use gums or not in baked goods will depend on what gluten-free flour blend you are using. Some gluten-free flour blends have xanthan or guar gum added already. A recipe should be tested and written using the specific homemade or store-bought gluten-free flour blend." —Richard Coppedge, CMB, Professor in Baking and Pastry at the Culinary Institute of America and author of *Gluten-Free Baking with The Culinary Institute of America*

TROUBLESHOOTING AND TIPS FOR GLUTEN-FREE BAKING

Grittiness

In foods made with all-purpose flour, the gluten bonds with the wheat starch, minimizing grittiness. Grittiness can be an issue when using gluten-free flours. Possible solutions include:

- Use a bit more water/liquid than normal.
- Give cake, quick bread, and pancake batters a 20- to 30-minute rest before baking or cooking to allow the starches and gums to fully hydrate.
- For cookie doughs, chill in the refrigerator for at least 2 hours (or overnight or more) to ensure all gums and starches are hydrated to their full potential; this also makes the batter less sticky, making it easier to work with.
- Allow cookies to cool on a wire rack (if using parchment paper, transfer the parchment paper with the cookies on it to a wire rack) as soon as possible so they don't get soggy and gummy (the starches and gums tend to hold on to moisture).
- Use nuts, purees, fresh and dried fruit, and chocolate to help achieve a more desirable texture with cookies and muffins.
- For crackers, experiment with using more liquid than seems necessary, not resting the batter, and cooking at a high temperature to help get rid of extra moisture and make the crackers crispier.

Gummy center

Reduce the oven temperature and increase the baking time. Start by increasing the baking time by 5 minutes to help get rid of the extra moisture that can cause a gummy texture. Record the cooking time for doneness so it is included in the recipe directions.

Pie dough

Decrease the amount of butter or oil used by 1 to 2 tablespoons to help the dough keep its shape. For pie doughs made with butter, melt it so the dough is hydrated more uniformly.

Muffins and cakes

Gluten-free batters tend to be sticky. To mitigate the stickiness, spray a spoon or scoop with cooking spray and drop cookie dough or muffin batter onto a cookie sheet or into muffin cups.

Mix the batter longer than usual to help aerate it (a stand mixer works well for this).

Bake cakes in a tube pan, as the additional surface area in the center helps provide structure (the cake won't sink in the middle), or a wide, shallow pan to make a thin sheet cake, which can then be rolled up or cut into layers.

Pancakes, waffles, and crepes

For pancakes, waffles, and crepes, experiment and develop recipes with any type of gluten-free flour or flour blend. Pancakes, waffles, and crepes don't require the same structure as other baked goods.

Use any amount of liquid desired, since the consistency of the batter doesn't matter.

For fluffier waffles and pancakes, use whole eggs: First, separate eggs and beat the whites until they are stiff; folding the whites into the batter will make them fluffier.

Always allow the batter to rest for 20 to 30 minutes.

Homemade Gluten-Free Flour Blends

You may choose to develop a baked good recipe using a specific store-bought gluten-free flour blend or try creating your own. Gluten-free flour blends are not created equal, so they don't work equally well in all recipes.

Understanding how all-purpose flour functions in a recipe will help you decide how to modify and make substitutions. Taking the time to develop your own blends can often make a difference. Using a combination of gluten-free flours and starches generally leads to better results in terms of replicating the functions of all-purpose flour, and including some rice flour also helps produce good results.

HOW TO DEVELOP YOUR OWN ALL-PURPOSE GLUTEN-FREE FLOUR BLEND

A good formula for an all-purpose gluten-free flour blend is:

- **Two-thirds gluten-free flour(s):** Two-thirds of the mixture should be a gluten-free flour on its own or a combination of gluten-free flours, such as amaranth, brown rice, buckwheat, chickpea, coconut, corn, millet, oat, quinoa, soy, sorghum, white rice, or teff.
- **One-third starch(es):** One-third of the mixture should be devoted to starch, either one on its own or a combination of starches, such as glutinous sweet rice flour, potato starch, tapioca starch, cornstarch, arrowroot starch.
- **Gums or strengtheners:** The amount needed will vary based on the type of baked good; options include xanthan gum, guar gum, flaxseed meal, psyllium, or dry milk powder.

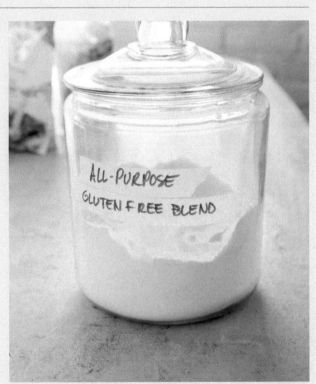

Gluten-Free Flour Blend Recipe Example

	Gluten-free ingredient	Weight	Volume measure estimate
Gluten-free flour	Millet flour	300 grams (10.6 ounces)	⅓ cup
Gluten-free flour	Brown rice flour	300 grams (10.6 ounces)	⅓ cup
Starches	Tapioca starch Sweet rice flour	150 grams (5.3 ounces) 150 grams (5.3 ounces)	⅓ cup
Gum	Xanthan gum	2.5 grams	About 1 teaspoon (for cookies or cakes, use ¼ to ½ teaspoon)

Adapted with permission from Dean Lavornia, associate professor, the International Baking & Pastry Institute at Johnson & Wales University's College of Food Innovation & Technology.

Photo courtesy of America's Test Kitchen

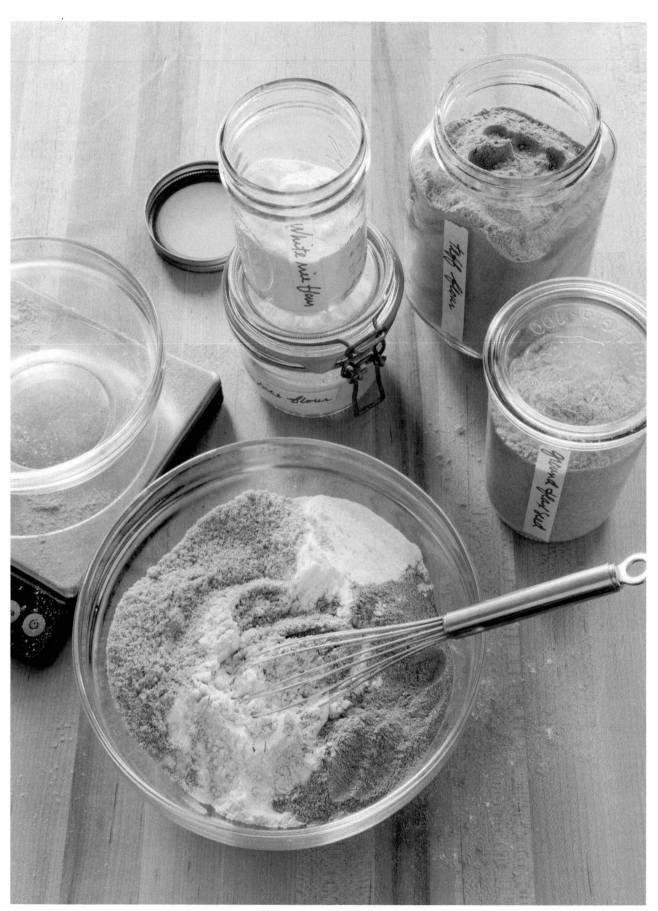

Photo courtesy of America's Test Kitchen

The gluten-free flour from America's Test Kitchen combines white and brown rice flours as a baseline for protein, starch, and flavor and includes two different starches—tapioca and potato—because different starches absorb water, swell, and gel at different temperatures. The milk powder helps add a bit more protein and contributes to the browning of baked goods.

Richard Coppedge's gluten-free blend is a whole grain alternative to the predominately refined gluten-free flour blends. White, brown, and sweet rice flour are commonly used in store-bought gluten-free blends, while this blend uses whole grain sorghum, whole grain buckwheat, and whole grain teff flour. The addition of a little white rice flour helps produce baked goods with a lighter texture.

Both gluten-free flour recipes are provided in weight and volume measurements since flours have different weights based on density and particle size per cup. Weighing flour is always the most accurate way to measure it.

America's Test Kitchen All-Purpose Gluten-Free Flour Blend

By America's Test Kitchen

Preparation time: 15 minutes
Yield: 9⅓ cups (42 ounces)

4½ cups plus ⅓ cup (24 ounces)
  white rice flour
1⅔ cups (7½ ounces) brown
  rice flour
1⅓ cups (7 ounces) potato starch
¾ cup (3 ounces) tapioca starch
3 tablespoons (¾ ounce) nonfat
  milk powder

Whisk all the ingredients together in a large bowl until well combined. Transfer to an airtight container and refrigerate for up to 3 months or freeze for up to 6 months. Bring to room temperature before using.

All-Purpose Whole Grain Gluten-Free Flour Blend

By Chef Richard Coppedge, CMB, professor in baking and pastry, Culinary Institute of America

Preparation time: 15 minutes
Yield: 8½ cups plus 2 tablespoons
(1.2 kilograms)

3¾ cups (425 grams) sorghum
  flour
2⅓ cups (340 grams) buckwheat
  flour
1 cup plus 5 tablespoons
  (195 grams) teff flour
1 cup plus 2 tablespoons
  (170 grams) white rice flour
¼ cup (28 grams) guar gum

Whisk all the ingredients together in a large bowl until well combined. Transfer to an airtight container and refrigerate for up to 3 months or freeze for up to 6 months. Bring to room temperature before using.

Recipe Example: Using a gluten-free flour blend for muffins

This recipe uses a mix of two-thirds white rice flour and one-third tapioca starch as a neutral gluten-free blend that works well in these banana muffins, as well as other cakes, cookies, and quick breads.

Gluten-Free Banana Muffins

By Cindy Ferron, MEd, CEPC, associate professor, Johnson & Wales University

Preparation time: 20 minutes
Cooking time: 25 to 30 minutes
Yield: 18 (3-ounce) muffins

1⅓ cups white rice flour
⅔ cup tapioca starch
1 teaspoon xanthan gum
1 teaspoon baking soda
1 teaspoon cinnamon
¼ teaspoon table salt
2 cups mashed bananas (about
    5 medium)
2 large eggs
¾ cup packed brown sugar
½ cup unsalted butter, melted

1. Heat the oven to 350° F. Sift the rice flour, tapioca starch, xanthan gum, baking soda, cinnamon, and salt into a small bowl.

2. Whisk the bananas, eggs, sugar, and butter together in a medium bowl. Gently fold the dry ingredients into the wet mixture and stir just until combined.

3. Spoon the batter into 18 muffin cups. Bake until the muffin tops spring back when pressed, 25 to 30 minutes.

Nutrition per muffin: 180 calories, 6 grams total fat, 3.5 grams saturated fat, 120 milligrams sodium, 32 grams carbohydrate, 1 gram fiber, 13 grams total sugar (9 grams added sugars), 2 grams protein

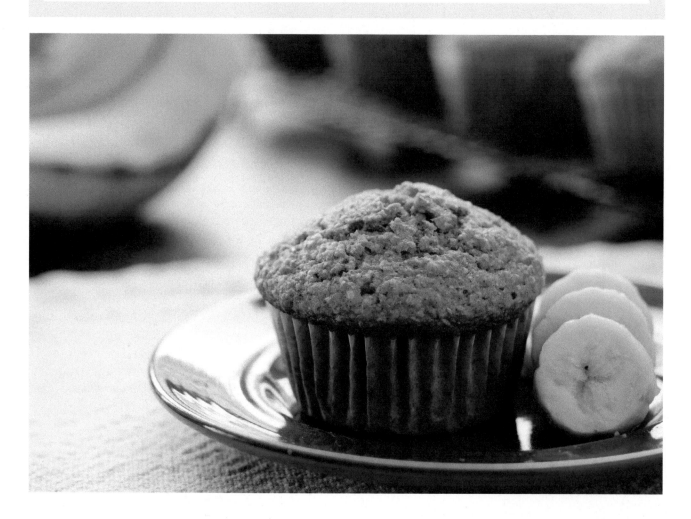

Developing Recipes for People With FODMAP Intolerance

Fermentable oligosaccharides, disaccharides, monosaccharides, and polyols—FODMAPs, for short—are a group of short-chain carbohydrates (sugars) that naturally occur in many foods. These short-chain carbohydrates cannot be completely digested or absorbed in the intestines, so in some individuals—particularly those who suffer from irritable bowel syndrome (IBS)—they trigger digestive distress.

F = Fermentable
Intestinal microflora (gut bacteria) ferment undigested carbohydrates.

O = Oligosaccharides
Fructo-oligosaccharides (fructans) are found in wheat- and rye-based foods, such as breads, cereals, and pastas, and also in onions, garlic, and other vegetables.

Galacto-oligosaccharides (galactans or GOS) are primarily found in beans, lentils, peas, and soy-based products.

D = Disaccharides
Lactose is a disaccharide found in dairy products like milk, soft cheeses, and ice cream.

M = Monosaccharides
Fructose is a natural fruit sugar found in many fruits (e.g., apples, mango, cherries, pears, watermelon) but also in honey, high-fructose corn syrup, and agave. When consumed in excess of glucose, it can be malabsorbed.

A = and

P = Polyols
Sorbitol, *mannitol*, *xylitol*, and *isomalt* are sugar alcohols that naturally occur in some fruits and vegetables (e.g., apples, pears, stone fruits, mushrooms, cauliflower). They are sometimes added to sugar-free foods and candies to sweeten them.

When the FODMAPs in foods reach the small intestine, they remain there and attract water. When they reach the large intestine, they are fermented by the bacteria found there. This results in excess gas production. This extra water and gas can lead to bloating, discomfort, and abdominal pain, as well as diarrhea, constipation, or both.

The FODMAP Diet

The low FODMAP diet, which was first developed by researchers at Australia's Monash University, is nuanced and complex, and it should be implemented and individualized for the patient by a registered dietitian nutritionist (RDN) who specializes in the diet. Because FODMAPs are found in hundreds of foods, the diet can be highly restrictive and can lead to nutritional deficiencies when some choose to eliminate entire categories of healthy foods because they are classified as being high FODMAP. In truth, not all FODMAPs are symptom triggers for all people with FODMAP intolerance; only those that are poorly absorbed by and cause symptoms in a particular person need to be restricted or eliminated. The FODMAP diet typically has three phases:

Phase 1: During this phase, all high FODMAP foods are restricted for 2 to 6 weeks to achieve total symptom relief. This diet phase is temporary, and during the phase, only low FODMAP alternatives are consumed instead of high FODMAP foods.

Phase 2: A 6- to 8-week phase during which one subgroup type (e.g., fructose, lactose, fructan, polyol, GOS) and amount of FODMAP foods at a time is reintroduced for a 3-day period to determine whether a person can tolerate the subgroup without experiencing symptoms (portion size matters). If symptoms occur when a particular FODMAP is reintroduced, a 3-day break is taken before testing the next food.

Phase 3: In this phase, the FODMAP diet is personalized to exclude only those foods that trigger symptoms.

Low FODMAP Recipes

A helpful starting point for low FODMAP recipe development is comparing high and low FODMAP foods and ingredients (see High FODMAP Ingredient Substitutions). For more detailed information, refer to a reliable source, such as the Monash University FODMAP Diet app or the FODMAP Friendly app. Both offer extensive databases of information about a wide variety of laboratory-tested foods and are updated frequently.

The USDA's FoodData Central resource includes data on lactose and fructose content for some foods, but that data is missing for many others, and it offers very limited data on other FODMAP short-chain carbohydrates (fructans and galactans) and sugar alcohols (polyols).

Keep in mind that a food can be high in one FODMAP but low in another. Just like with other types of healthy recipe development, modifying a food's serving size is one technique for creating low FODMAP recipes. It is possible to use high FODMAP ingredients in a recipe yet still yield a low FODMAP result if the ingredient amounts and serving sizes are monitored appropriately. A high FODMAP serving size is an amount that commonly triggers symptoms, and a low FODMAP serving size is an amount that is generally well tolerated by most individuals with IBS. Some foods are considered FODMAP free.

For example, an avocado can be classified as either a high, moderate, or low FODMAP food based on adjusting its serving size (see example from the Monash University FODMAP Diet app). Half an avocado (80 grams) is high in sorbitol, a polyol FODMAP, as indicated by the red dot in the image, so people who malabsorb sorbitol should avoid consuming this amount. However, if the serving size is reduced to ¼ avocado, the sorbitol level is considered moderate (yellow dot), and a further reduction to ⅛ avocado is considered low FODMAP (green dot). Since all of the other FODMAPs present in avocados are represented with green dots, this indicates that they are considered low at all three serving sizes.

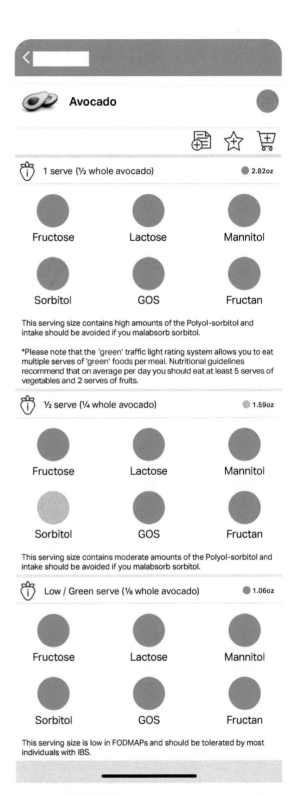

Images and FODMAP ratings information reproduced with permission from Monash University (monashFOD-MAP.com)

"FODMAPs dissolve in water, so they tend to leach out into the canning, soaking, and cooking water. This can be used to your advantage with beans. To minimize FODMAPs, choose canned, drained, rinsed beans. When cooking beans from scratch, discard the soaking and cooking water. If you will be consuming the cooking water in a bean soup or baked beans in a sauce, expect them to contain a lot of FODMAPs."

—Patsy Catsos, MS, RDN, LD, author of *The IBS Elimination Diet and Cookbook*

"Once you understand how to assess the FODMAP content of a single food at various serving sizes, you can approach the concept of FODMAP stacking. For example: if a yogurt parfait recipe uses low FODMAP lactose-free yogurt and then tops it with two foods that each have a low FODMAP fructans serving size—¼ cup (40 grams) for blueberries and approximately 30 berries (60 grams) of raspberries—you have stacked the fructans. Individually, blueberries and raspberries at these serving sizes are low FODMAP, but if you use them at the same time you have now created an overload of fructans by 'stacking' the same FODMAP. Alternatively, the low FODMAP yogurt could be topped with the blueberries or the raspberries along with a no FODMAP fruit, like strawberries or grapes, or a sprinkling of dried coconut. Dried coconut contains sorbitol, which is a FODMAP, but it doesn't contain fructans, so in this case, the FODMAPs would not be stacked." —Dédé Wilson, co-founder of fodmapeveryday.com and co-author of *The Low FODMAP Diet Step by Step*

HIGH FODMAP INGREDIENT SUBSTITUTIONS*

High FODMAP ingredients	Lower FODMAP ingredients (check for low FODMAP serving sizes)
Dairy and dairy alternative products	
Cow's milk, evaporated and sweetened condensed milk, buttermilk Soy milk (made from whole soybeans) Plant-based dairy products made with chicory root/inulin (read labels carefully)	Lactose-free milk Plant-based milks, including soy (only those made from soy protein), almond, rice, quinoa, hemp, macadamia, and coconut milk (canned)
Yogurt	Lactose-free or plant-based (e.g., soy, coconut) yogurt Lactose-free kefir
Cottage cheese, ricotta cheese	Aged cheeses such as cheddar, Swiss, and Parmesan
Ice cream	Lactose-free ice cream
Protein sources	
Silken tofu, whole soybeans Black, kidney, pinto, navy, fava, and lima beans and split peas	Plain/unseasoned meat, pork, chicken, lamb, fish, shellfish, canned tuna Eggs Firm tofu, soy cheese, tempeh, edamame Small portions of canned chickpeas and lentils

BOX CONTINUES >

High FODMAP ingredients	Lower FODMAP ingredients (check for low FODMAP serving sizes)

Fruits

Fruits that have a high fructose-to-glucose ratio and high polyols are not well tolerated:	Fruits that have a high glucose-to-fructose ratio and are usually well tolerated in small portions:

Apples	Watermelon	Bananas (firm, unripe)	Grapes
Apple juice	Boysenberries	Blueberries, raspberries, and strawberries	Kiwi
Bananas (ripe)	Blackberries		Oranges
Stone fruits (nectarines, peaches, apricot, plums, mango, cherries)	Pears	Cantaloupe	Papaya
	Dried fruits	Dried cranberries	Pineapple
		Grapefruit	Tamarind

Vegetables

Artichokes	Sun-dried tomatoes	Arugula	Lettuce
Asparagus	Onions	Beets	Parsnips
Cauliflower	White parts of green onions	Bell peppers	Potatoes
Mushrooms	Leeks	Bok choy	Radishes
Brussels sprouts	Shallots	Broccoli	Rutabagas
Green peas	Garlic	Cabbage	Spinach
Sugar snap peas		Carrots	Squash
		Cucumbers	Sweet potatoes
		Eggplant	Swiss chard
		Fennel bulb	Tomatoes
		Green beans	Zucchini
		Kale	

Grains and flours

Barley, rye, wheat; amaranth, coconut, and soy flours and food products made from these ingredients	Gluten-free grain flours and products made from the following ingredients: corn flour, polenta, corn tortillas, oats, rice, rice cakes, quinoa, buckwheat, sorghum, teff, and millet
Packaged grain products that contain chicory root extract (e.g., many granola bars)	Soba noodles made from 100% buckwheat
	Sourdough bread made with white, whole wheat, or spelt flour (the microbes in a sourdough starter consume some of the FODMAPs)
	Corn, potato, and tapioca starches

Nuts, seeds, and oils

Cashews and pistachios	Macadamia nuts, walnuts, hazelnuts, pecans, Brazil nuts, pine nuts, pepitas/pumpkin seeds, poppy seeds, sesame seeds, sunflower seeds, caraway seeds, chestnuts
	Peanuts or peanut butter, almonds or almond butter
	Chia seeds, flaxseed meal, hemp seeds
	Avocado oil, canola oil, coconut oil, olive oil, peanut oil, sesame oil, sunflower oil, vegetable oil

BOX CONTINUES >

High FODMAP ingredients	Lower FODMAP ingredients (check for low FODMAP serving sizes)	
Condiments and miscellaneous ingredients		
Read the ingredient label for packaged products that contain added high FODMAP ingredients	Mustard Ketchup Mayonnaise Soy sauce Worcestershire Vinegar	Capers Seaweed Note: Use a lab-tested low FODMAP serving size for any condiments that contain garlic or onion
Spices, herbs, and flavorings		
Garlic powder and garlic salt Onion powder and onion salt Note: Carefully read the labels of products that contain onion or garlic (e.g., jarred pasta sauce, canned broth, canned stock)	Fresh and dried spices and herbs Asafoetida powder (an Indian spice that adds an onion or leek-like flavor to foods) Green parts of green onions Chives Chili peppers Fresh ginger Lemon and lime juice and zest Garlic-infused oil (fructans are not fat soluble, so garlic-infused oil adds garlic flavor without adding FODMAPs) or sauté slivers of garlic in oil and then remove and discard them	
Sweeteners, sugars, and confectionary		
Agave, honey, molasses, and fruit juice concentrate Products that contain high FODMAP sugars and sweetener ingredients (read labels carefully—especially yogurt and cereal products): Isomalt — High-fructose corn syrup Fructose — Lactose Fructans (inulin, oligofructose, prebiotics, fructo-oligosaccharide) — Mannitol Fructose-glucose syrup — Sorbitol, Xylitol	Granulated sugar, brown sugar, confectioners' sugar, maple syrup, rice malt syrup, and stevia Cocoa powder Dark chocolate Vanilla extract	
Beverages		
Cow's milk–based drinks Fruit juices (most) Kombucha	All forms of alcohol except rum Coffee All forms of tea except chamomile and oolong Cranberry juice that does not contain high-fructose corn syrup	

* Some foods have low and high FODMAP portions, which is why there are differences in FODMAP food lists from different sources.
Sources: High and low FODMAP foods by Monash University: monashfodmap.com/about-fodmap-and-ibs/high-and-low-fodmap -foods | FODMAP Everyday: fodmapeveryday.com | FODMAP table: acronym, information and examples by FODMAP Friendly: fodmapfriendly.com/wp-content/uploads/2018/01/fodmap-table.pdf

Are grapes and bananas high or low FODMAP foods?

The FODMAP content of most fruits is affected by the fruit's water content and ripeness. For example, grapes are low FODMAP and raisins are high FODMAP, because when a fruit's water content decreases, its fructan content increases. This holds true with other dried fruits but may not for freeze-dried fruits. Bananas range from low FODMAP to high FODMAP depending on their level of ripeness: ripe bananas are high in fructans, but firm, unripe bananas are not.

Is soy a high or low FODMAP food?

The plant's maturity, the food's processing, and whether or not the food is fermented can impact the FODMAP content of soy foods.

Maturity: The FODMAPs in whole, mature soybeans include oligosaccharides: galacto-oligosaccharides and fructans. Edamame, which are soybeans that are harvested in an immature state, are lower FODMAP.

Processing: Soy yogurts and milks processed from soy protein (a protein isolated from soybeans) are lower in FODMAPs than soy yogurts and milks processed from whole soybeans. Firm tofu is low FODMAP because most of the water in the tofu is pressed out when it is processed, and when the water is expelled, the water-soluble galacto-oligosaccharide goes with it. Silken tofu, on the other hand, is high FODMAP because it has a higher water content and more remaining galacto-oligosaccharide. Remember: all FODMAPs are carbohydrates, and protein of any kind is not a FODMAP. If the protein is truly isolated from the soybean, it is low FODMAP. However, this does not apply to products like textured vegetable protein crumbles, which are not protein isolates and are instead made from soybeans.

Fermentation: Fermentation is another way to reduce the FODMAPs present in whole soybeans, which is why fermented soy products like miso, tempeh, and soy sauce are low FODMAP foods.

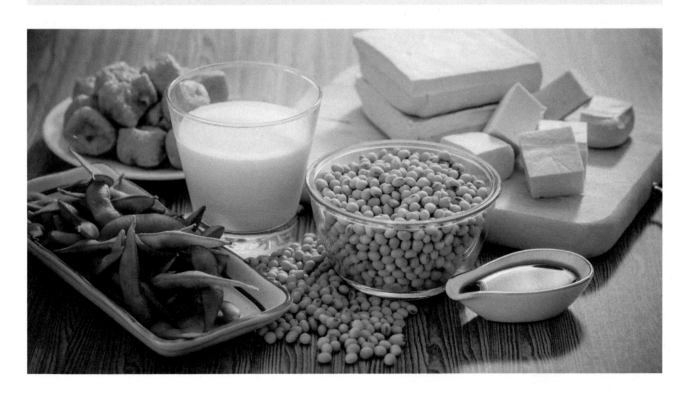

This pesto recipe uses garlic-infused oil, which can be enjoyed even during the elimination phase of the FODMAP diet since the fructans in garlic are not soluble in oil. While all nuts are not low FODMAP, pine nuts have been lab tested by Monash University and are low FODMAP in 14-gram portions. Always calculate the FODMAP load of the actual serving size per person. For this pesto recipe, a serving size of ⅓ cup (75 milliliters) or less is considered a low FODMAP portion.

Low FODMAP Basil Pesto

By Dédé Wilson, co-founder of fodmapeveryday.com and coauthor of The Low-FODMAP Diet Step by Step

Preparation time: 10 minutes
Yield: about 1⅔ cups, 405 milliliters (2 tablespoons per serving)

4 cups (96 grams) lightly packed basil leaves, washed, dried, and large stems removed
⅔ cup (165 milliliters) garlic-infused oil, plus more for storing the pesto
⅓ cup (44 grams) pine nuts, very lightly toasted
Generous ½ teaspoon kosher salt
⅔ cup (66 grams) finely grated Parmigiano-Reggiano cheese

1. Combine the basil, garlic oil, pine nuts, and salt in a food processor fitted with a metal blade. Pulse on and off a few times, then process until a paste forms, scraping down the bowl once or twice. Add the cheese and process until combined and somewhat smooth. It will remain a bit textured, which is fine.

2. Scrape into an airtight container and cover the top with a thin layer of additional oil to prevent discoloration. Refrigerate for up to 1 week. You can also divide into small freezer-safe containers and freeze for up to 1 month. Defrost in refrigerator overnight.

Nutrition per 2-tablespoon serving: 140 calories, 15 grams total fat, 2.5 grams saturated fat, 150 milligrams sodium, 1 gram carbohydrate, 0 grams fiber, 0 grams total sugar, 2 grams protein

This smoothie recipe uses low or moderately low FODMAP ingredients and limits the total amount of fruit. Try low FODMAP fruits such as 1 underripe banana; 1 orange; 1 cup pineapple, papaya, or grapes; and ¼ cup blueberries or raspberries. To increase the protein content, add a low FODMAP protein powder, a whey protein powder that is labeled "lactose free," or any plain egg white powder. Avoid soy- and pea-based protein powders unless they are certified as low FODMAP or FODMAP-friendly, and avoid protein powders containing high FODMAP ingredients like inulin (dietary fiber), fructo-oligosaccharides (FOS), or the sweeteners fructose and sorbitol.

Low FODMAP Smoothie

By Patsy Catsos, MS, RDN, LD, author of The IBS Elimination Diet and Cookbook *and editor of ibsfree.net*

Preparation time: 10 minutes
Yield: 1 serving (20 fluid ounces)

4 ice cubes (80 grams)
¾ cup (170 grams) lactose-free, low-fat plain yogurt (see Note)
½ cup (70 grams) strawberries, tops trimmed, sliced in half
2 kiwis (150 grams), peeled and cut into chunks
1 tablespoon (24 grams) dried egg white powder
1 tablespoon (11 grams) chia seeds
½ cup (18 grams) baby spinach or baby kale, optional
½-inch (3.5 grams) piece fresh ginger, peeled and chopped (about 1 teaspoon), optional
4 drops liquid stevia, optional

Combine all the ingredients in a blender container. Cover the container with the lid and puree on high speed until a uniform slushy texture. If the blender blades won't engage, add a little water. Enjoy immediately, or, if desired, allow the chia seeds to hydrate for a few minutes to thicken the smoothie. Alternatively, chill in the refrigerator or in an insulated beverage container for a few hours.

Note: *Almond milk may be substituted for the yogurt if you are allergic to or do not eat dairy.*

Nutrition per serving (including optional ingredients):
410 calories, 7 grams total fat, 2 grams saturated fat, 480 milligrams sodium, 57 grams carbohydrate, 11 grams fiber, 39 grams total sugar (8 grams added sugar), 32 grams protein

Gluten-Free and FODMAP Recipe Development Resources

In addition to the Recipe Development Resources listed in Chapters 1, 2, and 3, consult these websites and books when developing gluten-free and low FODMAP recipes.

Gluten-Free

Books

Cannelle et Vanille Bakes Simple: A New Way to Bake Gluten-Free, by Aran Goyoaga. 2021. Sasquatch Books.

Gluten-Free Flavor Flours: A New Way to Bake with Non-Wheat Flours, Including Rice, Nut, Coconut, Teff, Buckwheat, and Sorghum Flours, by Alice Medrich. 2017. Artisan.

The How Can It Be Gluten Free Cookbooks (Volume 1 and Volume 2), by America's Test Kitchen. 2014 and 2015. America's Test Kitchen.

Tartine All Day: Modern Recipes for the Home Cook, by Elisabeth Prueitt. 2017. Ten Speed Press.

Websites

Beyond Celiac:
beyondceliac.org

Celiac Disease Foundation:
celiac.org

Gluten-Free Living:
glutenfreeliving.com

Gluten Free Watchdog:
glutenfreewatchdog.org

The Gluten Intolerance Group:
gluten.org

National Celiac Association:
nationalceliac.org

FODMAPs

FODMAP Everyday:
fodmapeveryday.com

FODMAP Friendly:
fodmapfriendly.com

Monash University the Low FODMAP Diet:
monashfodmap.com/about-fodmap-and-ibs

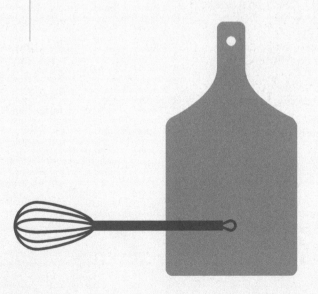

Bibliography

Gluten-Free/Celiac Disease

America's Test Kitchen. *The How Can It Be Gluten Free Cookbook: Revolutionary Techniques. Groundbreaking Recipes*. America's Test Kitchen; 2014.

Coppedge Jr RJ. *Gluten-Free Baking with The Culinary Institute of America: 150 Flavorful Recipes from the World's Premier Culinary College*. Adams Media; 2008.

Food labeling; gluten-free labeling of fermented or hydrolyzed foods. Federal Register website. August 13, 2020. Accessed June 30, 2021. federalregister.gov/documents/2020/08/13/2020-17088/food-labeling-gluten-free -labeling-of-fermented-or-hydrolyzed-foods

Gluten and food labeling. US Food & Drug Administration website. July 16, 2018. Accessed June 30, 2021. fda.gov/food/nutrition-education-resources-materials/gluten-and-food-labeling

Gluten-free labeling of food, Section 101.91. US Food & Drug Administration website. Accessed September 24, 2021. accessdata.fda.gov/scripts/cdrh/cfdocs/cfcfr/cfrsearch.cfm?fr=101.91

Goyoaga A. *Cannelle et Vanille Bakes Simple: A New Way to Bake Gluten-Free*. Sasquatch Books; 2021.

TTB ruling: gluten content statements in the labeling and advertising of wine, distilled spirits, and malt beverages. Alcohol and Tobacco Tax and Trade Bureau website. October 13, 2020. Accessed June 30, 2021. ttb.gov/rulings /r2020-2#

FODMAPs

Academy of Nutrition and Dietetics, Nutrition Care Manual. Low-FODMAP nutrition therapy. Accessed June 30, 2021. nutritioncaremanual.org/client_ed.cfm?ncm_client_ed_id=422

FODMAPs and irritable bowel syndrome. Monash University website. Accessed June 30, 2021. monashfodmap.com/about-fodmap-and-ibs

How are low FODMAP recipes created? FODMAP Everyday website. March 4, 2019. Accessed June 30, 2021. fodmapeveryday.com/how-are-low-fodmap-recipes-created

King K. What Is the Low FODMAP Diet? Academy of Nutrition and Dietetics website. Accessed June 30, 2021. eatright.org/health/allergies-and-intolerances/food-intolerances-and-sensitivities/what-is-the-low-fodmap-diet

Low FODMAP diet & food list. Epicured website. Accessed June 30, 2021. mmm.epicured.com/low -fodmap-food-list

Scarlata K, Wilson D. *The Low-FODMAP Diet Step by Step*. Da Capo Lifelong Books; 2017.

Vakil N. Dietary fermentable oligosaccharides, disaccharides, monosaccharides, and polyols (FODMAPs) and gastrointestinal disease. *Nutr Clin Pract*. 2018 Aug;33(4):468-475. doi:10.1002/ncp.10108

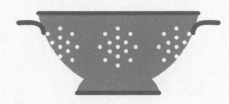

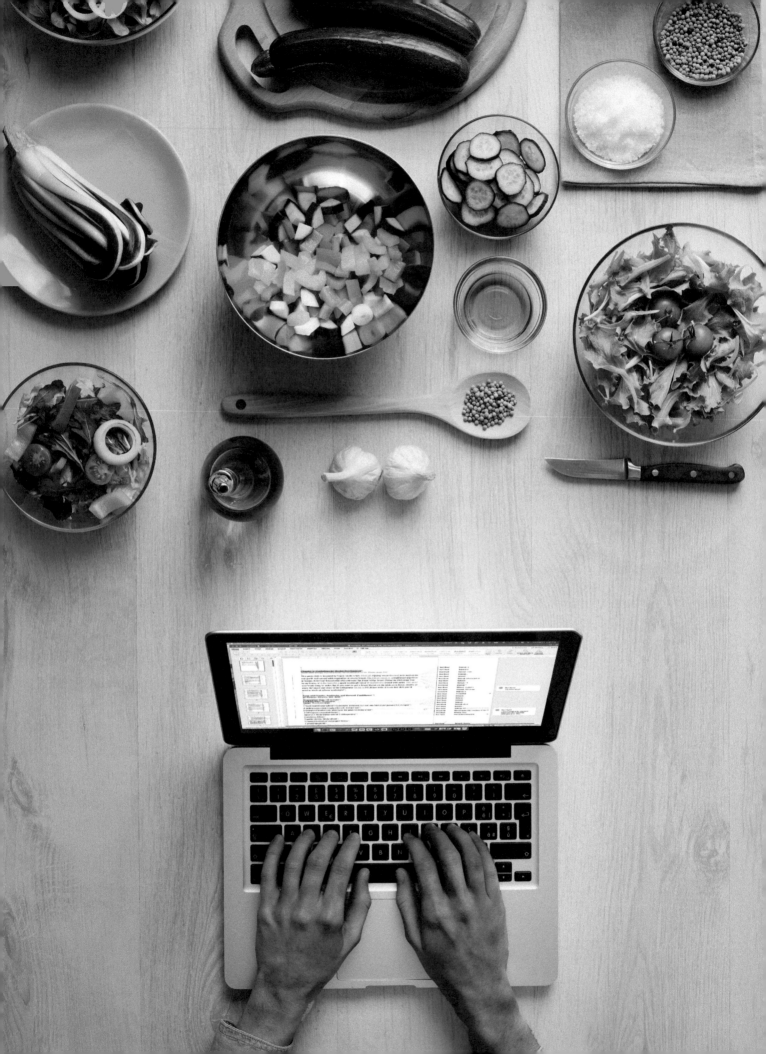

Chapter 7

Recipe Writing and Editing

While recipe development is an art and a science, recipe writing—translating the act of cooking food into words—is a literary skill that requires attention to detail and a solid grasp of culinary and kitchen language.

A well-written recipe should tell a clear story, be accurate, and use consistent language. The recipe should also act as a guide and a teacher, helping home cooks produce a successful dish regardless of their kitchen experience and culinary skill level. These parameters hold true regardless of where the recipe is published, whether it's in a newspaper, a cookbook, a digital or print magazine or newsletter, or on the back of a product's package.

Depending on where the recipe will be featured, different space constraints and ingredient and word count limits may ultimately affect the recipe writing process. If there are not clear guidelines for how much detail the recipe should include, think first about the audience (see Chapter 1). What do they need? What do they know? No matter who the recipe's intended audience may be, never assume that they have specific culinary knowledge.

A primary goal of recipe writing is to communicate a recipe in a way that readers can easily understand, ultimately allowing them to feel successful. It's always better to provide as much clarity as possible in the recipe's ingredient list and directions. Explain what to expect, how to complete a step (e.g., include a visual and estimated time), and, if possible, how to fix problems that could arise (e.g., what to do if the sauce is too thin or if a substitution needs to be made). When space and words are limited, you must learn to write more concisely. For readers who are already quite skilled, well-written recipes reinforce what they already know, lending the recipe writer more credibility as a culinary professional and recipe developer.

Recipe Format

Like all forms of writing, there is no one right way to write a recipe—the style or voice will vary depending on what works best for the audience. However, best practices and suggestions for how to write a recipe to ensure accuracy and clarity do exist. The foundation is in understanding the elements that comprise the basic structure of all recipes. Most well-written recipes contain the following elements, which are explained in more detail in this chapter (nutrition information is covered in more detail in Chapter 9):

- title
- headnote
- preparation and cooking time
- yield or servings
- ingredient list
- directions
- recipe notes or sidebars
- nutrition information

The Title

The recipe's title is the first chance to capture the reader's interest and attention. Titles should be descriptive and easily searchable in either an index or an online search. Include adjectives that are vivid, descriptive, and useful to the reader. Ultimately, the title must be clear. See Recipe Title Categories and Examples.

Titles to Avoid

Readers should be enticed by a recipe's title, not confused or misled by it. In general, try to avoid ambiguous, inaccurate, mysterious, or arbitrary titles.

Ambiguous titles Examples include "Loaded Cauliflower Casserole" (what's it loaded with?) and "Chocolate Cake" (not very descriptive). Better choices would be "Cauliflower and Broccoli Gratin with Garlic Breadcrumbs" and "Chocolate Layer Cake with Raspberry Filling."

Inaccurate titles Call a dish what it really is. For example, a chicken dish can't be called Chicken Francese if it does not contain chicken cutlets coated in a light batter of flour and egg, panfried and accompanied by a lemon, white wine, and butter sauce; a similar dish could be called Pan-Seared Chicken with Shallots and Wine. A dish isn't pasta carbonara if it doesn't include guanciale, pancetta, or another type of cured pork; an alternative title might be Creamy Pasta with Peas. Sometimes recipes that are similar to well-known dishes are titled with the similar dish in quotation marks, but this can still be misleading. For example, an eggless soufflé recipe titled Broccoli "Soufflé" requires explanation in the recipe headnote.

Overly cute or creative titles One example is "Holiday Mirror Glaze Poke Cake" (what is a holiday mirror glaze?). A better choice would be "Lime Poke Cake with Raspberry Frosting."

Titles including words in a foreign language Never assume your reader will know the translation of a recipe title into English. Either use the translated title or put the translation or more descriptive language in parenthesis. Titling a recipe "Pollo Diablo" assumes that readers will know *pollo* is the Spanish word for chicken, and that *diablo* (Spanish for devil) is often used in spicy dishes. A better choice would be Pollo Diablo (Garlicky and Spicy Fried Chicken). For more information on recipes and cultural sensitivity, see page 15.

Recipe attribute titles It's wonderful to give credit to a recipe's creator or source of inspiration, but consider how important the title is to the goal of making it findable for the reader. Instead of referencing individuals in recipe titles, include information about them in the recipe headnote. For example, better titles than Grandma Flo's Meat Loaf may include Three-Meat Meat Loaf or Balsamic Glazed Meat Loaf.

RECIPE TITLE GRAMMAR

In recipe titles, all words except articles, prepositions, and conjunctions should be capitalized.

- **Articles***: a, an, the
- **Prepositions:** at, by, in, for, on, to, with
- **Conjunctions:** and, but, or

Examples:

- Pigs in a Blanket
- Chicken Salad with Blue Cheese and Scallion Dressing
- Smoked Salmon and Dill Pasta Salad
- Patty Melt with Cabbage on Rye

* An exception is when the recipe title begins with an article.

RECIPE TITLE CATEGORIES AND EXAMPLES

Direct, descriptive titles

Avocado Toast with Smoked Salmon
Black Bean and Corn Quinoa Salad
Buttermilk Biscuits with Sausage Gravy
Buckwheat Soba Noodles with Tofu and
    Lemon-Ginger Dressing

Titles that highlight a cooking method

Roasted Cauliflower
Pork Tenderloin and Vegetable Stir-Fry
Grilled Sea Bass with Pickled Radish
Poached Chicken with Dill

Regional or cultural titles

New England Johnny Cakes
Persian Rice
California Avocado and Orange Salad
Lebanese Moussaka

Promotional titles

Best Chocolate Chip Cookies
Ultimate Fudge Brownies
Award-Winning Apple Pie
Favorite French Fries

Titles that highlight saving time

10-Minute Salad
Quick Chicken Curry
Make-Ahead Spinach Pasta Bake
No-Bake Trail Mix Bites

Ingredient- or health-focused titles

Gluten-Free Mac and Cheese
Reduced-Sugar Chocolate Mousse
Vegan Chocolate Chip Cookies
Healthy Oven-Baked "Fried" Chicken

The Headnote

Recipe writing is technical writing, but in the headnote, the recipe developer's personality can shine through. How much to write—anything from one sentence to multiple paragraphs—depends on space constraints. Recipes intended for the back of a package may not have space for a headnote, but headnotes for cookbooks or websites can be more accommodating.

Guidelines for Writing Recipe Headnotes

Give credit to the original source of the recipe. The headnote is the perfect place to discuss the inspiration of the recipe or its original author.

Share something informative or useful. Does the home cook need to use a special pan? Should the recipe be prepared or partially prepared ahead of when it's needed? Are there ingredient substitutions for those who follow special diets (e.g., vegetarian or gluten-free)? Why is a specific brand of ingredient used, and where can it be purchased?

Share something interesting. Interesting and engaging headnotes make a recipe more enjoyable to read.

Show, don't *tell*. A line like "This is the best grilled chicken ever" isn't very helpful. As an alternative, consider this: "Brushing the chicken breasts with a mixture of honey and salty miso before they're grilled helps create a caramelized grilled exterior. It's a sure-fire way to add a more complex and satisfying flavor to this simple weeknight meal."

Quick Tip

"Ask the publisher before you start writing your headnotes if there is a word limit. Some cookbook publishers limit a headnote to 75 words, forcing you to be succinct. Why? They don't want the recipe to carry over to a second page—that's where they may place the photo." —Rick Rodgers, culinary professional and cookbook author

Types of Headnotes

Credit or inspiration It's professional courtesy to give credit to the original person who inspired your recipe. Sample headnote for Chicken Curry:

> This wonderfully spicy chicken curry is inspired by a recipe from Madhur Jaffrey, an award-winning cookbook author and expert in Indian cuisine.

Cultural or historical The headnote is a great place to provide a cultural explanation or the historical context of a recipe or ingredient. Sample headnote for Southern Collard Greens:

> What's the difference between Southern food and soul food? According to Adrian Miller, a soul food scholar and author, Southern food is the mother cuisine of the American South. Several cuisines like Appalachian food, Creole food, and soul food claim heritage through its ingredients, technique, and tradition. Soul food, on the other hand, is the Southern food that Black Southerners modified after they settled in other parts of the country during the Great Migration (1910–1970). Both Southern and soul food dishes use lots of vegetables, especially cabbage, collards, mustard greens, turnip greens, and kale. This classic collard greens recipe has been served alongside fried chicken or smothered pork chops for over 250 years.

Instructional Instructional headnotes provide an explanation of an unfamiliar ingredient or technique or more detailed instruction on what the final dish should look like. Sample headnote for Spicy Thai Shrimp Salad:

> Makrut (also known as kaffir lime leaves) is the Thai and Southeast Asian cuisine equivalent of bay leaves in American cuisine. If you cannot find them fresh, frozen, or dried at an Asian supermarket, leave them out of the recipe. Nothing substitutes well for this distinctive aromatic herb.

Information on how to save time or use leftovers Sample headnote for Turkey Tetrazzini:

> You can double this recipe and divide into two casserole dishes; bake and serve one now and freeze the other for up to 2 months for an easy meal later. If you prepare it in a metal or ovenproof dish, the frozen casserole can go directly

from the freezer to the oven. Cook it at the same temperature you would if cooking it fresh, allowing for an extra 20 minutes to cook through.

Information on recipe preparation In the headnote, you can describe why the recipe (or part of it) is written as it is—for example, a portion of the recipe that requires advance preparation, or why something must be refrigerated before being fried. Sample headnote for Green Beans, Roasted Fennel, and Shallots:

> This recipe affords lots of flexibility for holiday preparation. The richly flavorful fennel and shallots can be roasted up to 2 days beforehand, and the beans can be steamed or blanched a day ahead. Refrigerate all vegetables until needed and ready to reheat.

Personal Readers want to imagine making a dish in their own kitchen. Ideally, they also want to make a pleasurable connection with you, the recipe writer, and others. Sample headnote for Sloppy Joe Casserole:

> Everyone faces the problem of finding enough time for the entire family to enjoy dinner together and talk over the day's happenings. This warm and comforting casserole will be ready to pop in the oven in 15 minutes, and dinner will be on the table about 20 minutes later.

Aspirational Everyone needs a little nudge to achieve their hopes and goals—even if it's just aspirational. Sample headnote for Molten Chocolate Cake:

> This decadent, romantic dessert takes only 20 minutes to prepare. Why not spend more time with your Valentine and less time in the kitchen?

Food memory Tell a story about a place, travel, flavor, or whatever you think will really bring in the reader. Sample headnote for Angel Food Cake with Strawberry Frosting:

> My mother used to make a terrific strawberry angel food cake that I still dream about. Maybe it's because she reserved it for times when strawberries were truly in season and filled with their unique and fragrant sweetness.

Quick Tip

"Always share the cultural history, context, and inspiration of where a recipe came from in either the recipe headnote, text of the publication, or during a live or online cooking lesson. And don't be afraid to reveal that the recipe is not completely your own, especially if the recipe is not from your cultural heritage. Attribution is very important—everyone's recipe starts somewhere." —Lisa Gross, founder and CEO of the League of Kitchens, a culturally immersive culinary experience where immigrants who are exceptional home cooks teach their family recipes and share their stories and culture

Quick Tip

"When writing a nutrition- or health–focused recipe headnote, make sure to adequately research the topic using reputable resources like the search engine PubMed to find professional peer-reviewed journal articles or reference online sites that end in .gov or .edu and are written by a MD, PhD, or RDN. If you are 'researching' and find information that is too good to be true . . . it probably is. Repeating misinformation doesn't make it true and will likely not get you hired for future work." —Ann Taylor Pittman, independent food writer and recipe developer and former *Cooking Light* Executive Editor

The Preparation and Cooking Time

If you decide to include information about preparation and cooking times, make sure it's accurate. Preparation and cooking times are critical tools that help the reader with planning and ultimately will tell them whether they have enough time to make the recipe. With that in mind, be realistic when giving preparation times. If a lot of vegetables need to be chopped for a recipe, a professional might be able to get it done in 5 minutes, but most will need 10 to 15 minutes. Time yourself, and then add on some extra time for novice cooks.

Many recipes make the claim that they can be ready in 15 to 30 minutes. Nothing will frustrate and make a cook feel more inadequate than finding out it takes them much longer than the stated time. In those cases, it's not the cook who's at fault: responsibility for the inaccuracy lies with the recipe writer. Unrealistic preparation and cooking times may lead to losing the reader's trust. Following are general guidelines for writing preparation and cooking times:

- State preparation time in increments of 5 minutes.

  Preparation time: 20 minutes.

- State cooking time in ranges of minutes.

  Cooking time: 10 to 12 minutes.

- Consider using additional descriptive times, which can provide the cook with helpful information.

  Baking time: 10 minutes
  Grilling time: 5 minutes on each side
  Marinating time: 2 hours
  Proofing time: 1 hour

The Yield or Servings

The term "recipe yield" refers to the total amount of a finished recipe. How the yield is stated depends on the recipe type. Often, the number of servings is stated as the yield, and some recipes provide the serving size, which helps to clarify how the number of servings is defined. The following examples illustrate how helpful a few details can be.

Less descriptive	More descriptive
Yield: Makes 1 (9-inch) loaf	Yield: Makes 1 (9-inch) loaf, serves 8
Yield: Enough frosting for double-layer cake	Yield: 3½ cups, enough to frost and fill 1 (9-inch) double-layer cake
Yield: 24 cookies	Yield: Makes 2 dozen cookies (2 cookies per serving)
Yield: Serves 4	Yield: Serves 4 (2 tacos per serving)
Yield: Serves 6	Yield: 12 cups or 6 (2-cup) servings

Guidelines for Providing Recipe Yield and Servings

Many recipes are designed to have a yield of four or six servings, so a cook can easily double the amount if more servings are needed (e.g., for leftovers or entertaining purposes). When a range of servings is provided, the nutrition analysis should always be calculated based on the smaller number of servings, and it should be clear to the reader that it was analyzed based on a specific number of servings (see Chapter 9).

Determining the number of servings and the serving size for a recipe can depend on various factors. For example, one determining factor may be a nutrient or calorie limit in a serving amount. See How to Determine Recipe Serving Sizes for several sources to consult.

In general, be consistent in how and where you provide yields and serving sizes in your recipes—either at the beginning or end—and pick a style or use the publisher's style to state the recipe yield. For example:

> Makes 8 servings
> Yield: 8 servings (1 cup per serving)
> Serves 8

Providing more detail with the yield, including the number of servings and serving size, makes it easier for the reader to know whether the recipe will produce enough food for the group it's intended for and whether the serving sizes are appropriate. For example:

> Pasta with Lentils and Kale, Yield: 6 servings (1¼ cup/291 grams per serving)

> Butternut Squash Soup, Total Yield: 7½ cups/ 1.7 liters, Makes 6 servings

Some nutrition-focused publishers or websites, such as *EatingWell.com*, may require specific details for yield and serving sizes to help provide an accurate nutrition analysis. For example:

> Total recipe yield and/or serving size in metric (grams or milliliters) and conventional units (cups, quarts, or gallons; weight in ounces and pounds)

> Serving sizes listed separately for each recipe component (e.g., a serving size listed for the main dish and a second listed for the accompanying garnish or side dish)

HOW TO DETERMINE RECIPE SERVING SIZES

There are no rules for choosing a serving size for a recipe, but several sources can be consulted, particularly for recipes with a focus on health and wellness.

Health and nutrition guidelines, such as the Dietary Guidelines for Americans, provide recommended daily (or weekly) amounts from each food group at various calorie levels. Although there are no "standard" serving sizes, these daily amounts can be referenced to help determine recipe serving sizes that fit within daily recommended food group amounts. When writing health-focused recipes that include any type of nutrition claim (e.g., low-calorie, high-fiber, or reduced-sodium), be sure the established definitions for these claims are met (see Chapter 2).

Food label serving sizes, established by the Food and Drug Administration (FDA), are based on the amounts of foods and beverages that people typically eat, not necessarily recommended amounts for better health. The FDA refers to the serving sizes on packaged products as "reference amounts customarily consumed (RACC) per eating occasion." These are used by food manufacturers so that serving sizes are consistent among similar products. Label serving sizes can be used as guidelines for recipes, but some label serving sizes may not be realistic for recipes. For example, a 16-ounce box of pasta has eight 2-ounce (1 cup cooked) servings. This serving size may or may not be appropriate for a pasta recipe depending on if it is being used in a side dish or main dish.

Restaurant serving sizes vary based on the chef's decision and factors such as food presentation, food cost, and customer expectations. Taking note of restaurant serving sizes can be helpful, but often restaurant serving sizes are generous compared to health and nutrition guidelines. For example, a restaurant serving size for steak might be 12 ounces; a similar recipe designed for home cooks might list a serving size closer to 5 to 6 ounces.

Cookbook and online recipe serving sizes. Reference serving sizes of similar recipes published in cookbooks or online, as well as your own personal experience in serving family or friends, to figure out the serving size based on how much of a recipe an individual is likely to consume. Be realistic based on the nature of the recipe. Some factors to consider include richness (a very rich dish may need a smaller serving size than a comparable lighter one) and purpose (an appetizer or first-course recipe will yield smaller servings than one for a main dish).

The Ingredient List

The purpose of the ingredient list is to help the reader understand what ingredients are needed and in what form they must be prepared to make the recipe. The ingredient list also serves as a shopping list and a quick preview of flavor combinations and familiarity with the ingredients. Guidelines for how the ingredient list should be written will depend on the publisher or the needs of the project. Regardless, the ingredients must be listed in a way that is accurate, clear, and consistent within the project. Following are some basic rules to follow, along with ideas for variations, when writing an ingredient list.

Ingredient List Organization

A well-organized ingredient list is logical and also helpful to the reader and your editor.

Order of Ingredients

A basic rule of recipe writing is to list the ingredients in the order they are used in the directions. After the recipe directions are completed, double-check that all ingredients in the list are included in the recipe directions and used in the order they are listed.

Ingredient list:
1 cup (120 grams) all-purpose flour
2 teaspoons baking powder
½ teaspoon fine sea salt or table salt

Directions:
Mix together the flour, baking powder, and salt in a medium bowl.

When the order of use doesn't matter or when ingredients are added at the same time, an alternative is to list the ingredients in descending order from the largest to the smallest quantity.

Ingredient list:
6 large eggs
3 medium zucchini (about 1 pound), thinly sliced
2 medium yellow onions, chopped
1 teaspoon dried thyme
½ teaspoon Morton kosher salt

Directions:
Whisk the eggs together in a large bowl. Add the zucchini, onions, thyme, and salt and continue whisking until well combined.

Divided Ingredients

Publishers or editors may specify how to list the same ingredient used more than once in a recipe. If there are no guidelines provided, list the total amount used in the recipe at the place in the ingredient list where it is first used. Place a comma after the ingredient and add "divided" or "divided use" after it, and note the amounts used at the different times in the recipe directions.

Ingredient list:
2½ cups all-purpose flour, divided

Directions:
"Sift 2 cups of the flour with the . . ." and later in recipe write, "add the remaining ½ cup of flour . . ."

If only a small amount is used at one point in the recipe, use a short description.

Ingredient list:
2 cups all-purpose flour, plus more to coat the pan

Directions:
"Grease and flour a 10-inch tube pan . . . " and later in the recipe write, "Sift 2 cups flour with the . . . "

If a recipe includes a subdivided ingredient list, such as for a crust and a filling, list each ingredient amount under the appropriate subhead.

When salt is used more than once in a recipe, especially when it is used in several increments, different methods can be used to list the ingredient. List the total amount at the place in the ingredient list where it is first used, then add "divided use."

Ingredient list:
1½ teaspoons kosher salt, divided use

Directions:
Toss zucchini and eggplant with oil on a baking sheet; season with 1 teaspoon of the salt.

Later step:
Add roasted vegetables, tomato, vinegar, thyme, and remaining ½ teaspoon salt.

Include an unspecified amount of salt in the ingredient list and then provide specific amounts in directions.

Ingredient list:

Kosher salt

Directions:

Stir the cheese into the breadcrumbs and season with ½ teaspoon salt.

Later step:

Transfer to a large bowl and stir in the sautéed vegetables and ¾ teaspoon salt.

Later step:

Meanwhile, cook pasta in a large pot of boiling salted water.

Another option, if permitted by the style guidelines you are following, is to include an unspecified amount as "add salt to taste." However, using this "salt to taste" convention assumes your reader is an experienced cook.

Ingredients List When Space is Limited

When space allows, it's always best to list each ingredient separately and on its own line, even when the same amount is used.

½ teaspoon table salt

½ teaspoon freshly ground black pepper

OR

1 small yellow onion, chopped (about ½ cup)

½ cup skim milk

½ cup (2 ounces) shredded mozzarella cheese

If the recipe has very tight space constraints—perhaps because it is being published in a newspaper or placed on a package—list ingredients used at the same time and in the same quantity together on the same line and highlight the word "each" in some way (e.g., capitalization, bold type, italics) so it is clear to the reader and no ingredients are missed.

½ teaspoon ***EACH***: table salt, freshly ground black pepper

½ cup ***EACH***: chopped yellow onion, skim milk, shredded mozzarella cheese

Ingredient List Subheads

If the main recipe includes subrecipes (e.g., a pie with a crust, filling, and topping), use subheads in the ingredient list to better organize the recipe for the reader.

Ingredient list:

CRUST

1 cup all-purpose flour . . .

FILLING

6 medium tart apples (such as Granny Smith), peeled and sliced . . .

TOPPING

1 cup halved walnuts or pecans . . .

For each subrecipe, the ingredients should be listed in the order the dish should be made (e.g., the crust first, followed by the filling, followed by the topping). See Recipe Example: Presenting a recipe with subrecipes on page 192. For more on how to write the directions for a recipe with subrecipes, see page 203.

Optional Ingredients

To indicate that an ingredient is not necessary for the success of the recipe, place a comma after the ingredient and write optional after it, or put optional in parentheses after the ingredient in the list to indicate that it can be left out.

Ingredient list:

Oil-packed sun-dried tomatoes, drained and chopped (optional)

Referring to Another Recipe

If a recipe's ingredient list includes another recipe that is located elsewhere—on another page, in a different section, or online—include it in the ingredient list in the order it is needed. Note that recipe titles are capitalized, so list them as such in your ingredient list.

Ingredient list:

1 pound dried pasta

Kosher salt

Walnut Pesto* (recipe follows) ***OR*** (page 000) ***OR*** ***IF ONLINE*** [hyperlink]

Halibut with Radicchio and Fennel

By Raeanne Sarazen, MA, RDN

Preparation time: 25 minutes
Cooking time: 8 minutes
Yield: 6 servings

VINAIGRETTE

½ cup sherry wine vinegar
2 teaspoons fresh lemon juice
1 small shallot, minced (about 2 tablespoons)
½ teaspoon kosher salt
¼ teaspoon freshly ground black pepper
½ cup extra-virgin olive oil

SALAD

1 medium fennel bulb, cored, thinly sliced
   (about 3 cups)
1 large shallot, diced (about ½ cup)
½ cup pomegranate seeds
½ cup chopped mango
¼ head radicchio, shredded (about 1 cup)
2 tablespoons chopped fresh parsley
Juice of ½ lemon
2 tablespoons extra-virgin olive oil
¼ teaspoon kosher salt

FISH

2 tablespoons extra-virgin olive oil
6 (5-ounce) halibut fillets, 1 to 1¼ inches thick
Kosher salt

1. For the vinaigrette, whisk together the vinegar, lemon juice, shallot, salt, and pepper. Whisk in the olive oil. Adjust seasoning to taste. (Makes 1¼ cups.)

2. For the salad, toss the fennel, shallot, pomegranate seeds, mango, radicchio, and parsley in a bowl. Add the lemon juice, olive oil, and salt and stir to combine.

3. For the fish, heat the oil in a large nonstick sauté pan over high heat. Season both sides of the fish with salt. Add the fish to the pan and cook for 3 to 4 minutes on one side. Turn the fish over, lower the heat, and cook until just cooked through, another 2 to 5 minutes, depending on the thickness of the fish. The fish is done when a metal skewer easily inserts into the fish and, when left in for 5 seconds, feels warm when touched to the hand.

4. To serve, arrange the salad on plates or large platter. Place the fish on top of the salad and spoon desired amount of vinaigrette on top; serve hot. (Refrigerate remaining vinaigrette for later use.)

Nutrition per serving (4½ ounces cooked fish, 1 cup salad, 2 tablespoons vinaigrette): 360 calories, 23 grams total fat, 3 grams saturated fat, 265 milligrams sodium, 10 grams carbohydrate, 2 grams fiber, 7 grams total sugar, 27 grams protein

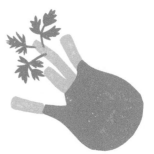

Quick Tip

"When writing recipes for a cookbook, keep in mind that publishers want consistent language. Check your ingredients lists, particularly. If you call for '1 large onion, chopped' in one recipe, don't write '1 cup chopped onion' in later recipes. Keep a style sheet so you can keep track of the language you've used." —Dianne Jacob, author, *Will Write for Food*

Ingredient Descriptions

Try to anticipate any questions that your reader may have about specific ingredients or substitutions. Remember, the more specifics you provide, the better.

Ingredient Type

If a certain type of an ingredient (e.g., salted butter) should be used, include the descriptor in the ingredient list. Some authors include information about their ingredient preferences or philosophies in the front matter of their cookbooks, but readers may miss it there.

> 1 cup (2 sticks) *salted* butter
> ¾ cup (62 grams) *superfine* almond flour
> 2 cups *whole* milk
> 1 cup packed *dark brown* sugar

For canned tomatoes, make sure to include information on whether they should be drained or not. When appropriate, note whether the tomatoes should be packed in juice or puree.

> 1 can (14½-ounce) diced tomatoes, drained
> 1 can (28 ounces) whole, peeled, plum tomatoes in puree

If a particular ingredient is easily confused with other types or varieties, be sure to point out clarifying details in the ingredient list.

> 2 tablespoons rice vinegar (not seasoned rice vinegar)
> 2 cups old-fashioned (rolled) oats (not instant oats)

Brand Names

Use the generic name of an ingredient whenever possible to allow for flexibility and personal preference. Include a specific ingredient brand or examples if you believe it matters or if a client requires it. Keep in mind that you can always list a specific product you prefer in the recipe headnote or in the ingredient list.

> 1 cup puffed rice cereal (such as Rice Krispies)

Substitutions

Specify ingredients that are readily accessible; if that's not possible, provide substitution suggestions. If the recipe requires a specific ingredient and you need space to explain why, do so in the headnote or in a note at the end of the recipe. Otherwise, provide a brief description in the ingredient list.

> 1 pound orecchiette or any shaped dried pasta, such as campagnola or farfalle
> 1 pound dried pinto beans or 5 (15- to 16-ounces) cans pinto beans, drained
> 2 large tomatoes, chopped, or 1 (16-ounces) can diced tomatoes, drained
> 2 tablespoons black soy sauce (or use 1 tablespoon balsamic vinegar and 1 tablespoon soy sauce)

Herbs and Spices

For spices, specify whether they should be whole or ground; for herbs, specify whether they should be fresh or dried, and provide suggestions for substitutions.

> 1 dried red chili pepper, broken into pieces, or ¼ teaspoon crushed red pepper
> 1 tablespoon fresh chopped sage leaves or 1 teaspoon dried sage

Quick Tip

"Terms like 'bittersweet' and 'semisweet' and 'dark' chocolate do not convey enough information in chocolate recipes. Make sure to call for a specific type of chocolate in the ingredient list. You may test a recipe using 70% bittersweet, but if the reader uses 60%, the results can be disastrous. The sugar and cocoa differences between 70% and 60% bittersweet are significant. The higher the cacao percentage, the less sugar and more dry cocoa in the chocolate. When any chocolate is melted and incorporated into a recipe, the sugar and dry cocoa in the chocolate interact with the other ingredients; any change of cacao percentage affects that interaction." —Alice Medrich, pastry chef and James Beard–Award-winning cookbook author

Ingredient List Amounts and Measurements

Associated Press (AP) Style, the style guide used by newspapers and magazines, and the Chicago Manual of Style (CMOS), which is generally used for cookbooks, both specify that measurements should be spelled out, with abbreviations used only when space constraints require them.

Best practices for listing amounts and measurements include:

- For clarity, spell out all measurements in the ingredient list. And if abbreviations must be used, periods are generally not included as the period could be misread as a stop in the sentence.

  1 teaspoon, **not** 1 tsp

- When two numbers appear next to each other, spell out the smaller number or enclose one of the numbers inside parentheses.

  One 3-inch cinnamon stick
  Makes 24 three-inch cookies
  Makes 1 (9-inch) double-layer cake

- Use the word "to" instead of an en dash or hyphen when indicating a range of ingredients, measurements, or time. Dashes and hyphens can be confusing.

  2 to 3 medium tomatoes, **not** 2–3 tomatoes

- When ingredient amounts do not equal an even quantity, list them as you would measure them, in the largest whole quantity first followed by smaller increments.

  ½ cup plus 3 tablespoons all-purpose flour, **not** 11 tablespoons all-purpose flour

- If a specific amount of water is required for a recipe, include it in the ingredient list. However, listing the quantities of water used to poach (such as chicken breasts or salmon) or boil (such as pasta, rice, or vegetables) foods is not necessary unless the publisher requires it to be included.

COMMON ABBREVIATIONS FOR UNITS OF MEASUREMENT IN RECIPES

Unit of measure	Abbreviation
teaspoon	t, tsp
tablespoon	T, tbsp
ounce	oz
pound	lb
cup	C, c
pint	pt
quart	qt
milliliter	mL, ml
liter	L, l
milligram	mg
gram	g
dozen	dz

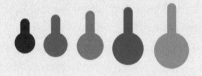

Descriptions of Ingredient Amounts

When it is important or helpful to do so, include an ingredient's size or descriptors in the ingredient list. If the size doesn't matter, it's best to give a range for the size and weight. The size or detailed descriptors can be included set off by a comma or placed in parentheses; whichever style you choose, remember to be consistent.

Fruits and vegetables Specify fruits and vegetables as small, medium, or large, and provide both a count and weight measurement.

  4 medium potatoes, peeled and quartered (about 2 pounds)

  1 large bunch broccoli, about 1½ pounds

  3 small globe eggplants, about 12 ounces each

Meat, poultry, fish, and seafood For meat, poultry, fish, and seafood, describe the piece of protein, its total weight, its weight by the piece, or a description of what to do with the piece.

>   1 beef tenderloin, 3½ to 4 pounds, silverskin trimmed
>
>   1 (4-rib) bone-in rib roast (about 10 pounds)
>
>   4 salmon fillets, about 6 ounces each
>
>   1 pound boneless, skinless chicken breast, cut into 1-inch cubes
>
>   16 cherrystone clams

Eggs For clarity, especially with baking recipes, include the size of the eggs in the ingredient list. Most recipes use large eggs, so eggs are presumed to be large unless otherwise specified.

>   2 eggs *(fine if savory recipe)* or
>
>   2 large eggs *(best if baking recipe)*
>
>   1 extra-large egg

Butter If a recipe uses 4 tablespoons (½ stick) or more of butter, include the stick amount.

>   3 tablespoons unsalted butter, melted
>
>   1 cup (2 sticks) unsalted butter

Milk When including milk or a milk alternative in an ingredient list, be sure to specify the type (e.g., whole, 2% [reduced-fat], 1% [low-fat], nonfat, soy, almond).

Cheese When listing grated or shredded cheese, include the weight and a conventional measurement.

>   8 ounces shredded mozzarella cheese (about 2 cups)
>
>   1 cup grated Parmigiano-Reggiano cheese* (about 4 ounces)

* When calling for "Parmesan," know that Parmesan cheese indicates a non-Italian version (which can be made anywhere) whereas "Parmigiano-Reggiano" is always produced in Italy.

Salt Whenever possible, specify the ideal type and amount of salt to use, as it is helpful guidance for the cook and also important to the accuracy of the nutrition analysis. The phrase "½ teaspoon kosher salt, plus more to taste" is much more useful than "salt, to taste."

Packaged products For packaged products, provide both an amount and a weight measurement. Keep in mind that manufacturers change package sizes often, so it's always wise to check online before you try to recall the package size from memory. Whenever possible, use the entire package or can of an ingredient in a recipe (e.g., chicken broth and other canned products). If the package contains more than what is needed for the recipe, use the headnote or a note at the end of the recipe to suggest uses for the remainder of the ingredient.

If the specific size is very important, provide it, but if not, offer a range.

>   1 (5-ounce) bag spinach leaves
>
>   One (5- to 9-ounce) bag spinach leaves

When canned ingredients are mentioned, list the number of cans first and then decide where to place the weight of the cans and whether to use parentheses. Whichever way you decide, be consistent.

>   2 cans (14.5 ounces each) chicken broth
>
>   2 (14.5-ounce) cans chicken broth
>
>   3 cans (14- to 16-ounce each) white beans, drained and rinsed

US Customary and Metric Measurements

Many publishers now ask recipe writers to include both US customary (e.g., tablespoons, cups, pounds, ounces) and metric (e.g., grams, liters) measurements in their recipes. Including both increases the global market for the recipes, as most people worldwide use the metric system, and it also allows all cooks to follow the recipe more precisely. As an added bonus, providing both measurements allows the recipe to be scaled up or down more easily. While many American cooks still measure ingredients by volume, providing the weights of ingredients is recommended, especially for baking recipes, which requires precision. The availability of metric measurements of ingredients can also make the recipe's nutrient analysis more accurate as well.

If your client or publisher specifies that your recipes should include both US customary and metric measurements, be sure to follow their style guidelines. Pay attention to their rounding rules, such as whether they want exact measures or cleaner, rounded numbers (e.g., 28.5 grams or 30 grams).

If no style guidelines are available, use these general rules:

- If the ingredient is a liquid, provide its metric measurement in milliliters or liters.

  ¼ cup (60 milliliters) olive oil, ***not*** ¼ cup (32 grams) olive oil

- Use teaspoons and tablespoons for amounts less than ¼ cup, which equals 4 tablespoons. Metric measurements are not generally used for small amounts.

  3 tablespoons finely grated fresh ginger, ***not*** 3 tablespoons (6 grams) finely grated fresh ginger

  2 teaspoons olive oil, ***not*** 2 teaspoons olive oil, (9 grams) olive oil

When including both US customary and metric measures in an ingredient list, make the layout as user friendly as possible. Keeping the list in an easy-to-read format is important; it shouldn't seem intimidating to the reader. Separate the measurements using brackets, columns, or even different colors (consult your recipe editor or designer for guidance). Following are a few suggestions for placement of US customary and metric measurements:

  1 cup/180 grams quinoa

  1 (½-inch [1.25 centimeter]) piece fresh ginger, peeled and coarsely chopped

  1 pound (455 grams) top sirloin

  3¾ cups | 450 grams coarsely chopped walnuts

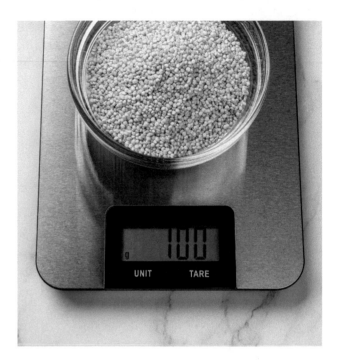

Quick Tip

"**Make your own personal list of weights and measures for commonly used ingredients, and then refer to this list for every project to avoid making mistakes. However, your publisher or client may have a required list that they have approved. This is especially true of cookbook publishers who want consistent measurements and weights across their catalogue. Do not depend on online sources for the final word, as they rarely agree, especially when it comes to flour weights and measures.**" —Rick Rodgers, cookbook author and recipe developer

Using a kitchen scale If you are required to provide both US customary and metric measurements in a recipe, the preferred method is to use a kitchen scale throughout the development process and document weight measurements at the time you are developing and testing the recipe. If you wait to convert the ingredients at a later time, the weight measurements will be less accurate. Volume-to-weight equivalency tables are not absolute; the volume measurement of an ingredient can fluctuate depending on how the measuring cup or spoon is packed (e.g., sifting, spooning, or dipping the ingredient affects its compressibility) and on the ingredient itself (e.g., how it is cut or milled, its density, its water content).

If it's not possible to document the weight measurements during development or testing, create and reference your own volume-to-metric equivalency chart, or use one developed by other culinary professionals. One option, for example, is using the appendix Common Ingredient Equivalencies and Conversions on page 349 for the volume and weight equivalents of frequently used recipe ingredients. FoodData Central (fdc.nal.usda.gov) is also a helpful site for finding volume and metric weight equivalents. Provide the conversion chart you use to the publisher to maintain consistency.

MEASURING VOLUME AND WEIGHT ACCURATELY

In addition to providing ingredients in US customary and metric measures, it's important to know how to use volume or weight measurements in recipe development, writing, and testing.

Weight

Weighing is the most accurate way to measure dry, solid, and semisolid ingredients (e.g., sour cream) and viscous liquids (e.g., honey). The advantage of weighing is that neither the variable moisture content of the ingredient nor how the ingredient is added to the bowl matters. When weighing ingredients, follow these guidelines:

- Place a bowl on the kitchen scale and press the "zero" or "tare" button. This accounts for the weight of the bowl and sets the scale back to zero. Add the first ingredient to the bowl in small increments until it reaches the desired weight in grams or ounces. When weighing multiple ingredients in the same bowl, zero out the scale each time you add an ingredient.

- When testing recipes or converting volume measurements to weight, document the weights either exactly (e.g., 112 g, 3.8 ounces) or rounded off (e.g., to the nearest whole number for ounces or to the nearest 5 or 10 for gram weights) based on the editor or publisher's guidelines.

Volume

Volume is a measure of how much space something takes up. Liquid ingredients measure at a consistent volume when using a liquid measuring cup. Some recipes—especially professional baking recipes—use gram weights for liquid ingredients instead of volume in milliliters because it makes it easier to measure all ingredients in a single bowl and also makes it easier to scale recipes up or down.

How to use liquid measuring cups: Place a liquid measuring cup on a stable, flat surface. Pour in the liquid until it reaches just below the desired measurement in cups, fluid ounces, or milliliters. Slowly add more of the liquid until the bottom of the meniscus (the concave surface of the liquid created by the surface tension) reaches the desired line.

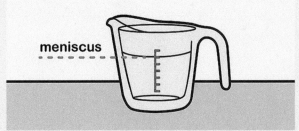

How to use dry measuring cups: To measure dry (e.g., flour, sugar) or semisolid ingredients (e.g., mayonnaise, nut butter) by volume, pour or spoon the ingredient into a dry measuring cup. These measures can vary in weight based on many factors, including the ingredient's moisture content and how it is scooped or poured into the measuring cup; this is especially true for flour, depending on the method used.

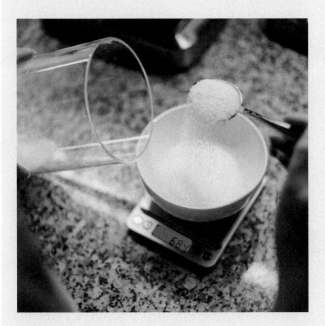

HOW TO MEASURE FLOUR

Measuring flour: In recipe writing, it's important to include a preferred measurement method for measuring flour in a recipe or a cookbook introduction and then consistently use the chosen method. A cup of all-purpose flour can weigh anywhere from 120 to 170 g, depending on the measurement method used. This discrepancy can make a difference in how baked goods turn out. (See the appendix Common Ingredient Equivalencies and Conversions on page 349.) For readers who prefer to use measuring cups for flour, one of the following methods should be described:

- **Spoon-and-sweep method** (recommended to lessen the risk of compacting the flour): Start by stirring the flour to loosen its naturally compact state. Spoon the flour into a measuring cup until heaping. Use a flat side of the knife or spoon handle to level off the flour so it's flush with the top of the measuring cup.
- **Dip-and-sweep method** (used most often by home cooks): Start by stirring the flour to loosen its naturally compact state. Gently dip the measuring cup into the flour, overfilling the cup. Use a flat side of a knife or the handle of a spoon to level off the flour so it's flush with the top of the measuring cup.

Spoon-and-sweep method   Dip-and-sweep method

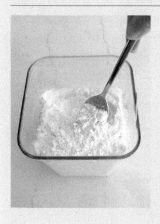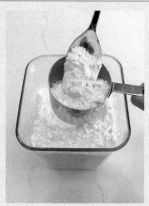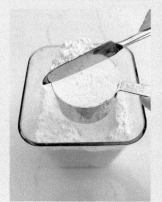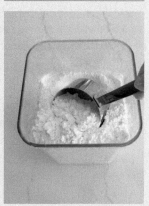

CLARIFYING OUNCES AS WEIGHT VERSUS VOLUME

Listing ingredient amounts in ounces can be confusing, since the term is used to denote both weight (weight ounces) and volume (fluid ounces) measurements. For example, if an ingredient list includes 4 ounces coconut flakes, the cook may question whether it should be measured in a ½-cup dry measuring cup (a volume measurement) or 4 ounces (a weight measurement) on a kitchen scale.

If the quantity of a **dry or semisolid ingredient** (e.g., coconut flakes, cookie crumbs, flour, rice, oats, chocolate chips) is listed in ounces, it is a unit of weight and should be measured using a scale. Metric measurements are listed in grams or milligrams.

If the quantity of a **liquid ingredient** (e.g., broth, water, milk, cream, oil) is listed in ounces, it is a unit of volume (fluid ounces) and should be measured using a liquid measuring cup. Metric measurements are listed in liters or milliliters.

Ingredient List Preparation Instructions

Assembling prepped ingredients before starting the cooking process—known as mise en place—is a streamlined practice to organize the cooking process.

If the preparation of an ingredient is straightforward and simple (e.g., chopped, drained), or helps the cook plan accordingly, include it in the ingredient list.

3 medium yellow onions, diced

1 large cauliflower, about 1½ pounds, broken into florets

1 tablespoon capers, drained

1 (9-ounce) box frozen chopped spinach, thawed

8 tablespoons (1 stick) unsalted butter, softened

Always use the correct culinary terms and understand their meaning. For example, while the terms "chop" and "dice" are often used interchangeably, they mean different things. Chop is a more casual term, while dice is more specific. Different-sized ingredients take different amounts of time to cook, which ultimately affects the final overall taste, texture, and visual appearance of the dish (see Culinary Terms for Recipe Writing on page 204 for definitions).

Indicating Order of Preparation

Preparation instructions for individual ingredients must be written in the appropriate order for clarity and accuracy. Everything that goes after a comma is a task the cook will perform after the ingredient is measured, and where you place the commas makes a difference!

5 large pears, peeled, cored, and chopped

1 large butternut squash, halved, seeds removed

1 pound Italian sausage, casings removed

The order of preparation instructions is important, especially when the overall amount changes based on how the ingredient is handled. Consider the following example.

1 cup walnuts, chopped

This instruction indicates that the cook should fill a dry 1-cup measure with whole walnuts and then chop them up.

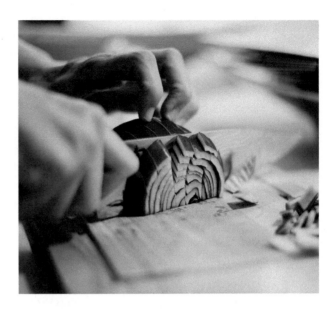

Now, consider this example:

1 cup chopped walnuts

This instruction indicates that the dry 1-cup measure should be filled with walnuts that have already been chopped. The prechopped walnuts will be a larger quantity than the whole walnuts that were chopped after being measured. The recipe editor should clarify with the recipe developer which amount is needed.

The same applies to any ingredient that requires dicing or mincing.

½ cup minced fresh cilantro

½ cup fresh cilantro leaves, minced

The ½ cup minced fresh cilantro will yield a larger quantity than the ½ cup fresh cilantro leaves, minced. See Writing Ingredient Instructions on page 200, for additional examples.

Complex Preparation Instructions

When preparation instructions for an ingredient become more complicated, they should be moved to the recipe directions or should be included in a note or an asterisk at the end of the recipe (another option is to reference preparation instructions that appear elsewhere in the publication, such as on a different page).

½ cup pine nuts, toasted (see note)

1 cup plain dried breadcrumbs*

4 large tomatoes, peeled, seeded, and chopped (see page 000)

No: 5 chopped medium carrots
Yes: 5 medium carrots, chopped

Why: *The instruction "5 carrots, chopped," clearly tells the reader what to do after gathering the carrots, but "5 chopped carrots" would give a reader pause due to its lack of clarity.*

No: 2 cups cooked chicken, shredded
Yes: 2 cups (5 ounces) cooked shredded chicken

Why: *The instruction "2 cups chicken, shredded" suggests measuring whole pieces of cooked chicken and then shredding it. This instruction is unclear. How is the chicken measured before shredding? Is it chopped? And how does a cook measure a whole piece of chicken in a measuring cup? Alternatively, "2 cups (5 ounces) cooked shredded chicken" explains to the reader that the cooked, shredded chicken must be measured in a dry measuring cup and can also be checked by weighing it on a kitchen scale.*

No: 3 tablespoons melted butter
Yes: 3 tablespoons butter, melted

Why: *The instruction "3 tablespoons melted butter" suggests that the reader should melt a larger quantity of butter and then measure out 3 tablespoons, which is inefficient. Alternatively, "3 tablespoons butter, melted" tells the reader to measure out 3 tablespoons of stick butter and then melt it.*

No: 1 cup chopped apples
Yes: 1 apple, peeled, cored, and chopped

Why: *Provide the whole ingredient amount when possible since this is what the reader buys at the store. Also, "1 apple, peeled, cored, and chopped" clarifies the order of preparation (peel the apple first, then core it, and finally, chop it). In "1 cup chopped apples," is the apple peeled? It's unclear.*

No: 1 (1-inch) piece fresh ginger, minced
Yes: 1 (1-inch) piece fresh ginger, peeled, minced (about 1 tablespoon)

Why: *If it's unclear whether the reader will have the knowledge needed to prepare a particular ingredient, be sure to include the details. Not everyone knows that fresh ginger should be peeled, so instead provide the clearer direction. It's not necessary to include peeling instructions for more common ingredients, such as onion or garlic, unless the recipe's target audience is people with little or no cooking experience.*

Be precise

1 cup sifted all-purpose flour
1 cup all-purpose flour, sifted

The placement of the word "sifted" is important. One cup sifted flour means the flour will be sifted first, before measuring. One cup flour, sifted means measuring the flour first, and then sifting it into a bowl. Flour sifted before measuring weighs much less than a cup of flour sifted after measuring—and this difference can make a big impact on the texture of baked goods. Be sure to specify exactly how the flour is measured and when (or if) it should be sifted.

1 cup whipping cream
1 cup whipping cream, whipped
1 cup whipped cream

These ingredients all describe different ingredients, quantities, or preparation so be sure to specify exactly what should be used.

Ingredient List Grammar and Style Rules

No ingredient amount When no amount is specified for an ingredient in the ingredient list, capitalize the ingredient's name or the first word of the ingredient description.

> Flour, for dredging
>
> Kosher salt, to taste
>
> Freshly ground black pepper, to taste

Two numbers next to each other When two numbers are listed next to each other in an ingredient entry, use parentheses or write out the first number in the ingredient list; no matter which style you choose, always be consistent.

> **No:** 2 7-ounce cans tuna
> **Yes:** 2 (7-ounce) cans tuna
>
> **No:** Two seven-ounce cans tuna
> **Yes:** 2 cans (7 ounces each) tuna

"To taste" phrase Some will argue that the characterization "to taste" should be considered an amount and should be included with the ingredients in the ingredient list; others believe it's merely a suggestion of how much to use, so it belongs in the recipe's directions. (And remember, specifying exact amounts is helpful to less experienced cooks, and for all those who don't know what "season to taste" is supposed to taste like.) Regardless, it is important that "to taste" should never be mentioned in both the ingredient list *and* the directions. Pick one or the other and be consistent.

> **Ingredient list:** Crushed red pepper
> **Directions:** Season to taste with the red pepper.
>
> **Ingredient list:** ½ to 1 teaspoon crushed red pepper
> **Directions:** Stir in the red pepper to taste.
>
> **Ingredient list:** Crushed red pepper, to taste
> **Directions:** Stir in the red pepper.

Repeated ingredients and phrases Be consistent with your characterization of a particular ingredient or repeated phrase throughout all the recipes contained in a particular project. Use the find and replace tools in word processing software to search for and identify each instance. Common inconsistencies that should be checked for include:

- olive oil/extra-virgin olive oil
- vegetable oil/canola oil
- heavy cream/heavy whipping cream
- salt/kosher salt
- eggs/large eggs

Quick Tip

"Recipe writing has evolved over time. Between 1800–1900s, recipe writers assumed everyone owned a bowl . . . and so no bowl is mentioned in a recipe direction. However, the further away we come from knowing how to cook, the more detail and direction is needed. I like to write the way I speak. No one talks like, 'In a medium bowl, combine . . . ' The goal is to be as succinct, complete, and clear as possible."

—Bonnie Benwick, former deputy food editor, *The Washington Post*

Quick Tip

"Some recipe writers today may put a bit 'too much of themselves' into the recipe, making it fun to read but hard to follow if you actually want to cook it. It's important to find a balance." —Carol Haddix, former food editor, *Chicago Tribune*

The Recipe Directions

There are no hard-and-fast rules for writing recipe directions, but recipe writing is similar to the act of teaching. Therefore, you should always try to put yourself in the shoes of a home cook who is not familiar with the recipe's ingredients, equipment, and preparation and cooking techniques. As you write the recipe's directions, anticipate what your readers will need to understand in each step and offer the same kind of useful and descriptive guidance you would provide if you were standing by their side in the kitchen.

Writing Style

Recipe directions can be presented in various styles. Sometimes, the style is specified by the publisher, editor, or client, or it may be left up to the recipe writer to decide. Either way, it's important to be consistent.

When recipes are edited, opinions may differ on how to best present the instructions. For example, when beginning a sentence in the recipe directions, some firmly believe that the equipment used should start the sentence (e.g., "In a medium bowl, combine the flour, salt, and sugar") and others believe a verb should always come at the beginning (e.g., "Combine the flour, salt, and sugar in a medium bowl."). Sometimes, it can be a matter of length. For example, with a long list of ingredients, it might be clearer to put the equipment first so that the reader knows what you are talking about.

Opinions, or choice of style, also differ as to whether recipe directions should include articles (e.g., a, an, the). For example, "Heat in medium saucepan" or "Heat in *a* medium saucepan." With cookbooks, it's more likely to include articles, whereas in magazines, and other places with space constraints, they are often left out. Some publishers or editors also differ on whether a comma should be used before the "and" or "or" in a list of three or more things, which is known as the serial or Oxford comma (e.g., mix the flour, sugar, and salt). *The Chicago Manual of Style* recommends it, but *Associated Press Stylebook* is vague about it, saying that the final comma should be used only if leaving it out would lead to confusion. This is a style choice; again, follow the guidelines of your publisher or editor or choose one method and be consistent. See more about Oxford commas and use of articles in Grammar and Punctuation for Recipe Directions on page 206.

The writer's voice is important. No one wants to read a boring recipe—especially nowadays when food is considered a form of entertainment. Yet it's also true that no one wants to read a confusing recipe. The recipe's context and its audience should drive the amount of detail and personality to include in the recipe directions, with the focus always placed on making those directions as clear and helpful as possible.

Style for the Recipe Steps

The recipe steps (another word for the directions) should be listed preceded by numbers or in a simple paragraph format. Either is appropriate, but each has its own pros and cons. Sometimes the publisher may decide, or the design of the book may influence this decision. Either way, choose one style, and be consistent.

Numbered steps Some writers believe that providing numbered steps gives the recipe a sense of order and that they help cooks keep track of where they are in the recipe.

Paragraph steps Some writers believe that skipping numbers and separating steps into paragraphs, with a space between each, makes the recipe seem more like a narrative and gives it a personal feel. Another option that can help readers is to capitalize or bold action verbs in the steps (e.g., "STIR together the flour, baking powder, and salt," "**Blend** the sugar and eggs . . . ").

Quick Tip

"I like numbered steps when the recipe is friendly and easy. Four steps work great as an organizing principle. When a recipe exceeds five or six numbered steps, using numbered steps can look daunting." —Sarah Billingsley, Executive Editor, Chronicle Books

Order of Recipe Directions

If there is one indisputable rule of recipe writing, it's that recipe directions should be written using the ingredients in the order they appear in the ingredient list. Likewise, the recipe directions must start by describing what the home cook has to do before cooking actually begins.

> Place the oven rack in the middle position and preheat the oven to 375° F.
>
> Grease a 9-inch loaf pan with butter and dust it with flour; set aside.

Heating directions are also of critical importance, as there must be enough time for the oven to heat or the water to boil. (It takes about 10 minutes to heat a large pot of water to a boil and 15 to 20 minutes to heat an oven to temperature.) Make sure that instructions such as "Preheat the oven . . . " and "Bring the water to a boil . . . " are located in the most logical place in the recipe directions. In some cases, oven heating instructions come at the very beginning of a recipe.

> Preheat the oven to 375° F. Combine the flour, baking powder, and salt . . .

In other recipes, a good bit of time passes between steps or stages, and it's best to place preheating instructions later in the directions just before it must be ready.

> Refrigerate the cookie dough for about 1 hour or longer.
>
> About 20 minutes before you're ready to bake the cookies, preheat the oven to 375° F.

Sentence Structure for Recipe Directions

Unlike other forms of writing, it is not always necessary to write recipe directions in complete sentences, but recipe directions should always be written as clearly and concisely as possible, and they should be written in the active voice. Avoid the passive voice as much as possible.

> **No:** After the fillets are dipped in flour, the excess should be shaken off. *(passive voice)*
>
> **Yes:** Dip each fillet in flour and shake off the excess. *(active voice)*

Sentences in recipe directions can begin in two different ways—with a description of the equipment used or with an action verb.

> **Description of the equipment used:** "In a medium bowl, beat the egg whites until stiff peaks form."
>
> **Action verb:** "Beat the egg whites in a medium bowl until stiff peaks form."

If space allows, add as much detail as possible, including a description of utensils or the desired appearance of the ingredients.

> Using a hand-held electric mixer set on medium speed, beat the egg whites in a clean medium bowl until foamy. Increase the speed to high and continue beating until they form stiff peaks.

Providing Subhead Directions

When a recipe has several subrecipes (e.g., a pie recipe that includes a recipe for the crust, the filling, and the topping), start the first step of each recipe with a directional phrase to orient the reader.

> To make the filling, stir together the condensed milk, sugar, and vanilla.
>
> To make the crust, pulse the flour, sugar, and salt in a food processor fitted with the metal blade.

Consistent Word Usage

When the same task is repeated twice in a recipe, use the same descriptive words for the task. For example, if an early step says, "Beat two of the eggs . . . " don't say later in the recipe, "Whisk the remaining eggs . . ." Stick with the same verb.

Likewise, when multiple terms can be used to describe the same item, be sure to use the same terms (whether it is a piece of equipment or an ingredient) throughout a recipe project. Decide which terms you prefer to use (e.g., confectioners' sugar or powdered sugar; Italian parsley or flat-leaf parsley; scallion or green onion; red pepper flakes or crushed red pepper) in your recipes and be consistent.

CULINARY TERMS FOR RECIPE WRITING

Many culinary terms have specific definitions and should be used accurately in recipes. If a word is unclear but central to the recipe, consider providing a definition of it in the recipe headnote. Most important, be consistent and clear with your choice of words when writing recipes.

Preparing

Listed from smallest to largest size.

Grate: Cut into tiny particles using small holes of grater or Microplane.

Mince: Cut into pieces that are random in shape and very tiny but are still discernible pieces (not mashed or pureed).

Finely chop: Cut into pieces that are random in shape and ⅛ to ¼ inch (3 mm to 0.5 cm) in size.

Dice: Cut into uniform cubes that are about ¼ to ¾ inch (0.5 to 1.5 cm) in size.

Cube: Cut into uniform cubes that are about ½ to 1 inch (1 to 2.5 cm) in size. (Only use this term for food that can actually be cut into cubes, like potatoes, not onions.)

Julienne: Cut into thin strips, matchstick-like pieces about ⅛ inch thick by 2 to 3 inches long (0.3 by 5 to 7.5 cm) in size.

Shred: Cut into thin pieces or slices using a fork, knife, hands, large holes of grater, or food processor.

Chop: Cut into pieces that are random in shape and ½ to ¾ inch (1 to 2 cm) in size.

Coarsely chop: Cut into pieces that are random in shape and ¾ to 1 inch (2 to 2.5 cm) in size.

Thinly slice: Cut into ⅛-inch thickness. (Suggest using a mandoline for paper-thin/ 1/16-inch slices.)

Slice: Cut into broad pieces of even thickness, as desirable, or on the bias (knife angle about 45 degrees).

Cut into chunks or pieces: Cut into larger pieces of no specific shape or size, but usually referring to 1½ to 2 inches in size.

Combining

Listed from gentlest to most vigorous methods.

Toss: Tumble ingredients with a lifting motion using hands or other utensil (e.g., tongs).

Fold: Gently combine two or more ingredients, usually with a rubber spatula, to create a uniform mixture. Usually done in two motions vertically through mixture and then across the bottom of the bowl and up the sides.

Cut in: Distribute solid fat, usually butter, into dry ingredients by using knives or a pastry blender.

Stir: Move ingredients, using a spoon or rubber spatula, in a repeated motion to combine ingredients together until a uniform consistency, or keep them moving so they do not burn if heating.

Mix: Combine in any way that distributes all ingredients evenly.

Combine: Mix two ingredients together. (Or, put all ingredients together and then mix.)

Knead: Press, fold, and stretch a dough using either your hands or the dough hook on an electric mixer.

Blend: Mix ingredients with a blender until they form a homogeneous, smooth, and uniform mixture.

Whisk: Use a wire whisk to combine ingredients or incorporate air into a mixture.

Cream : Combine sugar and a solid fat (such as butter) into a uniform mixture until smooth, light, and fluffy. Generally used in baking recipes (e.g., sugar is evenly dispersed in the fat for cookies and cakes).

Beat: Vigorously stir ingredients with a spoon, whisk, or electric mixer. Beating is generally done to incorporate air into a mixture or to develop gluten.

BOX CONTINUES >

Whip: Use a wire whisk or an electric mixer to vigorously beat ingredients, generally to incorporate air, as with egg whites and heavy cream.

Puree: Blend or process ingredients, using a blender or food processor, until they form a smooth, homogeneous mixture.

Cooking

Sauté: Cook quickly in fat over heat that can range from medium to medium-high to high.

Brown: Cook food until it changes color, usually in a small amount of fat over medium to high heat.

Caramelize: Cook to brown the sugars naturally found in fruits and vegetables until the food is the color of light or dark caramel. (Sugar by itself can be caramelized, e.g., caramel sauce.)

Bake: Cook, either covered or uncovered, in dry heat (usually between 300° F and 375° F).

Roast: Cook, uncovered, in hot (400° F or higher), dry heat, as in the oven or over an open fire. Roasting creates a browned and flavorful exterior.

Broil: Cook food directly under a heat source—traditionally done with broil setting in oven or toaster oven.

Steam: Cook food above, not in, water that is boiling or hot enough to produce steam.

Poach: Cook food submerged in liquid at a low simmer.

Braise: Cook slowly, covered, in moist heat, either in the oven or on top of the stove. Food does not need to be completely covered in liquid.

Simmer: Cook a liquid, or a food in a liquid, so that small bubbles break the surface at a slow but constant pace with the burner turned down as low as it will go.

Boil gently: Cook a liquid or a food in a liquid so that larger bubbles break the surface at a moderate pace. If stirred, bubbles will subside slightly, then resume as soon as stirring stops. Soups and stews are good examples of boiling gently.

Boil: Cook a liquid, or a food in a liquid, until bubbles rise continuously and break the surface at a rapid pace. Water for cooking pasta and grains are good examples of boiling.

Other

Drain: Remove liquid from a solid; a strainer or colander can be used to drain liquid from food (e.g., drain cooked pasta; drain juice from canned tomatoes).

Strain: Remove solids from a liquid; a porous (cheesecloth) or perforated device (strainer) can be used to separate out any solid or undesirable matter. Or, to press soft foods through the holes of a sieve, leaving a puree (e.g., strain stock).

Let stand or let sit: Cool food (or allow food to set) at room temperature before cutting or serving.

Chill: Place food inside the refrigerator until it gets cold.

Marinate: Soak foods in a seasoned, often acidic, liquid before cooking.

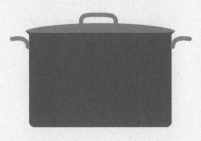

Using Descriptive Language

In recipe directions, it's best to describe the action versus using culinary terms. In most cases, a simple culinary term is appropriate (e.g., "mix," "stir"), but sometimes, the proper term is less familiar to most home cooks. When this occurs, be sure to provide clear instructions.

No: Deglaze the pan with wine.

Yes: Add the wine and stir to scrape up the browned bits from the bottom of the pan.

No: Reduce the balsamic vinegar.

Yes: Cook the balsamic vinegar over medium heat until it reduces by half.

No: Marinate chicken overnight. (This suggests that the chicken is then cooked first thing in the morning.)

Yes: Marinate the chicken in the refrigerator for 8 to 12 hours.

No: Dredge the chicken pieces in the flour.

Yes: Roll the chicken pieces in the flour until they are completely coated on all sides. Shake off the excess.

Be sure to always use the proper culinary term to describe the action, whether it's drain, strain, sauté, braise, or roast. (See Culinary Terms for Recipe Writing on page 204 for more information.)

Quick Tip

"If an item is set aside early in the recipe ('Set the chocolate aside to cool until it is tepid, but still liquid' or 'Set the breadcrumbs aside and cool completely'), make yourself a note to be sure it gets added to the recipe! It is an easy mistake to make, and even the best copy editors miss adding the 'set aside' ingredient to the recipe later, too." —Rick Rodgers, cookbook author and recipe developer

Grammar and Punctuation for Recipe Directions

Commas Depending on which style you or your publisher prefers, use the Oxford or serial comma (a comma placed before the "and" or "or" in a list of three or more things) or don't, and be consistent with your choice.

No Oxford comma: Add the remaining olive oil, onion and pepper to the pot.

Oxford comma: Add the flour, sugar, baking powder, and salt.

Articles (a, an, and the) Decide whether or not you will use them, and then be consistent. If space allows for their addition, articles make a recipe easier to read. The vast majority of cookbooks include articles for the ingredients in the directions; publications and publishing platforms that have more space constraints often do without articles.

No articles: Heat oil in large skillet.

Articles: Heat the oil in *a* large skillet.

No articles: Combine chicken, thyme, and garlic in 9-inch × 13-inch baking dish.

Articles: Arrange the chicken in a single layer in *a* 9-inch × 13-inch baking dish; sprinkle with the thyme and garlic.

Hyphens Be consistent in how you use hyphens throughout a recipe project. Use hyphens when compound adjectives are used to describe a noun (e.g., one 4-pound beef tenderloin; 1 bunch flat-leaf parsley). Following are several acceptable examples of hyphen usage to describe the same baking dish:

9 × 13-inch baking dish
9-by-13-inch baking dish
9-inch by 13-inch baking dish

Quick Tip

"When thinking about recipes for a cookbook proposal, try for as many different styles as possible: different lengths, cooking methods, technique, ingredients, spices, etc., to show your range." —Dianne Jacob, author, *Will Write for Food*

Equipment Instructions

Recommendations or suggestions for equipment or pans should be included in recipe directions. Some recipes require cookware or bakeware in a specific size, material, and dimensions or a specific kitchen tool or appliance. If it isn't necessary to have an exact match, suggest different choices, as guidance on cookware and bakeware helps home cooks replicate the recipe successfully. For example, if a recipe is written with instructions for using a rice cooker, include a note for a stovetop option for preparing the rice. Basic descriptions for cookware and bakeware in recipe directions should include:

- **Size:** small, medium, or large (provide exact size if necessary)

  Examples: medium skillet, 2-quart casserole dish, 8-quart stockpot

- **Dimensions, type, and shape:** square, round, or rectangular; shallow or deep

  Examples: casserole, Dutch oven, 8-inch square pan, or 9-inch × 13-inch baking dish

- **Material (if it makes a difference):** nonstick, copper, cast iron, glass, ovenproof

Avoid using an exact pan size unless it makes a difference in the recipe (see page 212 for common pan sizes).

> Heat ½ cup of the oil in a deep-sided skillet over medium-high heat.
>
> Heat the oil in a large nonstick skillet over medium-high heat until it is very hot but not smoking. Add the fish and cook . . .
>
> Transfer the pasta mixture to a 9 × 13-inch ovenproof baking dish.
>
> Transfer the cooked meat and vegetables into a 9-inch deep-dish pie pan or an 8- or 9-inch square baking dish.
>
> Divide the batter between six 6-ounce ramekins and chill for at least 4 hours.

Make note of how cookware is sold in stores and online and use similar terminology when describing the baking dish or pan size required for the recipe. For example, an instruction to use a "4-quart casserole" leaves questions in the reader's mind: Should it be shallow or deep? What are its dimensions? For more details, refer to Kitchen Equipment Used in Recipes on page 210.

Avoid suggesting a specific brand of equipment unless the recipe is for an equipment manufacturer. If the recipe has a direction to use an expensive piece of equipment that not every kitchen has on hand (e.g., a stand mixer or food processor), provide alternative instructions (e.g., using a hand mixer, a blender, a box grater) alongside it.

Additional Helpful Recipe Instructions

Recipe directions must always be detailed, descriptive, clear, and succinct—no matter how obvious an instruction may seem to the recipe writer. While what is helpful to one cook may seem obvious to the next, it's best to err on the side of providing more information than less, especially if no word count or space constraints are involved. For example, if a recipe calls for blind baking pie crust before the filling is added, make sure to instruct the reader to line the unbaked pie crust with aluminum foil or parchment paper before adding the pie weights or dried beans before baking.

Stovetop Directions

Each instruction that involves cooking on a stove top must also indicate the correct temperature level, and if the temperature is changed during the cooking process, specifics on the level the temperature should be raised or lowered should be included as well.

> Heat 2 tablespoons of the oil in a large skillet over **medium-high heat.** Add the onion and salt and cook, stirring occasionally, until the onion is lightly browned and softened, about 5 minutes. Reduce the heat to **medium-low** and continue cooking, stirring occasionally, until the onion is dark brown and caramelized, about 30 minutes.
>
> Heat the mixture to a boil. Reduce the heat to **low** and simmer for 6 to 8 minutes or until the vegetables are tender when pierced with a knife.

Doneness Directions

Several factors will affect cooking and baking times, such as the following:

- The size of the food being prepared (consider how much longer a large chicken breast takes to cook through than a small one)
- Differences in cooking equipment (e.g., size, material, brand)
- Variations with gas, induction, or electric stovetop; gas versus electric oven (often varies by brand as well)
- For grilling, cooking in the summer versus the winter and grill performance

For these reasons, it's important to help guide the reader through a recipe by clearly conveying visual cues about what the food should look like when it's done alongside estimated times. Food safety guidance and its relationship to doneness are important as well (see page 213 for more on food safety). **Both visual descriptions and cooking times should be included in the recipe instructions.**

> **No:** Bake the brownies for 40 minutes.
>
> **Yes:** Bake the brownies until the top is shiny and a wooden toothpick inserted in the center of the brownie comes out with a moist crumb, about 40 minutes.

> **No:** Cook chicken about 4 minutes.
>
> **Yes:** Cook chicken, turning halfway through cooking, until golden brown on both sides, about 4 minutes.

> **No:** Cook, stirring frequently, until the vegetables are tender.
>
> **Yes:** Cook, stirring frequently, until the vegetables are tender and just beginning to brown, 10 to 12 minutes.

Helpful Information in Recipe Directions

Extra helpful details After the recipe is written, read through the directions and think about what additional details should be added, including information that seems obvious or second nature.

> Allow the pancake batter to sit at room temperature for about 5 minutes before making the pancakes.

> Pour the pie filling into the baked and cooled pie crust.

> Remove and discard the bay leaf before serving.

> Heat an empty cast iron skillet over high heat before adding the oil.

> Heat the oil in a nonstick skillet over medium heat and then add the fish. (Be careful: heating a nonstick skillet while it's empty can damage the pan.)

When considering how much additional information to provide, think about details that could help the home cook avoid problems or challenges with the recipe.

> **No:** Puree soup in batches.
>
> **Yes:** Allow soup to cool slightly before pureeing. Working in batches, add enough soup to fill blender ½ to ¾ full and puree until smooth.

Make-ahead advice Give make-ahead advice whenever helpful. Tell the reader to what point a dish can be prepared ahead, how it should be stored, and how long it can be stored before finishing it.

> The vegetable mixture can be refrigerated up to 3 days. Reheat slowly in a saucepan, adding additional liquid (water or broth) as needed.

> Chill cake, uncovered, 1 hour or up to 8 hours to allow pudding layer to firm up.

> This soup can be frozen in freezer-safe containers for up to 3 months. When ready to use, defrost soup overnight in the refrigerator or run container under cool water.

Serving or storing information Provide helpful instructions on serving or storing cooked food at the end of the recipe.

> Cool pie completely, which may take up to 5 hours, then reheat slices or whole pie just slightly before serving. (Don't serve hot because juices will be too fluid.)

> Cookies will keep at room temperature in an airtight container for 4 to 5 days.

> Store leftover whoopee pies layered between sheets of wax paper or parchment in an airtight container at room temperature.

Notes and Sidebars in Recipe Directions

Notes or sidebars can be used to include important information that doesn't fit in the recipe's headnote, ingredient list, or directions. Notes and sidebars can be placed alongside a recipe or at its end, after the directions.

Tips for where to find unusual ingredients:

Ingredient list:
4 ounces guanciale, chopped (see Note)

Note: Guanciale (cured pork jowls) can be purchased at many specialty butchers and Italian delicatessens. Although guanciale (pronounced gwan-chi-ah-lay) has a stronger flavor, pancetta (cured pork belly) works well as a substitute.

Tips for ingredient substitution:

Ingredient list:
2 tablespoons butter (see Note)

Note: To make this recipe dairy-free, substitute vegetable or coconut oil for the butter. Unrefined coconut oil will produce a mild coconut flavor.

Explanation of a technique or short preparation instructions:

Ingredient list:
1 head garlic, roasted (see Note)

Note: Heat the oven to 425° F. Remove the outer layer of papery skin from the garlic and cut a ½-inch-thick slice from the top of the head. Place the garlic on foil and coat with 1 tablespoon olive oil; close and seal the foil. Roast until soft, about 40 minutes.

Alternative cooking instructions:

Note: If you don't have a grill, use your broiler. Set your oven rack about 4 inches from the heat source and turn on the broiler about 5 minutes before ready to use. Broil, turning once, until slightly charred, about 8 minutes total.

Using leftovers:

Note: You can dice up the leftover chicken and make a chicken tetrazzini casserole or thinly slice it for delicious panini.

Storing and reheating instructions:

Note: On serving day, remove the roasted fennel, shallots, and beans from the refrigerator and allow them to come to room temperature. Heat the oven to 400° F and line a baking sheet with nonstick aluminum foil or parchment paper. Spread the vegetables on the sheet, drizzle 2 tablespoons olive oil over them, and toss until well coated. Place in the oven until heated through, about 10 minutes, depending on the temperature of the vegetables.

Suggestions for beverage accompaniments:

Note: Start your Thanksgiving meal with a sparkling wine. It's an elegant choice that pairs well with turkey and stuffing!

KITCHEN EQUIPMENT USED IN RECIPES

It's important to indicate the proper type of prep tools, cookware, and appliances when writing recipes—especially when a specific finish or pan size affects the cooking or baking time or amount of liquid needed for the recipe. Whether or not conventional and/or metric sizes are stated will depend on your style guide.

Cutting and peeling

Cutting board: A durable surface most often made from wood or polypropylene; used for many kitchen prep tasks, from chopping vegetables to trimming meat

Chef's knife: 8- to 10-inch blade; for most kitchen prep tasks (chopping, slicing, dicing, mincing)

Paring knife: 3- to 4-inch blade; for peeling and slicing small fruits and vegetables

Bread knife: Long, serrated blade; to cut through bread and any other soft food with a tough crust or skin

Kitchen shears: For trimming poultry, snipping herbs, and opening packaged food

Grater (or Microplane): For zesting citrus fruits and grating cheese

Vegetable peeler: For peeling skin from firm fruits and vegetables

Silicone basting or pastry brush: For smoothly applying sauce, glaze, or melted butter on food. Heat-resistant silicone bristles make for easy cleaning

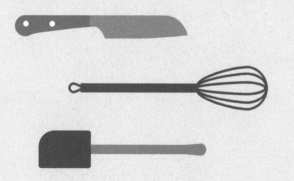

Combining and measuring

Measuring cups: ¼-, ⅓-, ½-, and 1-cup sizes for dry ingredients; 1-, 2-, and 4-cup sizes for liquid ingredients

Measuring spoons: ¼-teaspoon, ½-teaspoon, 1-teaspoon, and 1-tablespoon sizes

Mixing bowls: Small, medium, and large; typically glass or stainless steel

Tongs: For panfrying, sautéing, lifting, turning, tossing, and more

Large spoons: For mixing, combining, stirring, serving

Whisk: For eggs, whipped cream, mixing vinaigrettes, combining dry ingredients for baking, removing lumps from sauces and gravies

Rubber spatula: For scraping down bowls, folding, mixing

Spatula: For lifting, flipping, and removing food from cookware

Potato masher: For mashing potatoes (also a ricer and food mill, but both less commonly used)

Colander: For rinsing and draining hot or cold foods

Fine-mesh sieve/stainless-steel strainer: For straining stocks, soups, sauces; designed to fit over pots and mixing bowls

Hand mixer: For blending batters, mixing cookie doughs, beating egg whites

Stand mixer: Professional or high horsepower; for blending batters, mixing and kneading bread, mixing cookie doughs, beating egg whites; 3½- to 7-quart bowls; a variety of mixer attachments are available

BOX CONTINUES >

Immersion blender: Also known as a stick blender; for blending and pureeing food in the container it is being prepared in

Blender: 48- to 64-ounce; for smoothies, sauces, dips, soups, and more

Food processor: Mini (3½- to 5-cup) or regular (7- to 16-cup); for chopping and pureeing soups, pesto, salsa, nuts, breadcrumbs, vegetables, and more

Cookware

Skillet: Shallow pans with slanted sides, sometimes referred to as frying pans; often used for high heat, fast cooking and does not have a lid; available in nonstick; a deep skillet has higher sides than a typical skillet but still no lid

- small: 8-inch diameter
- medium: 10-inch diameter
- large: 12-inch diameter

Sauté pan: A pan with straight sides and a wide, flat bottom, usually deeper than a skillet; comes with a lid; performs better than a skillet for cooking sauces, braising meat, and shallow frying

- medium: 3-quart (10-inch diameter)
- large: 4- to 6-quart (11- to 14-inch diameter)

Cast-iron pan: Heavyweight cast iron with incredible heat retention; great for searing/browning; used on the stovetop and in the oven; sizes vary, but most common is 12 inches in diameter

Saucepan: Tall, deep, round pans with straight sides, a long handle, and a lid

- small: 1- to 3-quart (for sauces, steaming vegetables, cooking grains)
- medium: 4-quart
- large (saucepan or pot): 5- to 6½-quart (for boiling pasta)

Stockpot: Tall, deep, large pot with two handles and a lid; sizes range from 8- to 16-quart; 12-quart is a typical and good all-around size to cook broths, soups, sauces, lobsters, corn on the cob

Dutch oven: Oval or round enameled cast-iron pot

- mini: 1-cup
- small: 3- to 4-quart
- medium: 5- to 6-quart (great all-purpose size)
- large: 9-quart (for soups, stews, one-pot, slow cooking meals, etc.)

Casserole and baking dish: Oven-to-table glass or ceramic baking dishes (Food baked in glass baking dishes needs about a 25° F oven temperature decrease.)

Large casserole or baking dish: Sometimes known as a rectangular baking dish or baking pan; 13 × 9 × 2-inch (3½-quart/3.3 liters)

Small casserole or baking dish: Sometimes known as a square baking dish; 8 × 8 × 2-inch (2-quart/1.9 liters); or 9 × 9 × 2-inch (2½-quart/2.4 liters)

Oval or round casserole or baking dish: Variety of baking dish and casserole sizes available (usually a deep dish with high edges); typical sizes:

- 1-quart (0.95 liters)
- 1½-quart (1.5 liters)
- 2-quart (1.8 liters)
- 2½-quart (2.5 liters)
- 3-quart (2.7 liters)
- 4-quart (3.6 liters)

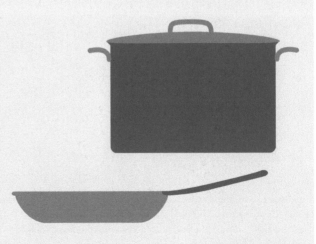

BOX CONTINUES >

Gratin dish: Shallow, most often oval, baking dishes; typical sizes:

- 1-quart (9½ inches)
- 2-quart (12½ inches)
- 4-quart (14 inches)

Ramekin: A variety of sizes can be used interchangeably with custard cups (flared sides) versus ramekins (straight sides); typical sizes, allowing ¼ to ½ inch of space left over when filled:

- 4- or 5-ounce (approximately: ½ cup, 3-inch diameter by 2 inches high)
- 6- or 7-ounce (approximately: ¾-cup, 3½-inch diameter by 2½ inches high)
- 8- or 10-ounce (approximately: 1 cup, 4-inch diameter by 2½ inches high)

Roasting pan:

- small: 14 × 12 × 3-inch; holds up to a 15-pound turkey
- large: 16 × 13 × 3-inch; holds up to a 20-pound turkey

Sheet pan: Rimmed baking sheets used for everything from roasting meat and vegetables to baking bread

- quarter-sheet pan: 13 × 9 × 1-inch
- half-sheet pan (most often used for home cooking): 18 × 13 × 1-inch
- full-sheet pan (generally too large for home cooking): 26 × 18 × 1-inch

Appliances

- **Slow cooker**
- **Instant Pot**
- **Pressure cooker**
- **Air fryer**

Bakeware

Loaf pans:

- 8 × 4-inch (20 × 10-cm)
- 9 × 5-inch (23 × 12.5-cm)

Round baking pans:

- 8-inch (20 centimeters)
- 9-inch (23 centimeters)

Springform pan: Type of cake pan that is made in two parts; has a bottom with a removable ring that serves as the side of the pan

- 7-inch (18 centimeters)
- 8-inch (20 centimeters)
- 9-inch (23 centimeters)
- 10-inch (25 centimeters)

Pie/quiche dish:

- 8-inch (20 centimeters)
- 9-inch (23 centimeters)
- 10-inch (25 centimeters) deep dish

Tube pan: 10-inch (25 centimeters)

Bundt pan: 10-inch (25 centimeters)

Square metal or glass baking pan:

- 8-inch (20 centimeters)
- 9-inch (23 centimeters)

Rectangular metal or glass baking pan: 13 × 9-inch (33 × 23-cm)

Muffin pans:

- mini: 12 or 24 small built-in cups, 1¾ by 1 inch deep (4.5 × 2-cm; about 2-ounce/30 milliliters)
- standard: 6 or 12 standard-size built-in cups, 2¾ by 1⅛ inches deep (7 × 3-centimeters; about 4-ounce/60 milliliters)
- jumbo: 6 larger built-in cups, 4 by 1¾ inches deep (10 × 4.5-centimeters; about 8-ounce/12 milliliters)

Sources: Substitutions for baking pan sizes by Catherine Boeckmann: almanac.com/content/substitutions-baking-pan-sizes | Baking pan sizes by Joy of Baking: joyofbaking.com/PanSizes.html | Casserole dish sizes by Cook's Info: cooksinfo.com/casserole-dish-sizes | Williams Sonoma: williams-sonoma.com/shop/cookware/?cm_type=gnav | Sur La Table: surlatable.com/products/cookware

Promoting Food Safety in Recipes

Well-written recipes include food safety information in the recipe instructions, including everything from safety warnings to proper food handling. According to the Partnership for Food Safety Education, consumers who use recipes that include basic food safety instructions are more likely to adhere to safe food handling practices in their home kitchens.

Safety Warnings

Safety warnings about hazards like splattering hot liquids, boiling over, and scalding steam—anything that might be a pitfall for a beginner cook or someone following the recipe for the first time—should be included in the recipe directions.

> When opening the steam valve on the pressure cooker, be sure it is pointing away from you to prevent getting burned from the hot steam.

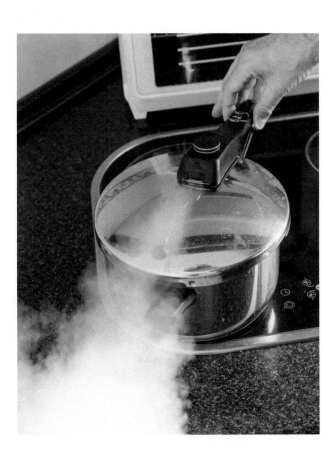

Quick Tip

"Recipes are messages. Take care what you write." —Shelley Feist, former executive director, Partnership for Food Safety Education

Safe Food Handling

Whenever possible, include food safety information in recipes to teach proper food handling in home kitchens, especially when writing recipes for kids or individuals learning to cook. Alternatively, include food safety basics in the front of a cookbook or as introductory copy in a recipe headnote or in an article featuring recipes.

Foodsafety.gov offers hands-on guidance for food safety in the home based on four core practices: clean, separate, cook, and chill. See the appendix Food Safety Instructions in Recipes on page 379 for examples of how to include food safety practices in recipe writing.

Raw or Undercooked Food

If a recipe includes the use of raw or undercooked food, consider including a disclaimer in the recipe note or in its place of publication (e.g., cookbook, digital or print publication).

> Consuming raw or undercooked meats, poultry, seafood, shellfish, or eggs may increase your risk of foodborne illness, especially if you have a medical condition.

If an ingredient in a recipe is intended to be used raw, suggest an alternative for it or provide a warning about the potential risk of foodborne illness. A good example is raw or undercooked eggs:

Ingredients
2 large eggs*

Note at the end of the recipe
* To minimize the risk of salmonella, use pasteurized eggs for the Caesar dressing

OR

* If you are concerned about the safety of using raw eggs, substitute pasteurized eggs in the shell or ¼ cup (60 milliliters) pasteurized liquid whole eggs.

Using a Food Thermometer

A food thermometer is an essential kitchen tool for taking the guesswork out of cooking and ensuring the safety of certain prepared foods. Measuring the internal temperature of cooked meat and poultry, egg dishes, and reheated foods ensures that a safe temperature has been reached and that harmful bacteria have been destroyed. Bacteria thrive and grow rapidly in temperatures ranging between 40° F and 140° F, the "danger zone," especially if the food remains in that zone for more than 2 hours. Raw meats that have been mishandled (e.g., cross-contaminated or allowed to stay in the danger zone for too long) could contain hazardous bacteria that produce toxins that can cause foodborne illness. Some toxins are heat resistant and may not be destroyed by cooking. This means that cooked meat and poultry mishandled in the raw state may not be safe to eat, even after proper preparation.

When Is It Done?

The USDA Food Safety and Inspection Service (FSIS) recommends cooking foods that may contain pathogens that cause foodborne illness to safe minimum internal temperatures (see Safe Minimum Internal Temperatures).

Steaks, chops, and roasts The FSIS recommends a minimum internal temperature of 145° F for beef, pork, veal, and lamb roasts, steaks, and chops. However, some chefs, cookbook authors, and other culinary professionals have their preferred doneness temperatures for rare and medium-rare whole cuts, believing that the temperatures recommended by FSIS produce overcooked meats. Searing the outside of a whole piece of meat helps destroy any bacteria on the surface.

Ground meats Because bacteria may live on the outer surface of whole cuts of meat, any bacteria present on the surface will get distributed into ground meat during the grinding process. To kill the bacteria, ground beef, pork, and lamb must be cooked to an internal temperature of 160° F (71° C) to be considered safe to eat; ground chicken and turkey should be cooked to 165° F.

Where do harmful bacteria come from? Some of the more common pathogens that cause foodborne illness, such as *E. coli* and *Salmonella*, are found in animal (and occasionally human) waste or sometimes on their skin, fur, and feathers. Contamination can occur at various points in the food production chain, such as during processing and preparation. Although commercial sanitation measures are designed to prevent contamination during processing, equipment and surfaces can be contaminated with dangerous bacteria from an animal's intestines, hide, feathers, or feet. During preparation, bacteria from a person's hands can contaminate foods, and cross-contamination can occur—such as between raw meats and produce—if the same utensils or cutting boards are used for both.

IMPORTANT POINTS TO SHARE IN MEAT RECIPES

Always use an instant-read or meat thermometer to obtain the internal temperature of meat. Insert the thermometer through the side of the meat until the tip reaches the center (without touching bone or fat).

Remove the meat from the heat when the meat thermometer registers a temperature that is 5° F (for steaks) to 10° F (for roasts) lower than the desired final temperature; the exact temperature depends on the thickness of the meat.

Allow the meat to rest, and the temperature will continue to rise while it rests.

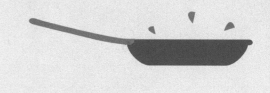

SAFE MINIMUM INTERNAL TEMPERATURES

Food item	Minimum internal temperature (measured with a food thermometer)
Beef, pork, veal, and lamb roasts, steaks, and chops	145° F, allow to rest at least 3 minutes **Note:** Professional chefs often use different internal temperatures and remove meat from the heat several degrees lower to allow temperatures to rise during resting. For example: For beef and lamb (roasts, steaks, chops) • Rare: 125° F • Medium rare: 130° F • Medium: 140° F • Medium well: 155° F • Well done: 160° F For pork (chops, roasts, loins, and tenderloins) • Medium: 145° F
Ground beef, pork, veal, lamb	160° F
Ham (uncooked/cooked)	145° F, allow to rest at least 3 minutes Reheat cooked ham to 165° F
Poultry (whole, parts, and ground/stuffing)	165° F
Eggs and egg dishes	160° F for sauces and custards; for eggs, cook until the whites are completely set and the yolks begin to thicken
Finfish and shellfish	145° F For clams, oysters, and mussels, cook until shells open during cooking For shrimp, lobster, and crab, cook until flesh is pearly and opaque For scallops, cook until flesh is milky white, opaque, and firm
Leftovers	Reheat to 165° F

Adapted from: Safe minimum cooking temperatures chart, Foodsafety.gov:. foodsafety.gov/keep/charts/mintemp.html

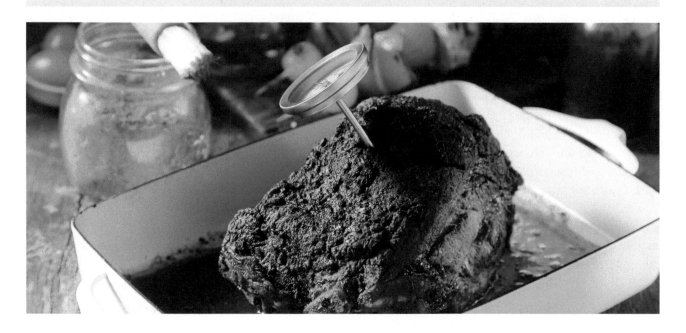

Recipe Style Guides

In recipe writing, the style that's followed for a project is dependent on preferences—what works for the author, the audience, the project, or the publisher. This chapter covers a variety of options for writing recipes, but most professional food writers, recipe developers, food editors, copy editors, and proofreaders typically rely on recipe-writing style guides. Formal style guides help ensure that the language and recipe style choices are consistent within a project and that the recipes are accurate, clear, and concise. When writing recipes that will appear together—whether they're on the back of a package, on a website, or in a cookbook—it's very important to follow a single writing style. Style guides are indispensable aids.

Most publishing companies, magazines, newspapers, food companies, restaurant groups, and food nonprofits have their own recipe style guides that must be followed, so if you are involved in a recipe development project for a client, ask the client to supply their style guide. If the client is unable to supply a style guide, review an array of the client's published recipes, take note of how their recipes are written, and create a style guide for your own use. Having the guide handy as you work will prevent additional work later on and will ensure that the recipes are written correctly and consistently (for examples, see the appendix Recipe Writing Style Guides on page 362).

Recipe style guides can vary considerably. Some are little more than a formatted recipe template describing how recipes should be written, with a few notes about writing rules. Others are very lengthy and detailed, with specifics on headnote requirements, grammar and punctuation rules, measurement rules, correct usage of commonly written phrases, and even long lists of preferred names and spellings for terms. All style guides, no matter their source, are working documents that regularly require updates based on new products and evolving culinary words, terminology, and phrases. For most recipe writers, a style guide is an invaluable editorial cheat sheet.

Each time a change is made or additions or deletions occur, rename the style guide document and include the date it was updated. Following are some examples of why style guide updates are useful.

Package sizes Manufacturers often downsize packages to improve cost margins. As these changes occur, update your style guide so package size changes are reflected in your recipes. For example, a recipe may have been created with a 19-ounce can of beans that its manufacturer now packages in a 15-ounce can.

Frequently used common weights and measurements of recipe ingredients For example, if you often use freshly squeezed lemon juice in recipes, having the measurement equivalents in your style guide will be very helpful (e.g., freshly squeezed juice of 1 lemon [about 2 tablespoons]).

Repetitive ingredient descriptions, instruction phrases, or notes in recipe directions For example, when a recipe calls for breadcrumbs, storing a note on how to make homemade breadcrumbs in your style guide will be helpful.

Quick Tip

"Each of the brands that the Meredith Test Kitchens serve maintains their own recipe writing style, which seems to be a continual work in progress as we try to make recipes as easy to understand with as few words as possible. For example, *Better Homes and Gardens* monthly magazine begins with 'In a small bowl stir together . . . ,' 'In a large saucepan . . . ,' 'On a lightly floured surface . . . ,' whereas some of our other titles start with an action: "Stir together flour, baking powder . . . in a medium bowl.' Much is dictated by the space we are given in print. We have a checklist that we use in our kitchen as we develop and test recipes. It is our job to ensure all the data is correct in the recipe. The food editors and copy editors then fit the recipes for the space in print."

—Lynn Blanchard, Test Kitchen Director, Dotdash Meredith

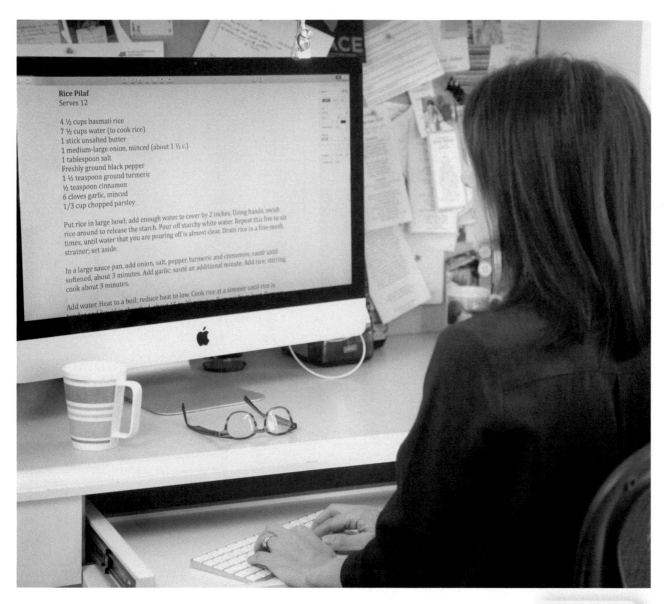

Rice Pilaf
Serves 12

4 ½ cups basmati rice
7 ½ cups water (to cook rice)
1 stick unsalted butter
1 medium-large onion, minced (about 1 ½ c.)
1 tablespoon salt
Freshly ground black pepper
1 ½ teaspoon ground turmeric
½ teaspoon cinnamon
6 cloves garlic, minced
1/3 cup chopped parsley

Put rice in large bowl; add enough water to cover by 2 inches. Using hands, swish rice around to release the starch. Pour off starchy white water. Repeat this five to six times, until water that you are pouring off is almost clear. Drain rice in a fine-mesh strainer; set aside.

In a large sauce pan, add onion, salt, pepper, turmeric and cinnamon; sauté until softened, about 3 minutes. Add garlic; sauté an additional minute. Add rice; stirring cook about 3 minutes.

Add water. Heat to a boil; reduce heat to low. Cook rice at a simmer until rice is

"When writing a style guide, use subheads for each of the categories (e.g., spelling, grammar, measurements, abbreviations) and turn it in with your manuscript so the editor and copy editor can see your wishes specific to the project. Ultimately, the reader benefits by having a set of well-written recipes to follow." —Rick Rodgers, cookbook author and recipe developer

"At the very beginning, I ask authors to send sample text and sample recipes for their book. I complete very detailed line edits on their recipes. I find this most useful. The writer now models my recipe style for all future recipes and uses this as their guide. I do give a style sheet, but I find this detailed first edit works best. And if an author prefers another recipe style, I am happy to hear their thoughts on it and make a change."

—Sarah Billingsley, Executive Editor, Chronicle Books

The following recipe is an example of a draft recipe that needs translating for a consumer publication. Text in red refers to editor questions or suggested changes.

Chilled Carrot Bisque *(Consider including the orange-forward flavor in the title, e.g., Chilled Carrot and Orange Bisque? Will reader know what makes this a bisque? Change to "Soup" instead? Add a recipe headnote.)*

Yield: 1 gallon *(Most home cooks have difficulty visualizing 1 gallon of soup; in addition to total yield, give number of servings and serving size; also give prep, chilling, and cooking time.)*

1 ounce minced shallots *(Provide number of shallots and a measurement in tablespoons. Chopped is fine since pureeing in soup.)*

2 each garlic cloves, minced *(delete "each.")*

1 ounce minced ginger *(Provide a measurement in tablespoons and the size of the piece of ginger; mention that it should be peeled.)*

¼ pounds minced white onion *(Provide a measurement in cups and the size and number of onions needed. Chopped is fine since pureeing in soup.)*

3 Tbsp butter *(Do not abbreviate tablespoon; salted or unsalted butter?)*

3½ pounds carrots sliced thinly *(Provide a measurement in cups and whether they should be peeled. Description should be "thinly sliced," not "sliced thinly." Measurements seem off. Quantity seems large. Check when retesting recipe and adjust other ingredients as necessary.)*

2 cups carrot juice (or water) *(Store-bought or homemade carrot juice?)*

2½ qts water *(Do not use an abbreviation for quart, and include the number of cups after the 2 quarts instead of the fraction 1/2. Check amount in testing. Too much?)*

2 ounce white wine *(Provide a conventional measurement.)*

½ tsp ground cardamom *(Spell out teaspoon.)*

1 quart orange juice *(Freshly squeezed? Check amount in testing. Too much?)*

7 ounce yogurt *(Provide a measurement in cups and a suggestion for a size to purchase at the store, if appropriate. Should the yogurt be plain or vanilla flavored? Regular or Greek? Nonfat, low fat, or whole milk?)*

salt and pepper to taste *(Provide a measurement in teaspoons for salt and pepper, and specify the type preferred [e.g., kosher, table salt, freshly ground black].)*

1 cup heavy cream, whipped into soft peaks *(Some cooks may miss that this is part of the garnish; create garnish recipe; provide whipped cream instructions in steps.)*

4 tablespoons chopped chives *(Garnish recipe and add "fresh." Once you hit 4 tablespoons, the volume measurement should change to cups [in this case, 1/4 cup chopped fresh chives.])*

1. Sweat shallots, ginger, garlic, and onion in the butter on low heat until they are soft, approximately ten minutes *(Provide a suggestion for pot size. "Sweat" is not a commonly used culinary term among consumers; use cook as an alternative term. Directions are not in the same order that ingredients are listed—which order is correct, the ingredient list or the directions? Use "about" instead of "approximately." The time—10 minutes—seems long; please check.)*

2. Add carrots, wine, cardamom, and orange juice. Simmer on low-medium heat until carrots are tender, approximately 30 minutes. *(Water is mentioned in the ingredient list but not in the step; should it be added here? The ingredients list is not in the correct order, as the carrot juice not used until Step 4. Should the simmer time be covered or uncovered? Include an instruction to remove the pot from the heat to cool. Again, "about" not "approximately.")*

3. Puree in a blender to a smooth texture and chill well in refrigerator. *(Add a note about pureeing hot soup in a blender in batches, as a gallon of soup could not be pureed all at once. Include directions for transferring the soup to a container before refrigerating it. Give chilling time.)*

4. Finish by whisking in the yogurt. Thin with the carrot juice and adjust the seasoning. *(Is the yogurt whisked into the container, blender, or pot? Describe how to adjust seasoning.)*

5. Serve in chilled soup bowls and garnish with a chive whipped cream (mix both ingredients). *(How do you chill the bowls? Describe how in the headnote. Provide more instruction on making the garnish; give whipping cream instructions in this step.)*

Chilled Carrot and Orange Soup

Serve this smooth and creamy carrot soup as an elegant appetizer. For a nice touch, if you have the time and refrigerator space, chill or freeze the bowls for 30 minutes or so to help keep the soup cold during serving.

Preparation time: 25 minutes
Cooking time: 50 minutes
Chilling time: 2 hours
Yield: 6 servings (7 cups; generous 1 cup per serving)

3 tablespoons unsalted butter
1 small white onion, chopped
1 small shallot, chopped (about 2 tablespoons)
2 cloves garlic, minced
1 (3-inch) piece fresh ginger, peeled and minced (about 2 tablespoons)
1¾ pounds carrots, peeled and thinly sliced (about 4½ cups)
5 cups water or vegetable stock
2 cups 100% orange juice (not from concentrate)
2 tablespoons white wine
¼ teaspoon ground cardamom
1 teaspoon kosher salt, plus more to taste
¼ teaspoon freshly ground black pepper
1 (5.3-ounce) container (about ¾ cup) plain low-fat or whole-milk yogurt
Up to 1 cup store-bought fresh carrot juice

CHIVE CREAM GARNISH
½ cup heavy whipping cream
¼ cup chopped fresh chives

1. Melt the butter in a large pot over medium-low heat. Add the onion and shallot and cook, covered and stirring occasionally, until softened, about 8 minutes. Stir in the garlic and ginger and cook for 1 minute. Stir in the carrots, water, orange juice, wine, cardamom, salt, and pepper. Bring to a boil, then reduce the heat and simmer, partially covered, until the carrots are very tender, about 40 minutes. Remove from the heat and let the soup cool slightly in the pot, about 10 minutes.

2. In batches, puree the soup in a blender until smooth, keeping the lid of the blender slightly ajar so steam can escape. Transfer the soup to a medium bowl, cover, and refrigerate until chilled, at least 2 hours.

3. Before serving, whisk in the yogurt. Thin the soup to desired consistency with carrot juice. Taste for salt and season with more if needed.

4. For the chive cream, using an electric hand mixer or whisk, whip the cream in a small bowl to soft peaks (the tips of the cream will curl and flop over immediately when beaters are lifted). Fold in the chives.

5. To serve, ladle the soup into bowls and garnish each serving with a dollop of chive cream.

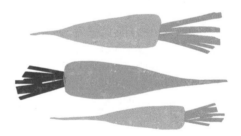

Digital Recipe Organization and Storage

Some food companies and food-service establishments use a recipe software storage platform or hire developers to create a customized recipe database that can be regularly maintained and updated. These databases allow the company to customize recipes according to specific needs. Publishing companies, food companies, culinary consultants, and chefs manage and organize their recipes in different ways. Examples include:

- Word processing digital files and folders (Microsoft Word or Apple's Pages)

- Spreadsheet documents (Microsoft Excel and Apple's Numbers)

- Evernote note-taking app

- Dropbox file-sharing service

- Google Drive file-sharing service (and Google Docs for sharing individual recipe files)

- Paprika Recipe Manager app: A cloud-based app that helps organize recipes, make meal plans, and create grocery lists. A licensing fee is required.

- Scrivener app for text and recipe organization: Scrivener is a manuscript-management system that allows you to have separate files for written content and recipe index cards that can be pinned to a board. The order of the cards can be rearranged by simply dragging and dropping their icons, making reordering easy if the structure of the book changes. A licensing fee is required.

Recipe Database Fields

Use database fields to digitally manage, categorize, or access recipes. A recipe template can be created by using any of the following customizable fields:

- recipe developer name
- development date
- version number
- category
- cuisine
- skill level (e.g., beginner, intermediate, advanced)
- brand(s)
- title
- alternate title
- headnote
- prep time
- bake time
- cook time
- yield
- serving size
- ingredients (fields include open text for ingredients or branded ingredients, amounts, preset units of measurement)
- method/directions
- nutrition information
- developer notes
- photos (e.g., embed images: step-by-step, final)
- video (embed)
- allergies and intolerances (e.g., peanut-free, soy-free, egg-free, wheat-free, gluten-free)
- dietary restrictions (e.g., low-carb, sugar-free, low-fat, FODMAP-friendly)

RECIPE WEBSITE PLUG-INS

Publishing recipes online is possible in any format, but recipe-card plug-ins for your website give you access to templates that are nice looking, easy to read and print, and designed for search engine optimization (SEO). Because technology changes fast, stay abreast of any new and improved plug-ins that emerge in the future. See Chapter 9 for recipe plug-ins that offer nutrition analysis.

Examples of WordPress plug-ins include Meal Planner Pro, EasyRecipe, Easy Recipe Plus, ZipList, WP Tasty Recipes, WP Ultimate Recipe, WP Recipe Maker, Recipe Card Blocks, Zip Recipes, and Cooked.

Recipe Writing and Editing Resources

Use the following reference books on style, grammar, spelling, and punctuation for additional guidance on recipe writing. Also, see the appendix Recipe Writing Style Guides on page 362.

Food References

The Food Substitutions Bible, 3rd Edition, by David Joachim. 2022. Robert Rose.

Larousse Gastronomique: The World's Greatest Culinary Encyclopedia by Librarie Larousse. 2009. Clarkson Potter.

The New Food Lover's Companion, 5th Edition, by Sharon Tyler Herbst and Ron Herbst. 2013. Sourcebooks.

The Oxford Companion to Food, 3rd Edition, by Alan Davidson and Tom Jaine. 2014. Oxford University Press.

Recipe Writing and Editing

Recipes into Type: A Handbook for Cookbook Writers and Editors by Joan Whitman and Dolores Simon. 1993. HarperCollins.

The Recipe Writer's Handbook by Barbara Gibbs Ostmann and Jane L. Baker. 2001. Harvest.

Will Write for Food by Dianne Jacob. 2021. Hachette Go.

Style Books

The Associated Press Stylebook (published every other year). Basic Books. [Includes a food guidelines and recipe style section.]

The Chicago Manual of Style, 17th Edition. 2017. University of Chicago Press.

The Elements of Style (annotated edition) by William Strunk Jr. and E.B. White. 2020. Auroch Press.

Bibliography

FoodKeeper App. Foodsafety.gov website. Accessed June 14, 2021. foodsafety.gov/keep/foodkeeperapp/index.html

Four steps to food safety. Foodsafety.gov website. Accessed June 14, 2021. foodsafety.gov/keep-food-safe/4-steps-to-food-safety

Gisslen W. *Professional Cooking*. 8th Ed. Wiley; 2018.

How to convert recipes from cups to weights. Alice Medrich website. Accessed June 14, 2021. alicemedrich.com/blog

Ingredient weight chart. King Arthur Flour website. Accessed June 14, 2021. kingarthurflour.com/learn/ingredient-weight-chart.html

Lopez-Alt JK. *The Food Lab: Better Home Cooking Through Science*. W. W. Norton & Co.; 2015.

Lynch FT. *The Book of Yields: Accuracy in Food Costing and Purchasing*. 8th Ed. John Wiley & Sons; 2010.

Partnership for Food Safety Education. The core four practices. Partnership for Food Safety Education website. Accessed April 27, 2022. fightbac.org/food-safety-basics/the-core-four-practices

Safe Minimum Cooking Temperatures Chart. Foodsafety.gov website. Accessed June 14, 2021. foodsafety.gov/keep/charts/mintemp.html

Whitman J, Simon D. *Recipes Into Type: A Handbook for Cookbook Writers and Editors*. Harper Collins; 1993.

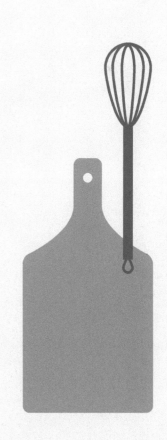

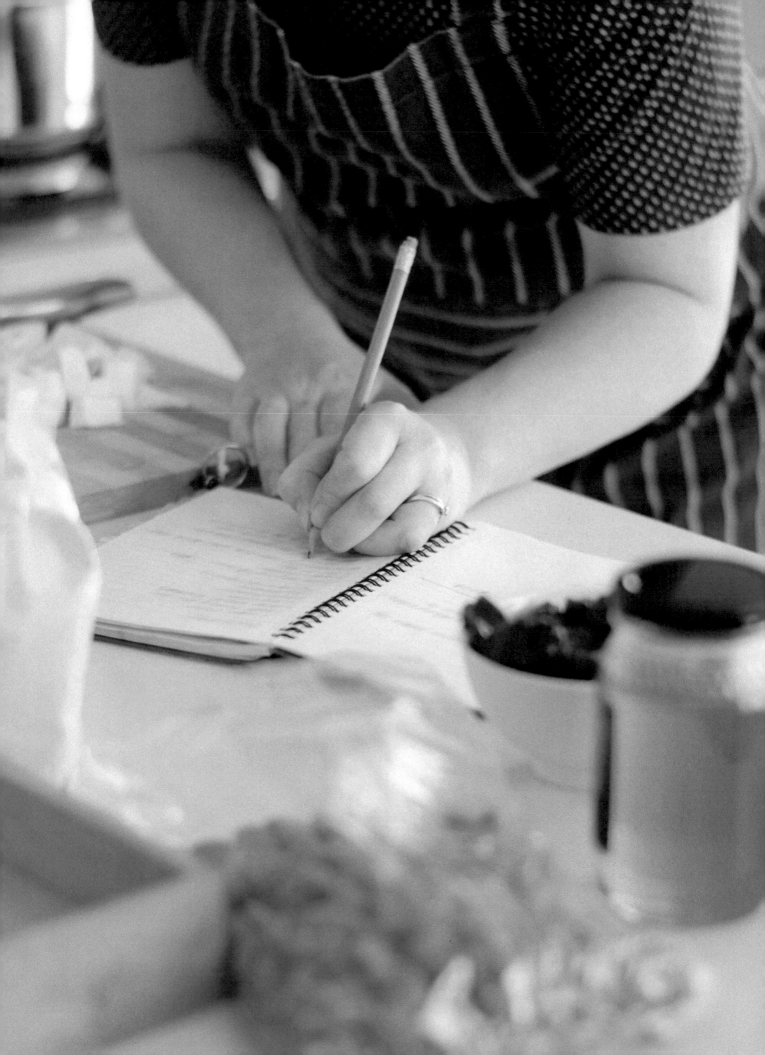

Chapter 8
Recipe Testing

IN THIS CHAPTER, LEARN ABOUT:

- Why recipe testing is important for a successful recipe

- Step-by-step guidelines for recipe testing

- How to capture, document, and evaluate information before, during, and after recipe testing

- Advice for using home cook recipe testers

Recipe testing is an important yet often overlooked—or even skipped altogether— step in a recipe's journey from development to publication. If a recipe is written and tested well, providing a clear road map for the home cook, any person should be able to successfully prepare it. A recipe's ideal outcome is to deliver what is promised and to leave the person preparing the recipe feeling successful and competent in the kitchen. The guidelines presented in this chapter align closely with the recipe writing principles covered in Chapter 7.

Unlike the creative process of recipe development, recipe testing is all about precision, accuracy, and thoroughness. Professional recipe testers, who may or may not be the same individuals who develop and write the recipe, work in a variety of settings, including food company test kitchens; newspaper, magazine, or digital food publication test kitchens; restaurant group or food-service test kitchens; or in their own kitchens. Regardless of the setting, the skills a professional recipe tester should possess include:

- patience
- attention to detail
- the ability to objectively work through a recipe, leaving personal taste preferences aside
- an understanding of the end user (the recipe's audience)
- a breadth and depth of experience in ingredient use, culinary techniques, and culinary problem-solving skills

Some recipe testers "road test" recipes before publication. These testers are usually home cooks who volunteer or are hired by a publisher or cookbook author to capture any pitfalls the recipe may have for a novice or average cook, and their feedback can be invaluable. They may not have culinary training, but ideally, they should be detail oriented.

Why Test Recipes?

Marketing strategy and accuracy are the two primary reasons for testing recipes. There's also the obvious need to test for one's personal and professional reputation, whether the recipe is being created for use in a cookbook, social media post, or article or written for a client/food company. A recipe that doesn't work reflects poorly on its developer.

Marketing Strategy

A content marketing strategy that includes recipes must answer the needs of the target audience while simultaneously helping build brand awareness and reputation. Testing helps in assessing whether marketing strategy efforts are being met by answering the following questions:

- Does the recipe meet the overall project strategy, project goals, and project guidelines?

- Does it meet the major selling points (e.g., a quick, one-pot dish) that are desired?

- Does it highlight what makes the recipe unique or better than its competitors?

- Does it meet and satisfy the intended audience's needs?

- Does it adequately showcase a highlighted ingredient, product, or appliance?

- Does it teach the home cook how to use the highlighted ingredient, product, or appliance?

- Can the recipe be easily adapted for different uses and platforms (e.g., the back of a food package, a website, social media, a cooking demonstration)?

Recipe Accuracy

Cooking and recipe testing are entirely different things. When professionals cook, they often instinctively adjust recipes to produce the best results, but the average cook should not be expected to do the same. That's why a recipe must be tested, tasted, tweaked, and tested again until the outcome is desirable and consistent. Translating kitchen notes into a recipe that readers can follow and replicate successfully is more time-consuming than it sounds, but this step should never be skipped if you intend to create a successful recipe.

FOODSERVICE RECIPE TESTING

In a foodservice kitchen, the process of testing recipes is focused on clarity and accuracy, but often, testing recipes for food service may also involve vetting a culinary operational procedure, determining cost effectiveness, or making modifications to meet nutritional parameters.

Testing foodservice recipes as part of a recipe standardization process also helps ensure continuity of quality when prepared by different employees. Other factors include testing for:

- accuracy of ingredient amounts

- predictability of yields and food costs

- correct procedures for preparation of ingredients and cooking (provides a guide for kitchen staff)

- consistent quality and customer satisfaction

See page 19 for more on developing standardized recipes for foodservice operations.

The Stages of Recipe Testing

Recipe testing is done at different times in a recipe's journey before publication, including during the development stage, during the draft stage, and, once the recipe is finalized, during the period immediately prior to publication. The processes or protocols for recipe testing may differ depending on whether testing is done in a professional test kitchen or in a home kitchen for a cookbook, online publication, website, or social media. Regardless of where, why, and how the recipe testing is completed, **the overall goal of all recipe testing is the same—the recipe should work as written for the audience it is intended for, it should be reproducible with consistent results and yields every time, and it should taste delicious!**

Testing During Recipe Development

During the first stage of recipe testing, a recipe developer might start with an idea for a recipe, which may include a working ingredient list and general quantity amounts and directions. They will test the recipe until it meets their overall recipe goals and desired flavor profile. During this stage, the recipe developer's culinary skills are put to work testing ideas, refining the recipe, and ultimately translating the raw ideas into a final draft or "working" recipe.

This creative stage of the process could be brief, with only a few tests, or lengthy, with twenty or more tests; there is no hard and fast rule. It all depends on how much research and experimentation is needed to get to a final successful recipe. The research might require testing many versions of a recipe to determine which variables and factors are essential to create the new recipe. Throughout the process, the recipe developer will test, taste, refine, revise, and edit the recipe until a final draft of the recipe comes into focus.

Testing of "raw" chef recipes may also occur in the recipe development stage. In these instances, recipe testers are given an incomplete recipe and asked to test it, translate it, and do their best to retain the chef's intent. Many expert recipe developers/testers are known for this skill.

Testing the Working Recipe

During the second stage of recipe testing, the "final" working recipe is tweaked as it undergoes several tests. The main purpose of testing a working recipe is not necessarily to make it more creative; instead, it is intended to note and fix any problems with the ingredients and instructions. The working recipe is tested, tasted, tweaked, revised, and edited until it is ready for final recipe testing. Professional recipe testers know how to do this well and are able to quickly apply their culinary skills to create a clear and reproducible recipe. See Chapter 7 for more on recipe writing and editing.

Testing the Final Recipe

During the last stage of testing, the final recipe is tested by a professional recipe tester or a home cook exactly as written. Recipe testers in a food company test kitchen might also perform tolerance testing during this final testing stage, in which the recipe is tested under a variety of different conditions to ensure it always works. This may include testing the recipe with a range of oven temperatures (e.g., 325° F instead of 350° F, since consumer oven temperatures vary) or testing with alternate ingredients that consumers might be likely to use on their own (e.g., nonfat instead of whole milk).

After the final testing is completed, the recipe is updated with any changes that were noted, and if needed, the recipe is tested again with the changes. Once all final changes are made, the recipe is ready for the next stage, which may include copy editing, photography, and video.

Documenting Recipe Testing Notes

In each stage of recipe testing, it's critical to take copious notes and document *everything* from ingredient tweaks and technique changes to evaluating cooking or baking times and yields. During testing, record comments on flavor, texture, and color, and possibly suggest ideas for the recipe's headnote. After the revisions are documented, the recipe is ready for retesting.

It's also important to keep track of all tests and recipe versions by dating and numbering each test version. Every professional or company has their own

system of documentation: some use recipe testing sheets, while others make notations and edits directly on a hard copy of the recipe (see pages 237 and 238 for examples).

Once the documentation is complete, it should be stored properly. Testing sheets or marked-up hard copy recipes should be filed with all other relevant recipe development paperwork; if the documentation is digital, you can store all documents (including photos and videos) in a single folder (e.g., Google Docs, Evernote, Pages, or Microsoft Word, or a proprietary or online content management system).

Documentation of a recipe from its origin point—ideation, inspiration, or adaptation—on through to recipe testing leaves behind a helpful paper trail that can be revisited any time during the writing and editing process, during the recipe pitch, or after the recipe is published. Include as many details as possible on each testing sheet, and if testing an ingredient variation, use a new sheet to record and annotate the results.

During testing, take photographs of the recipe process. Having a visual representation of the recipe, no matter how humble it may be, can help facilitate the editorial process, generate content ideas for the recipe's headnote, and provide the food stylist and photographer with ideas for shot selection.

How to Test Recipes

The steps for testing and the type of information collected during the testing process will vary based on the nature of the project, expectations of the editor or client, and the stage of testing. Is the recipe being tested for an online publication, a website, a social media platform, a cookbook, a magazine, a restaurant, a food company, a package label, or a use and care manual? Does the editor want you to test the recipe exactly as written? Or does the editor want you to use your culinary knowledge and skills to improve the recipe while testing it and then document why these changes are needed? Your recipe testing approach may also vary depending on whether testing is done during the development stage, the "working" recipe stage, or the final recipe stage just before publication. Regardless of the type of project and the stage of recipe testing, it is critical to always take detailed notes.

The necessary recipe testing information can be captured in many different ways. Use the guidelines in this chapter as a framework.

Step 1: Read through the Recipe from Start to Finish

Reading through a recipe thoroughly can be considered a form of editorial recipe testing. Before entering the kitchen, read the recipe all the way through two to three times, and keep in mind the intended audience for and purpose of the recipe. While reading, think through the recipe as if you are already in the kitchen. Identify any areas where you foresee a potential problem or where a reader might have questions, and add your initial comments to the document containing the recipe or the recipe testing sheet. While you are reading, and before you start the first round of testing, ask the following questions:

- Is the recipe suitable for its intended audience? Will they have the cooking skills or equipment needed to prepare it?
- Does it meet the defined requirements created by you or by the client?
- Is the title clear?
- Are the ingredient descriptions and amounts clear and written in the order they are used in the directions?

- Is there a preferable culinary method or technique?
- Does the cooking time and temperature appear accurate?
- Does it contain confusing wording or terminology?

Step 2: Set Up a Recipe Testing Station

After reading through the recipe several times and making editorial testing notes, it's time to set up a testing station. First, gather the recipe ingredients in the correct quantities (a process known by the French term *mise en place*, which means put in place) and the equipment needed to test the recipe, which may include part or all of the following:

- recipe ingredients
- large cutting board(s)
- knives (e.g., paring, chef, or a santoku [an all-purpose knife])
- measuring utensils (e.g., several sets of measuring cups and spoons)
- ramekins and bowls of different sizes to accurately measure or weigh ingredients
- mixing bowls
- mixing utensils (rubber spatula, wooden spoons, whisk)
- cookware and bakeware in the specific types and sizes needed
- ruler for measuring and ensuring the correct pan size
- tasting spoons
- digital kitchen scale
- instant-read thermometer
- oven thermometer
- kitchen timer (or smartphone timer)
- red or other nonblack pen (if making notes on a hard copy of the recipe) or a computer if making notes digitally (use the Track Changes feature)
- pad of paper
- camera (a smartphone camera is handy)

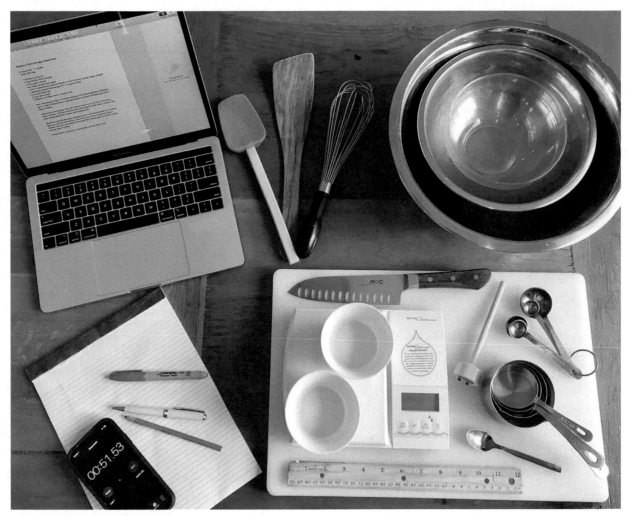

Typical items needed for a recipe testing station.

Step 3: Record Recipe Testing Notes

Throughout the testing process, you must capture, document, and evaluate all of the information you collect every step of the way. It's always better to document more information than you really need during the initial recipe testing process. For all recipe testing, keep the following tips in mind:

- While recording testing notes, focus on precision, accuracy, and thoroughness. Write or input these notes directly on a printed copy or digital version of the recipe, a recipe testing sheet, or a recipe testing spreadsheet. Be sure to number each version of the recipe that is tested. See pages 237 and 238 for examples.

- Evaluate whether the recipe is accurate, replicable, and easy to follow for the intended audience.

- Never wait until a test is finished to record notes, as it's very easy to forget something. Taking pictures—process shots or even just a final finished shot—is very helpful, as they can be used by the editorial and design team to inform photography decisions.

- Never make a change to the recipe that is not tested.

- Test recipes in the same environment where the audience will use them. For example, if you are testing a recipe intended for a home cook in a professional kitchen with access to high-end or commercial equipment, the cooking times and temperatures may not be the same (e.g., an induction burner in a professional kitchen may boil water or reduce a sauce in significantly less time than an electric burner in a home kitchen).

THERMOMETERS AND SCALES FOR RECIPE TESTING

Instant-read thermometer

Used to test the doneness of meat and poultry or to test the temperature of hot foods in steam trays or foods or sauces as they cool

Brands and models include ThermoWorks ThermoPop or Thermapen; Thermo Pro Thermapen; Lavatools Javelin Pro; and Taylor Precision

Candy and deep-frying thermometer

Measures the temperature of ingredients when making candies or for heating oil for deep-frying; clips to the edge of a pot

Brands include ThermoWorks ChefAlarm, Polder, Taylor Precision, and Oxo

Oven thermometer

Confirms the oven temperature, which tend to vary

Brands include Cooper Atkins, Rubbermaid Commercial, Taylor Classic, AcuRite, and Farberware

Digital kitchen food scale

Precisely measures the weight of ingredients

Brands and models include Escali Primo Digital, Etekcity Multifunction, Ozeri Pronto Digital Multifunction, Wireless Perfect Bake Pro Smart Kitchen, and My Weight

What to Capture in Recipe Testing Notes

While you are testing recipes, many details must be considered and evaluated. The initial editorial recipe testing step involves flagging issues and noting questions, but specific details are captured during the tests themselves. To ensure consistent results, always follow the same testing guidelines and approach for each project. This section provides more detail on what should be captured in recipe testing notes; refer to Chapter 7 for best practices for writing a recipe to ensure accuracy and clarity.

Recipe Testing Notes on Ingredient Measurements and Descriptions

As you begin, focus first on the recipe's ingredient measurements and descriptions. Share your suggestions (or edits) on how to describe the amounts and descriptions of ingredients more clearly.

Measurements

- Make sure measurement abbreviations are clearly written. In your notes, spell out terms of measurement (e.g., grams or teaspoons versus g or tsp) to ensure clarity when reviewing notes at a later date.

- Weigh, measure, and record everything, and make detailed notes about how this is done. Place each measured ingredient in small bowls before beginning each test (gathering all ingredients before starting a test is very important).

- For ingredients, record the count when appropriate (e.g., 2 medium onions), the weight in US customary and metric measures (e.g., ounces, pounds, grams, milliliters), and a common volume measure (e.g., cups, teaspoons).

- Record ingredients' volume in both US customary (fluid ounces, cups, tablespoons, teaspoons) and metric (milliliters, grams) measures.

- Decide on the best method to record metric measures (many publishers round metrics off to the nearest increment of 0 or 5).

- Record any package sizes of ingredients in ounces, pounds, and grams, and note all of the variations available.

- If the recipe uses only a small portion of an ingredient that the consumer must buy in a larger quantity (e.g., can or package), note the issue and specify whether this is necessary. Can the remaining amount of the ingredient be used in the recipe or easily stored?

Ingredient Descriptions and Availability

- Note the exact brands of ingredients used in testing; naturally, if you are testing for a food company, use their brand.

- Note how accessible the ingredients are. Are they easy to obtain?

- Note whether more clarity is needed for the ingredients' descriptions. For example, if the recipe calls for broth, does it specify whether beef, vegetable, or chicken broth should be used or if the broth should be homemade or canned? What color onion should be used—yellow, white, or red?

- Note whether the preparation of ingredients should be described more clearly. For example, should the eggplant be left unpeeled or peeled before slicing? Note your recommendation.

- Test ingredients that are in season, if possible. If ingredients in the recipe are tested when they are out of season, make note of their quality, and if necessary, make note of any substitutions you use.

Cost

- If appropriate, note the cost of all ingredients, as well as the overall per-serving cost of the recipe, to help evaluate the recipe's cost effectiveness.

CRITERIA TO EVALUATE WHEN RECIPE TESTING

Recipe testing is performed to confirm that a recipe works as written by evaluating it according to the following criteria.

Ingredients: The ingredients are listed in order of use and provide accurate descriptions, including package size, preparation instructions, and correct amounts or weights for each.

Directions: The directions are clear and the flow of preparation should be efficient; the method and culinary techniques should work as written or should include further explanation or clarifications on technique.

Prep and cooking time: The preparation and cooking times are accurate.

Doneness: The temperature, time, and visual doneness cues are provided.

Yield: The recipe's total yield and serving sizes are included and verified.

Taste: The recipe should offer a balance of taste, texture, temperature, and mouthfeel.

Visual: The presentation and visual appearance is appealing. The recipe offers serving suggestions, if appropriate.

Reproducibility: The recipe should be able to yield consistent results when different cooks prepare the same recipe.

Nutrition information: The ingredient amounts, total yield, and serving size are clear and verified for the nutrition analysis.

Food safety: Proper food handling and ingredient usage tips are included.

Storage: The recipe offers make-ahead and freezing recommendations, if appropriate.

Tolerance (abuse) testing: The recipe is successful with a variety of ingredient, equipment, and cooking technique changes that might occur in a home or foodservice kitchen.

Cost: The recipe meets requirements for cost per serving, if applicable.

Recipe Testing Notes on Specific Ingredients

Dairy and Eggs

- Confirm or provide a weight measure and cup measure for shredded or grated cheese. International recipes usually require measurements for cheese to be given in both ounces and grams (e.g., 8 ounces/226 grams), while most recipes developed for use in the United States provide measurements in cups and ounces (e.g., 2 cups [about 8 ounces]).

Weight: 8 ounces (226 grams) shredded sharp cheddar cheese
Measure: 2 cups shredded sharp cheddar cheese

Weight: 1¾ ounces (50 grams) Parmigiano-Reggiano cheese
Measure: ½ cup freshly grated Parmigiano-Reggiano cheese

Additional guidelines:

- Use full-fat dairy ingredients (e.g., milk, yogurt, sour cream, half-and-half, cheese, cottage cheese), unless the recipe indicates that low-fat, reduced-fat (2% or 1%), or nonfat versions should be used. An exception is buttermilk, which is generally only available at grocery stores in a low-fat version.

- Specify the type of milk used if not using whole (e.g., nonfat, 1%, 2%, milk alternatives).

- If cream is used, specify the type (e.g., heavy, half-and-half).

- For butter, note the proper temperature to be used (e.g., cold, softened/room temperature) and whether it should be salted or unsalted.

- For eggs, use large, unless otherwise specified (e.g., medium, extra-large).

- Note whether eggs must be beaten before adding to other ingredients (e.g., 2 large eggs, lightly beaten).

Meats, Poultry, Fish, and Seafood

- Confirm or provide the count when appropriate (e.g., 2 [5-ounce] fillets), the raw and cooked weights (in grams/kilograms, ounces/pounds), and the thickness (e.g., 1 inch). This information is helpful when determining the recipe's serving size and also simplifies the ingredient shopping process.

Raw weight: 1 pound (454 grams) pork tenderloin, silverskin removed
Cooked weight: 12 ounces (340 grams)
Serving size: 3 ounces (85 grams)

Number: 1 whole roasted chicken
Raw weight: 2½ pounds (1.2 kilograms) chicken
Cooked weight, bones removed: 1½ pounds (680 grams)
Measured amount: 4 cups diced chicken

Number: 6 pork chops
Thickness: 1 inch (2.5 cm) thick, each
Raw weight: 2¾ pounds (1.3 kilograms) total; 7 ounces (198 grams) each
Cooked weight: 5 ounces (142 grams), each

- For shrimp, note the desired size and whether they should be peeled and deveined.

Jumbo: 21–25 count per pound (about 23 shrimp)
Large: 31–35 count per pound (about 33 shrimp)
Medium: 41–50 count per pound (about 45 shrimp)
Small: 51–60 count per pound (about 55 shrimp)

- For scallops, indicate whether they should be small bay scallops or large sea scallops.

- For oysters and clams, note the type, as it denotes the size (e.g., littleneck, middleneck, cherrystone, chowder, Manila, quahogs) and whether they should be in the shell or shucked.

Additional guidelines:

- Provide details on the cut of meat (e.g., for beef, top round, sirloin, tenderloin; for poultry, wing, thigh, breast; for fish, fillet or steak).

- Specify whether the meat or poultry should be bone in or boneless, and whether poultry should be skin on or skinless.

- If meat or poultry must be browned, note whether fat should be drained from the pan after browning.

- Indicate whether canned tuna should be in oil or water and whether it should be drained or undrained.

- For frozen fish, note whether it should be thawed first or cooked from frozen.

Pasta, Rice, and Grains

- List the type of pasta used in testing and provide suggested alternatives—e.g., 1 pound tube-shaped pasta, such as ziti, rigatoni, or penne.

- Note the package size and whether it's dried or fresh (e.g., 16 ounces dried pasta or 12 ounces fresh pasta).

- Note the cooked yield in parentheses—e.g., 1 pound elbow macaroni (yields 4 cups cooked).

- Specify whether the recipe requires cooked or uncooked pasta, rice, or grains; assume that it is uncooked unless stated otherwise (e.g., 3 cups cooked white rice).

- If the recipe directions indicate that the ingredient should be cooked according to the package directions, note whether fresh or dried is used and anything unusual about the process.

- Provide the type of rice used (e.g., white, Thai jasmine, basmati, arborio, brown, wild, black) and whether it is instant or quick cooking.

- For pita bread, tortillas, or wraps, provide the desired diameter.

- For breadcrumbs, indicate whether fresh, dried, or seasoned is used, and if texture matters, specify fine or coarse crumbs.

Fruits and Vegetables

- Confirm or provide the count when appropriate, the as-purchased fruit or vegetable weight, and the prepared ingredient measurement and weight.

  Purchased count: 2 broccoli stalks
  Purchased weight: 1½ pounds (640 grams)
  Prepared measure and weight (yield):
  4 cups broccoli florets (365 grams)

  Purchased count: 6 medium baking potatoes
  Purchased weight: 3 pounds (1.37 kilograms)
  Prepared measure and weight (yield):
  5 cups diced (1.13 kilograms)

  Purchased count: 1 medium yellow onion
  Purchased weight: 8 ounces (250 grams)
  Prepared amount and weight (yield):
  1 cup diced (150 grams)

Additional guidelines:

- Use consistent standards for size (e.g., define a "small" onion or "medium" apple).

- Specify use of the white and/or green portions of scallions (i.e., green onions).

- Clarify whether a fruit or vegetable should be peeled (e.g., potatoes, carrots, eggplant).

- For frozen fruits or vegetables, indicate whether it should be thawed or partially thawed.

- Clarify whether no-salt-added or no-sugar-added canned fruits or vegetables should be used.

- Specify whether canned fruits or vegetables should be drained or used with their juice or syrup.

- Specify exactly which type of canned tomato should be used and note whether the tomatoes should be used with their juices or drained. If relevant, indicate whether the no-salt-added variety should be used. Canned tomatoes come in a wide variety of options, including whole, crushed, and diced, as well as tomato paste, puree, and sauce.

- Note the seasonality of fruits or vegetables if the testing is completed when they are out of season.

Seasonings

- Use fresh or dried herbs as specified, and note whether they are ground, crushed, chopped, or whole.

- Use kosher salt unless table or flaky sea salt is specified; for kosher salt, document whether Morton or Diamond Crystal is used.

- Use freshly ground black pepper unless otherwise noted (e.g., white pepper).

Baking Ingredients

- Use approximately 70% cacao for bittersweet chocolate, unless otherwise specified.

- Be specific about the type of chocolate used (e.g., unsweetened, semisweet, milk chocolate).

- Clarify whether Dutch process or natural cocoa powder should be used.

- Specify light or dark brown sugar, and unless otherwise noted, densely pack the brown sugar.

- Clarify the type of yeast used: fresh (compressed or cake), active dry, instant, rapid rise, or quick rising.

- Use unbleached all-purpose flour (unless bleached all-purpose, cake, or whole wheat flour is specified).

- Make note of how flour is measured using an asterisk or parenthetical notation—especially if the flour is not being weighed—and test accordingly. The average home cook uses a dip-and-sweep method, despite the fact that the spoon-and-sweep method is usually a more accurate measurement. See page 198 in Chapter 7 for more on measuring flour.

Recipe Testing Notes on Directions

Recipe testers ensure that a recipe's details—including kitchen equipment, cooking techniques, descriptions and order of steps, and timing—are written clearly and with enough specificity to produce a great-tasting dish, no matter who makes the recipe. If something in the recipe's directions does not make sense or if you believe it should be done differently, explain why in your notes, and make suggestions and edits accordingly.

Kitchen Equipment
- Record all kitchen tools used during each step of the recipe directions (e.g., wooden spoon, rubber spatula).

- Record the specific size, type, finish, and materials of cookware, bakeware, and appliances used in testing (e.g., a medium stainless bowl, a large nonstick skillet, a 4-quart soufflé dish, an 8-inch square aluminum or glass baking pan, an immersion blender).

- Note whether the size or capacity of cookware and bakeware called for is correct.

- Indicate whether the kitchen equipment called for is readily available to the consumer or likely to be on hand in the average kitchen.

- Note whether an alternative piece of equipment can be used in the recipe (e.g., a blender versus a food processor, a wooden spoon versus a hand mixer) and be sure to test the recipe using the alternative.

Cooking
- Eliminate any ambiguity in the recipe directions. Write down all observations, including sensory cues, from the cooking process and clarify the instructions if necessary.

- Make suggestions or comments on culinary techniques used. Note whether a culinary technique needs further explanation.

- Fix ingredient amount errors ahead of time if appropriate. For example, a recipe for béchamel sauce that calls for the addition of ½ cup flour to thicken 2 cups of milk is clearly in error (a more appropriate amount would be about 3 tablespoons). Flag the error and correct it immediately instead of following the recipe faithfully just to report in your testing results that the sauce was too thick.

- If a recipe provides ingredient substitution options, test the substitution if possible (e.g., for a blueberry pie that specifies the use of fresh berries, with frozen as a substitution option).

- Make suggestions for better and more efficient flows in the preparation and cooking processes.

- Offer time-saving tips or ideas for simplifying the recipe.

- Note any potential ways to make the recipe more user-friendly to the home cook.

- Record the recipe's yield to ensure consistent results during multiple testing rounds or when it is prepared by different cooks. For each test, note how the end result turns out.

Food Safety
- Note whether proper food handling and ingredient usage is included in the recipe instructions.

- Note whether the food is cooked to recommended minimum internal temperatures (see Chapter 7).

Timing
- Place an oven thermometer in the center of the oven to verify the correct temperature and to

ensure the cooking time is correct based on this temperature.

- Use a kitchen or smartphone timer to accurately record preparation and cooking times.

- Be consistent when documenting preparation and cooking times by starting a timer each time you begin a task. For example, for ingredient preparation, start timing as you start gathering ingredients, measuring, and chopping. And for cooking, record the time once the food is placed in the pan or in the oven.

- Be consistent when recording cooking time in conjunction with visual observations (e.g., is the onion softening, becoming translucent, or browning at 3 minutes or 6 minutes)?

- Record the cooking temperature along with the cooking time (e.g., simmer on low heat for 3 minutes, bake at 350° F for 10 to 12 minutes).

- Be precise and record every unexpected result that occurs—e.g., still uncooked at the stated time (cooked for an additional 10 minutes); sauce never thickened (needs an additional 15 minutes); too salty; needs more liquid.

- Some clients or companies request that different baking times be recorded when testing with a variety of baking pan finishes (e.g., a dark versus a shiny pan). If no specific type of pan is called for, apply your culinary knowledge to choose the appropriate type for testing and get it right on the first try.

Doneness

- Record the temperature, time, and visual indications for when a food is properly cooked.

- Whenever helpful, give descriptive visual indications for a step of the recipe (e.g., toast nuts until golden brown).

- Offer descriptors that indicate doneness, along with an estimated time, to make the recipe easier to follow (e.g., bake until the top of the cake springs back gently when touched and an inserted

toothpick comes out clean, about 25 to 30 minutes. Alternatively, bake until the cake pulls back from the sides of the pan, 25 to 30 minutes).

Yield

- Never assume that halving or doubling a test recipe will provide an accurate yield.

- Provide the total yield and serving size for the recipe (e.g., the number of pieces; weight [grams, ounces]; measurement [cups, tablespoons, teaspoons]. These specific yield measurements also help ensure accurate nutrition analysis (see Chapter 9).

- If several recipes are combined into one (e.g., angel food cake, whipped cream, strawberry topping), record the yield for each component.

- Ensure that the amounts yielded by each component of the recipe are sufficient to create the final product. For example, is 1 quart of marinara sauce sufficient to coat 1 pound of cooked pasta? Is 3 cups of frosting enough to frost a 9-inch three-layer cake?

- Factor the total yield and serving size into the overall recipe cost, if needed.

Taste

- Approach the testing with an objective palate; set aside all flavor biases and food prejudices.

- Make note of the balance in flavor, texture, temperature, mouthfeel, and color.

- Taste each component of a recipe separately, and then taste them together to evaluate how they complement each other.

- Be accurate in your flavor descriptions, and avoid subjective language. This will help in making taste comparisons from each test.

- Provide additional tasting comments that will help provide ideas for the recipe's headnote.

- Note whether the recipe met your expectations and whether you would make the recipe again.

- If possible, assemble a tasting panel to evaluate the final test using a taste panel worksheet (see sample below).

Visual

- Evaluate how the dish looks in its final prepared state. If it doesn't look appealing, suggest ways to improve its visual presentation—or how to make it more photogenic.

- During the tests, consider photographing each stage of the cooking or baking process, the finished dish, and the plated presentation. These photos can help those who will make the final photos of the recipe—art directors, food stylists, prop stylists, and photographers—as they decide on a final shot list.

Make-Ahead and Storage

- Note whether part of or the entire recipe can be prepared in advance. If making ahead is an option, offer suggestions for how the food should be stored, how long it can be safely stored, and its ideal storage conditions.

- Record any flavor, texture, or appearance changes that occur when the recipe or parts of it are made ahead; note whether there are any differences in storing it at room temperature, in the refrigerator, or in the freezer.

- If a freezer storage test is completed, thaw out and taste the food once the maximum time recommended for freezing it has passed. If that length of time is not possible, perform a shorter and more realistic freezer storage test.

CREATE A TASTE PANEL WORKSHEET

Engaging a tasting panel—ideally composed of people who fit the target audience for the recipe—is a good final step in recipe testing. If you cannot assemble a formal or consistent tasting team to evaluate and provide feedback on the test results, ask anyone who is available to taste the food. Create a tasting sheet for the project and use these notes to make further adjustments if needed. The following is an example of what can be included in a tasting sheet.

Sample Tasting Sheet

Recipe Name: _____

Tasting Date: _____

Did you like the dish? Yes   No

If no, please explain: _____

Rank the recipe in each of the following areas from 1 to 5, with 1 being the lowest and 5 being the highest rank. Provide comments on each ranking.

Appearance: 1 2 3 4 5 _____

Taste: 1 2 3 4 5 _____

Texture: 1 2 3 4 5 _____

Additional tasting comments: _____

_____

_____

Tolerance Testing

Tolerance testing is commonly done in food company test kitchens. Companies want to make sure their recipes always work and can be trusted, even if the consumer decides to make their own changes.

Tolerance testing involves testing a recipe according to several different ingredient, equipment, and cooking variabilities. Testing a recipe under a variety of conditions allows you to judge how the changes affect the end result and also allows you to instruct the cook on how to make adjustments. Following are several different options that test kitchen professionals often follow for tolerance testing:

- using fresh herbs and their dried equivalent

- using a variety of milk types, such as nonfat, low-fat, whole, half-and-half, and heavy whipping cream

- using fresh, frozen, or canned fruits or vegetables

- using both a gas and an electric oven or stove

- using variations on the oven temperature (e.g., 350° F versus 375° F)

- using different-sized or differently finished pans or dishes—for example, dark versus shiny cookie sheets; 1-inch-deep versus 4-inch-deep metal roasting pans; or 9 × 13-inch versus 8-inch square glass or ceramic baking dishes

- testing with a variety of appliances or techniques (e.g., pureeing soup in a regular blender versus a high-performance blender or mixing cookie dough or cake batter using a stand mixer, a hand mixer, and by hand)

- testing the results when certain ingredients are not measured exactly by the cook (e.g., decreasing or increasing the baking soda, baking powder, flour, or liquid or failing to drain a can of tomatoes) to determine how much wiggle room the recipe has before the end product is affected

Recording Recipe Testing Notes

Capture recipe testing information throughout the testing process and document your notes on a recipe testing sheet or directly on the recipe (see examples on pages 237 and 238). The recipe testing sheet is an example of what might be used by a professional recipe tester. Create your own testing sheet based on your company or project.

Quick Tip

"The advice I give to recipe testers: feel free to note any comments or questions on cooking techniques, instructions, or the order of recipe steps. If the recipe and instructions do not make sense to you, explain why, then tell me how you decided to interpret it. If the recipe is not specific enough and you must second guess or make assumptions about what the author meant, note that you are doing so. Add specific words and descriptions that might help the reader, even if you know the answers. For example: Should the lemon juice be strained? Should the nutmeg be freshly grated? How should the mixture be stored, covered? Can a step be done in advance; if so, how long in advance? And if something unexpected happens with the recipe—tell me how you dealt with it."

—Mary-Frances Heck, Senior Brand Director, *Outside* magazine; former senior food editor, *Food & Wine* magazine

RECIPE TESTING SHEET

Tester's Name	**Date**
Recipe	**Project**
Test #	**Preparation Time**
Marinating/Chilling/Rest Time	**Cook/Bake Time**
Stovetop Burner (circle one) Gas Electric Induction	**Oven (circle one)** Gas Electric **Temperature** _____
Total Yield	**# of Servings**

Ingredient Comments: Add detailed notes directly in the recipe, including the brands and package sizes used. Provide any additional comments here.

Preparation Comments: Add any details, include mixing and cooking times with visual notes for doneness, directly in the recipe, and provide any additional comments here.

Equipment Notes: Include type, sizes, pan material (e.g., nonstick/aluminum), pan preparation (e.g., greased/ungreased), utensils used, and any additional comments.

Yield Details: Include total yield and number of servings: US customary measures and metric weights. Include subrecipe yields (e.g., frosting, marinades).

Make Ahead/Storage Notes: Provide detailed instructions.

Tasting Comments: Be specific about flavor and texture, including comments on salt, sugar, and acid.

Additional Comments: Suggestions for headnote writing, photography, or video.

Next Steps: Ready for editing or retesting? What further testing is needed?

Tester: R. Sarazen
Date: 3/20/23
Test: #1

Seven Layer Bars
Prep time: 10 min
Cook time: 35 min
Yield: 40 bars

Amount and bag sizes not given

1 can sweetened condensed milk *(14 oz)*

chopped pecans *- used 1 cup*

1 bag butterscotch morsels *(typical bag size is 11 oz ~); suggest changing to #1 cup butterscotch morsel*

1 bag milk chocolate morsels *(typical bag size is 9-12 oz); #1 cup chocolate morsels — chips falling off the top*

1 bag *sweetened* coconut flakes *- bag sizes are variable; — suggest #1½ cup*

1 stick unsalted butter *(½ cup)*

2 cups graham cracker crumbs *(about 15 full size crackers)*

Not typical size; tested in 9x13

Preheat the oven to 350. Take a 9x11 pyrex pan and butter and line it
with parchment. I leave an overhang of parchment for easier removal
later. Melt 1 stick of unsalted butter on stove top. *over low heat. (or, melt in microwave in small glass bowl)* Mix with graham
cracker crumbs *(mixture is crumbly)* to create a base layer for the pan. After creating the *↘ Add to prepared pan and press crumbs into bottom of pan.*
base layer, layer on coconut flakes, butterscotch morsels, chocolate
morsels. *and nuts* Then pour the can of condensed milk on top. Cover with
chopped pecans. Bake for 35-40 minutes. Let cool completely before
removing from pan. Cut into small bars. *↘ until golden brown, about 30 min. → store in airtight container.*
↘ Suggest to add: Chill in refrigerator or freezer for easier cutting.

Tasted great with changes made!
Recipe needs editing - ingredients are not in order of use. Suggest decreasing chips to 1 cup each and 1½ c. sweetened coconut flakes. This amount is plenty — test again with correct amounts.

Recipe Testing by Home Cooks

Professional recipe testers know how to fix a recipe, making it reproducible, accurate, and delicious. While professional testers can test the final version of recipes before their publication, many cookbook authors and recipe content creators prefer to have home cooks test recipes at this stage. Keep in mind that while using home cooks to test your recipes may have benefits, it also has drawbacks.

Home cook testers can help you discover where consumers might struggle or have questions with the recipe, allowing you time to address these issues before the recipe is published. Consumers are likely to complain online if a recipe doesn't work properly, so this is a way to gain that sort of feedback in advance. On the other hand, home cooks often make mistakes—most notably, in not following the recipe exactly as it's written. Recruiting testers and managing the testing process is also time-consuming and can be challenging.

Following are tips for how to get started with recipe testing by home cooks:

- Create a spreadsheet that organizes your recipes for testing (see the example).

- Locate testers and assign recipes to them.

- When you send the recipes to testers, clarify your recipe testing parameters and share a set of recipe testing guidelines and testing sheets.

- Input tester feedback into the recipe. Use the feedback to edit it, to retest it (if needed), or to decide whether to drop it altogether.

- Send each tester a note of thanks.

SPREADSHEET FOR ORGANIZING HOME COOK RECIPE TESTING

Create a spreadsheet to organize and help manage the testing process. In the spreadsheet, list the recipes that need testing, who will be testing them, and when their feedback is due and received. Consider using an online platform that makes it easy to share content, such as Google Docs or Evernote, and set up a separate email account for direct communication with recipe testers.

Recipe	Tester 1 (name, email address, date submitted)	Feedback Received (date)	Tester 2 (name, email address, date submitted)	Feedback Received (date)	Tester 3 (name, email address, date submitted)	Feedback Received (date)
Spaghetti with meatballs						
Garlic bread						
Minestrone soup						

Finding Home Cooks to Test Recipes

The number of recipe testers you will need depends on the number of recipes you are testing, how many different people you want to test each recipe, and if recipe testers will test more than one recipe. Ideally, each recipe should be tested by at least two or three different testers. It can be challenging to find people who have the time and interest to help, especially if testers are not compensated for their effort. With that said, some ways to find potential home cook testers include:

- Reach out to enlist friends and family, including those who rarely cook.

- Use social media, which has a broad reach, to find new testers.

- Ask for help using a targeted mailing list.

- Create a landing page on your website that describes the recipe testing project and ask people to sign up by filling out a form.

In all cases, make sure to ask your potential testers a set of questions related to the specific recipes in either an email or an online survey form. It's best to create a template that can be edited and reused for each new testing project. The more specific your questions are, the more time you'll save with testing in the long run. Ideas for questions include:

- **Deadline:** *Can you test the recipe by [provide specific date]?* The testing process should take about 3 to 4 weeks.

- **Dietary restrictions:** *Do you have any dietary restrictions or allergies? If yes, please list them (e.g., vegetarian, gluten intolerance, peanut allergy).* This will ensure that they can taste the food they cook.

- **Kitchen equipment:** *Do you own a slow cooker/ stand mixer/food mill/popover pan?* Neglecting to ask whether a tester owns a piece of necessary equipment early on could compromise your timeline if they contact you weeks later to say that they couldn't complete the recipe. It could compromise the results of your test if a tester decides to use an alternate piece of equipment and assumes it's okay.

- **Testing preferences:** *How many recipes are you willing to test? Do you prefer sweet or savory recipes?*

If you have the time and location is not a problem, it's best to train any home cook tester(s) in your own kitchen to receive the most benefit. If this isn't possible, record a short training session and share the video clip with your testers.

Home Cook Recipe Testing Parameters

Once you have found home cook recipe testers and gathered their preferences and restrictions, you can assign recipes to each tester and input their names into your testing spreadsheet (or an alternative organizational system). If testers will be taking on more than one recipe, try to assign them recipes that use overlapping ingredients. For example, if one recipe requires a small amount of an ingredient (e.g., soy sauce, Dijon mustard, fish sauce), include a second recipe that uses the same ingredient to help hold down the testers' grocery costs.

When sending out the recipes to testers, be sure to restate their deadlines and include any financial and recipe usage agreement terms. Depending on the situation, this may involve a nondisclosure agreement, a letter, or a casual, verbal explanation. Consider communicating part or all of the following to your testers:

- **Deadline and process for submittal:** provide your testers with a deadline to turn in the forms you have provided via a cloud-based platform that will allow them to share files quickly and simply.

  Completed recipe testing sheets must be submitted by Tuesday, February 8 via Google Drive.

- **Anticipated grocery and equipment costs:** it costs money to buy ingredients and equipment, so be clear about whether you are reimbursing testers. For example:

  All groceries and equipment expenses are the tester's responsibility.

  Testers will receive up to $30 per recipe to cover the cost of ingredients.

- **Recipe testing compensation:** recipe testing takes time, so be clear about whether or how testers are compensated. Either look for volunteers who are willing to test for free or offer testers some form of acknowledgment or compensation for their time. For example:

Testers will not receive compensation for recipe testing, but they will receive credit in the book's acknowledgments page and a copy of the book after publication.

Although I cannot reimburse you for your ingredients, please know how much I appreciate your help, and I'll include your name on the acknowledgments page.

Testers will receive $50 for each recipe tested and $65 for recipes that include two to three sub-recipes (e.g., a recipe for a cake, its frosting, and a chocolate sauce that is poured over it).

- **Confidentiality requirements:** if you wish to keep your recipe testing project private, you should share that, but if you want to be certain of confidentiality, ask your testers to sign a nondisclosure agreement. It will protect you and your recipes.

Please do not share these recipes with others.

Do not post photos or videos of the recipe testing process or provide commentary about the recipe online or in other media until the final recipe is published by me.

Instructions for Home Cook Testers

Along with communication that clarifies the recipe testing deadline and process for submittal, compensation, and confidentiality, include the recipes, instructions, and a testing sheet (see Recipe Testing Instructions for Home Cooks on page 242 and Recipe Testing Sheet for Home Cooks on page 243 for examples). Recipe testing instructions, just like recipe testing sheets, may differ based on the type of recipes being tested. Testing forms for baking, cooking, and health-focused recipes often include unique questions. You can also create a straightforward and short online survey with questions that require yes/no answers. Or create a longer testing form with a combination of yes/no answers with space for written comments.

Quick Tip

"The first recipe test is always done by me. I want my hands in every one of my cookbooks. I then have my assistant test recipes, or I invite friends over to test them. I give my friends a testing worksheet that describes how the testing should be done—including something basic like, 'Read the entire recipe through and ask me any questions before you begin.' After the testing is done, we sit down at my kitchen table, share testing notes, and taste the food—making corrections on the spot for each recipe. And while recipes may be moving away from perfection and more toward a casual recipe that leaves room for the home cook to improvise, a recipe in a cookbook should work, and that comes from testing." —Joan Nathan, cookbook author of 11 cookbooks, including *Jewish Cooking in America* and *King Solomon's Table*

Quick Tip

"If you have a blog, include a section on book corrections or new thoughts about a recipe. Readers can be directed to it from other social media such as Instagram. People really appreciate this." —Rose Levy Beranbaum, baking expert, cookbook author of 12 books, including *The Cake Bible* and *The Pie and Pastry Bible*

Receiving and Implementing Feedback

As you receive completed forms from your testers, be sure to update your spreadsheet with their feedback, and then edit the recipe. If needed, retest it. If you receive poor feedback from two to three testers on the same recipe, consider dropping the recipe altogether, putting it aside to rework later, or using it to develop something different. If the feedback you receive for a recipe is mixed, remind yourself that palates and preferences differ. Once the testing stage is completed, be sure to send your testers a thank-you message via email or a handwritten note—especially if they were not compensated.

RECIPE TESTING INSTRUCTIONS FOR HOME COOKS

The following examples illustrate the types of instructions to include when working with home cook recipe testers. Create your own set of recipe testing instructions based on your recipe project--or use a variation of the instructions that follow.

1. Test the recipe at a time when you're not rushed or multitasking. Accurate testing requires focus!

2. Before you begin, read through the recipe in its entirety at least once and ideally twice.

3. Contact me if anything in the recipe needs clarification. Don't guess.

4. Gather all of your ingredients in the proper amounts and place them on your work surface before you start cooking.

5. Use metal or plastic measuring cups and spoons for dry ingredients and glass measuring cups for liquids to carefully measure all ingredients before you start testing.

6. When you are measuring out dry ingredients using measuring cups, be sure to overfill the measuring cup, and then level off the top by scraping off the excess with a knife or other straight edge.

7. When measuring flour or cocoa powder, use the dip-and-sweep method. First, use a large spoon to fluff up the ingredient in its container. Then, dip a measuring cup into the container and overfill it; scrape the excess back into the container using a straight edge or knife. [Alternatively, ask them to test the recipe using the spoon-and-sweep method and provide these instructions.]

8. Please prepare the recipe exactly as it is written. Otherwise, you're not really testing the recipe.

9. As you're testing, check off each ingredient as you use it in the recipe.

10. Use the exact size and type of cookware or baking dish called for in the recipe. If that is not possible and you have to use something different, make a note of what you use. Measure the pan instead of guessing.

11. Use a kitchen timer or smartphone to keep track of preparation or cooking/baking time.

12. Take lots of notes throughout your testing. I want to hear all your feedback!

13. Take a picture of the final dish. It's okay if it doesn't look perfect!

14. Fill out the testing form while your testing results and your thoughts about the recipe are fresh in your mind.

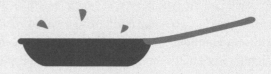

RECIPE TESTING SHEET FOR HOME COOKS

Tester Name: _____

Date Tested: _____

Recipe Name: _____

Were the ingredients readily available? Yes   No

  If no, please comment and share whether you made a substitution. _____
  _____

Were the kitchen tools and equipment needed for this recipe readily accessible? Yes   No

  If no, please comment and share whether you made a substitution. _____
  _____

Were the measurements clear? Yes   No

  If no, please share any questions you have. _____
  _____

Were the instructions clear? Yes   No

  If no, please share any questions you have; include which section or step of the recipe your question
  relates to. _____
  _____

Did you make any changes to the recipe? Yes   No

  If so, what did you change? _____

Were the preparation time and cooking time correct? Yes   No

  If no, please share the correct time. _____

How many servings did this recipe claim to make? _____

How many servings did this recipe actually make? _____

Would you make this recipe again or share it with a friend? Yes   No

  If no, please explain. _____

Would other people who tasted the recipe want you to make it again? Yes   No

  If no, please explain. _____

Rate this recipe on a scale from 1 to 10 (with 1 being horrible and would never make again and
10 being best) on taste, texture, appearance, and overall appeal:

Taste _____   Texture _____   Appearance _____Overall appeal: _____

Any other feedback? _____
_____
_____

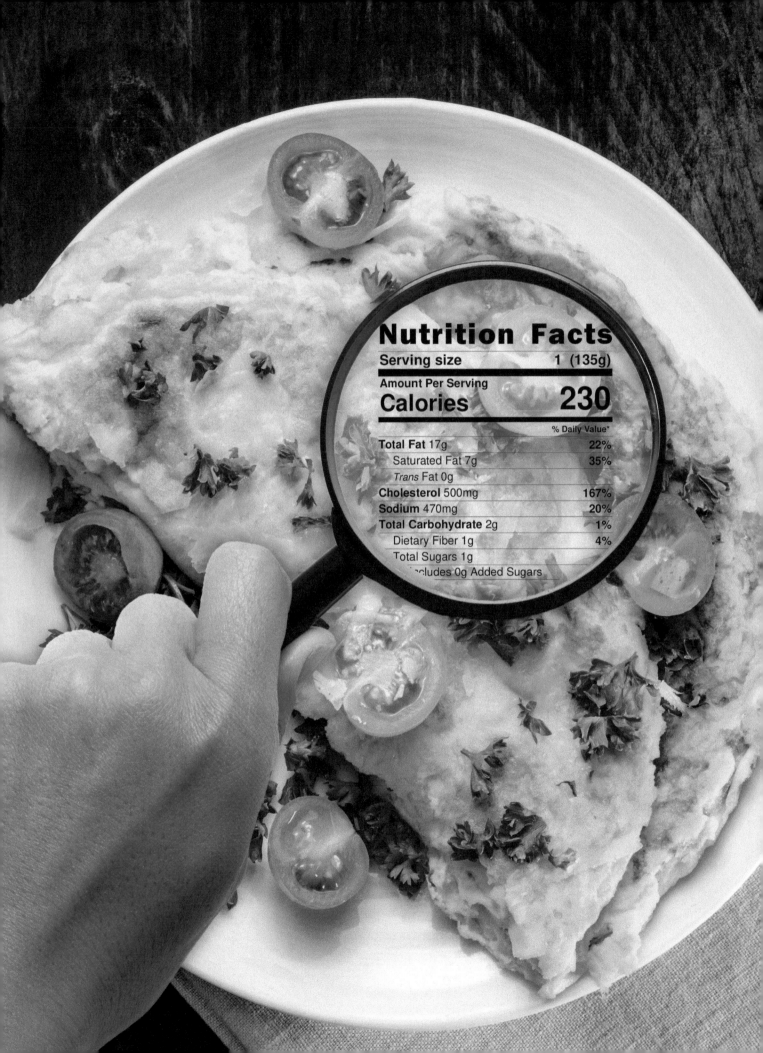

Nutrition Facts

Serving size	1 (135g)

Amount Per Serving

Calories 230

% Daily Value*

Total Fat 17g	22%
Saturated Fat 7g	35%
Trans Fat 0g	
Cholesterol 500mg	167%
Sodium 470mg	20%
Total Carbohydrate 2g	1%
Dietary Fiber 1g	4%
Total Sugars 1g	
Includes 0g Added Sugars	

Chapter 9

Nutrition Analysis of Recipes

IN THIS CHAPTER, LEARN ABOUT:

- Nutrition analysis options for recipes: laboratory analysis, software analysis, application program interfaces, and website plug-ins

- Evaluating and working with an independent laboratory

- Evaluating and choosing a nutrition analysis software program

- How to analyze recipes using a nutrition analysis software program

- Guidelines for analyzing recipes with complex ingredients, preparation methods, or cooking methods

Health-conscious consumers demand nutrition information for published recipes and for prepared menu items they select while eating out. They want transparency to help make more informed food decisions. This is especially true for recipes and menu items that are health-focused (e.g., low in saturated fat, high in fiber, reduced in sodium).

When developing and testing recipes, you may be asked by your client—perhaps a publisher, food company, or restaurant group—to provide or manage the nutrition analysis. Food professionals must understand the types of analysis options that are available and how to evaluate them as well as when to consider hiring an experienced food and nutrition expert to oversee and analyze the recipes.

Purpose of Nutrition Analysis

In addition to helping consumers make informed food choices, nutrition analysis is performed for other purposes, including:

- to estimate the nutritional content of the food during recipe development, which can support the process of improving the nutrient profile through recipe modification

- to substantiate a health or nutrient content claim (see Chapter 2) for recipes found on websites, digital and print publications, social media platforms, and cookbooks

- to serve as a marketing tool and improve online search engine optimization (SEO)

- to create government compliant Nutrition Facts labels, which are required by the US Food and Drug Administration (FDA) on all consumer-packaged foods

- to provide nutrition information for menu items of restaurants with twenty or more locations in the United States, including Puerto Rico and Guam (required by the FDA)

SHOULD ALL RECIPES INCLUDE NUTRITION INFORMATION?

Food professionals and publishers have differing opinions as to whether all recipes should include nutrition information. On one hand, some believe that if a health claim is not associated with a recipe, then nutrition information is not necessary and the focus should be on eating and enjoying food, regardless of its nutrient amounts. Conversely, others argue that nutrition information is often where people begin when they want to improve their eating habits. Regardless, nutrition information can help consumers make more informed food choices to support their health goals, such as losing weight or managing diabetes, high blood pressure, and other health conditions.

Nutrition Analysis Methods

There are two primary methods used for determining the nutrient content for packaged food products, restaurant menu items, and published recipes:

- **chemical analysis** (also known as laboratory analysis)
- **calculated analysis** using a nutrient database, which may be performed using nutrition analysis software

Using either or both of these methods is accepted by the FDA for Nutrition Facts labels and restaurant menu labeling. There are no rules for calculating or publishing nutrition information in cookbooks or on social media platforms, websites, blogs, and digital newsletters, but there are professional best practices based on regulations and guidelines of the FDA.

In a *chemical analysis* (referred to in this chapter as a laboratory analysis), the food products or samples are sent to a laboratory. There, samples are prepped and analyzed using various scientific instruments and techniques to yield nutrient data for that specific food or meal item.

In a *calculated analysis*, recipe nutrition information is calculated using nutrition analysis software or a nutrition API (application program interface) that gathers data from a food and ingredient composition database. Some software allows users to add new product nutrition information, modify current food and ingredient nutrition information in the database, and make adjustments for cooking process nutrient changes. See page 284 for more information on selecting a nutrition analysis software program. See page 249 for more on APIs, automated calculators, and website plug-ins.

Using a combination of chemical and calculated analysis methods may be necessary due to budget and efficiency reasons or because a nutrient or ingredient cannot be accurately analyzed using only one method. For example, a food company may offer several ice cream flavors that all use the same vanilla base. The company can send out the vanilla ice cream base for laboratory analysis and then use a software analysis to include nutrient data for the ingredients added to the base to create different flavors.

Many factors can influence which method is best for a project. Nutrition Analysis Methods: Advantages and Disadvantages provides an overview of advantages and disadvantages of each nutrition analysis method.

NUTRITION ANALYSIS METHODS: ADVANTAGES AND DISADVANTAGES

Laboratory analysis

Advantages	Disadvantages
Creates regulatory-compliant food labels and information needed to verify nutrient content claims; can also produce ingredient and allergen statements Preferred and more accurate method for: • food product recipes that are difficult to analyze, such as dehydrated, brewed, fermented, deep-fried, pickled, or brined foods • food products and recipes with unique ingredients for which nutrition data is not available Useful for determining nutrient stability (e.g., loss of vitamins) during a food product's shelf life to assess accuracy of nutrient claims; often done during research and development and product development stages Independent and unbiased; not dependent on the accuracy of a nutrient database or product supplier nutrition information Additional services available for specific food allergen, gluten, and shelf-life testing	Relatively expensive, especially in comparison to using software Offers a one-time snapshot of nutrient information If an ingredient changes in the recipe or product, the laboratory analysis is no longer relevant Analyzes for total sugars but cannot analyze for added sugars in a food product or recipe; a laboratory analysis cannot distinguish the difference between sugars added during food processing and naturally occurring sugars found in milk products, fruit, and vegetables Does not show how each ingredient contributes to the total nutrient profile Results are not immediate (requires 2 weeks to 1 month)

BOX CONTINUES >

Calculated (Software) Analysis*

Advantages	Disadvantages
Creates regulatory-compliant food labels and information needed to verify a nutrient content claim; many applications can also produce ingredient and allergen statement	May be less accurate than a laboratory analysis, particularly if a recipe has inaccurate measurements for recipes with preparation methods that make it difficult to analyze, including deep-frying, pickling, marinating, fermenting, and dehydrating
Helpful during the initial stages of recipe development, especially if trying to meet specific nutrient targets and during reformulation of a food product or recipe	Accuracy of analysis dependent on accuracy of the software's database
Useful for accurately analyzing consumer recipes for publication	Final analysis accuracy is dependent on the skills of the professional performing the calculation.
Nutrient analysis report shows how each ingredient contributes to the final nutrient content profile	
Allows users to make ingredient and recipe modifications as needed; eliminates the time and cost of sending out for laboratory analysis	
Enables the addition of an unlimited number of new foods, ingredients, allergens, and suppliers to the nutrient database	
Allows for calculation of the amount of added sugar	
Manages all ingredients, recipes, and formulations in one place; many are able to calculate recipe yield and cost	
Cost-effective and efficient	

Automated Calculator Analysis

Advantages	Disadvantages
Useful for analyzing a large volume of consumer recipes, where speed is more important than accuracy	Cannot be used to create regulatory-compliant food labels
Can provide a general estimate of a recipe's nutrient information quickly and at a relatively low price (applies to more powerful calculators)	Source and accuracy of nutrition information for an ingredient or product often unknown and may not be identical or similar to what is used in the recipe
	In general, tends to underreport nutrient values (especially sodium)
	Possibility of no standards or parameters built into the automated calculator for difficult-to-analyze recipes
	Not all allow a user to edit incorrect data or make adjustments in nutrients or cooking method

* Based on software with robust features and extensive food and ingredient databases for accurate and comprehensive nutrition analysis.

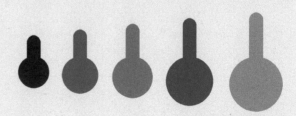

Automated Calculators and Application Programming Interfaces

A nutrition API (application programming interface) is a computer interface that interacts with a nutrient database to perform an automated nutrition analysis for a recipe. Many consumer recipes available on blogs, online publications, and websites are analyzed using an automated calculator on an app or a website plug-in. These apps and plug-ins are developed using a nutrition API to calculate the nutrition analysis.

Nutrition analysis APIs use specialized technology that allows them to perform automated nutrient calculations of hundreds or thousands of recipes very quickly (e.g., for websites with extensive libraries of recipes). A nutrition analysis API can be an appropriate choice for large jobs like these, as it can provide a *reasonable* estimate of a recipe's nutrient information quickly and cost-effectively.

Analyzing recipes using an API usually involves a monthly licensing fee. More powerful APIs may offer other applications, including menu planning, scaling recipes, and converting measurements.

Limitations of Automated Calculators

The accuracy of automated calculators varies widely due to many factors, including the database source and how the calculator was developed. Although analyses performed using calculators or APIs are similar to software analyses, using an automated calculator will not yield results as reliable as an analysis performed by an experienced food and nutrition professional using a robust nutrition analysis software program.

APIs provide ballpark estimations for nutrition information, and generally, they tend to underreport nutrient values (especially sodium). APIs don't claim to be error free, and food professionals should assume responsibility for information that is published about their recipes. Investing in reputable nutrient analysis software is recommended to get the most accurate nutrition information, especially if the recipes being analyzed are for people who manage their chronic health conditions through diet.

WEBSITE RECIPE PLUG-INS

Plug-ins are software applications that add a specific feature to an existing website. In addition to providing templates for easy-to-read formatting, searching, and filtering of recipes, many recipe plug-ins offer the functionality of automated nutrition analysis. Another benefit of using a plug-in is that the metadata can improve search engine optimization (SEO) and attract more visitors to a website.

How accurate are recipe plug-ins?

Nutrition information automatically calculated by recipe plug-ins can vary widely. Plug-ins send data to an API, which tries to match the recipe's ingredients with ingredients stored in a database. The first match the API finds is typically the one that is used unless the plug-in allows you to manually view and select ingredient choices. Nutrition information can vary widely across different brands, so the product used in a recipe might differ from the one stored in the plug-in's database. Some plug-ins allow you to create a custom food item and input the data manually, which helps yield a more accurate result.

Quick Tip

"For recipes where FDA compliance is not required and the focus is on analyzing large volumes of recipes or real time nutrition analysis, consider an automated calculator. This can approximate the accuracy of the human performing nutrition analysis by using natural language processing—mapping how humans speak to get to the right recipe ingredient and default to specific ones when necessary." —Victor Penev, founder and CEO of Edamam

Why Nutrition Analysis Is an Estimate

Nutrition analysis of the nutrient content of food products, restaurant menu items, and recipes is not an exact science. This is true whether the analysis is done by laboratory analysis or by calculation using software or a nutrition API/recipe plug-in. Nutrition analysis results must be considered an e*stimate* and may vary from the *actual* nutrient composition for several key reasons, including the following:

- the inherent nutrient variability of foods
- any changes that cooks may make during preparation of a recipe
- the limitations of the nutrition analysis method used

Nutrient Variability of Foods

Many factors can impact the nutritional content of food. The composition of foods is variable as a result of many environmental factors, including, but not limited to, soil and growing conditions, ripeness at time of harvest, the diet of animals, and length of storage. For example, tomatoes of the same varietal that are grown in Indiana and California can have slightly different nutritional values due to the different nutrient levels in the soil, or the amount of fat or marbling in a steak can differ depending on the specific diet of the cow it came from.

Changes Made during Recipe Preparation

Variations or changes in the preparation and cooking of food can result in nutrient gain or loss. For example, changes in the cooking method, cooking temperature, and cooking time can affect fat, vitamin, and mineral content. Examples of methods that produce nutritional differences include boiling or steaming vegetables, panfrying or grilling fish, and cooking meats or soups at a low or high temperature for varying amounts of time, which produces differences in the dish's final volume and weight.

It's important to remember that recipes are not always followed exactly as directed, and that alone is a reason why nutrition analysis is an estimate. Cooks often deviate from recipes by adding, deleting, or substituting ingredients and by changing preparation methods, cooking procedures, cooking times, and portion sizes. This is true regardless of whether the recipe is prepared by a home cook or in a foodservice establishment.

Another reason why results vary is that cooks may not always use the same brands of ingredients. For example, different brands of Dijon mustard have different formulations; subsequently, they have different nutrient composition (sodium content, in particular, often varies significantly among brands). In addition, manufacturers may change their product formulations, so results from when a recipe was initially analyzed may not remain accurate after changes are made.

Limitations of Methods Used for Analysis

Each method of nutrition analysis has its own limitations, which can result in inaccurate results. For example, a calculated analysis is more nuanced than just entering types of foods and ingredients into a software program. Factors that influence these results include the software program's database and the person performing the analysis. While accurate and reliable nutrition information is possible when an experienced food and nutrition professional uses a robust nutrition analysis software program—not all software programs and recipe analysts are equal. Inaccurate results can occur when a software application uses inaccurate, out-of-date, or incomplete data. And if the recipe analyst lacks knowledge and experience with nutrition analysis software, errors can result from inaccurate ingredient selections from the database and from not following nutrition analysis standards or using consistent recipe assumptions. Limitations of laboratory analysis and automated calculators are discussed on page 248.

Quick Tip

"[The] FDA requires values on Nutrition Facts labels to be accurate within the tolerances specified in the Code of Federal Regulations but does not require a specific method of analysis to determine the values. When performed correctly, database analysis is typically a better predictor for nutrient values as it uses the statistical average for commodity ingredients." —Karen Duester, Founder, Food Consulting Company

Nutrition Analysis Method: Laboratory Analysis

Laboratory analysis, also referred to as chemical analysis, is considered to be the most accurate method of nutrient analysis. It's often referred to as the "gold standard" for nutrition analysis, but it's also relatively expensive. As a result, laboratory analysis is not always practical or possible. For this reason, laboratory analysis is typically used by large food manufacturers, restaurant chains, retailers, and foodservice establishments. Small companies and individual restaurants often rely on nutrition analysis software (see Recipe Nutrition Analysis Software and Databases page 287). Understanding laboratory analysis, in general, is helpful when working in recipe development, new product development, or nutrition regulatory and labeling compliance for a food manufacturer or restaurant company.

When to Use Laboratory Analysis

Laboratory analysis is often the preferred method for validation of nutrient content and compliance with FDA labeling rules. The most common circumstances for sending food to a laboratory for a chemical analysis include the following:

- ensuring regulatory compliance by documenting that nutrient and allergen statements and claims are correct and not misleading or untruthful
- adding a food's precise and essential nutrient data to an existing nutrient database (e.g., the US Department of Agriculture [USDA] FoodData Central database or proprietary nutrient analysis software)
- analyzing a product or recipe that is difficult to accurately analyze using software—especially those that are prepared in a way that is inherently complex to analyze, such as:

  - fried foods and coated fried foods that may absorb fat and lose moisture during the frying process
  - cooked proteins that lose fat during cooking

  - marinated, braised, brined, pickled, fermented, or dehydrated foods
  - made-from-scratch broths, stocks, strained soups, juices, and steeped beverages
  - recipes with reduced and simmered sauces
  - alcohol-containing recipes that are cooked down or reduced (e.g., red wine reduction)
  - recipes or products that include an ingredient with no available nutrient data (e.g., an exotic ingredient used in a formulation or recipe)

The best practice for these types of food is to send them to a laboratory to obtain the most accurate nutrient analysis. If this is not possible, refer to page 256 for best practices when analyzing these types of foods using nutrition analysis software.

Quick Tip

"There are some nutrients and foods that are difficult to calculate by software—like the sodium in pickles or foods such as kombucha and dehydrated meat (jerkies). The database calculation cannot accurately capture the nutrient changes that happen with some processed foods, and it is recommended that these products be sent to a lab for a COA (Certificate of Analysis) test. And some foods like pickled vegetables can be sent for lab analysis for sodium only. This will save money versus asking for a full lab analysis." —Wendy Hess, MS, RDN, nutrition analysis consultant

Quick Tip

"Keep a record of each sample that is sent to the lab—after receiving a nutrition report, your notes and pictures of the sample will help to remind you what food sample was sent to know exactly what the results represent." —Andrea Custer, MS, RDN, Technical Sales Coordinator, Mérieux NutriSciences

How to Choose a Laboratory

The first step in choosing an independent laboratory is assessing whether the laboratory meets all of the project's needs, including the budget, the nutrients that must be analyzed, and any additional services that are necessary. Once these factors are established, it's also important to ensure that the laboratory utilizes Association of Official Analytical Chemists (AOAC) methods, as this assures that the lab's testing procedures are current. In addition, the laboratory should be ISO 17025 accredited, which demonstrates that it is technically proficient and able to produce precise and accurate tests and calibration data.

Working With a Laboratory

Laboratory analysis for food labeling involves sending in physical samples of prepared food items to a laboratory for chemical analysis. Labs usually require a minimum of 1 pound (454 grams) of the food in question, but most recommend that solid food samples weigh 3 to 4 pounds and liquid samples must be 16 ounces or more to successfully complete an analysis. FDA protocols recommend that the sample should be a composite of 12 randomly selected subsamples (consumer units). For example, prepared samples of a restaurant menu item may come from several different locations to account for variations in how the food is prepared and the amounts of fat absorbed by each batch. Samples may be prepared in and collected from restaurant test or control kitchens as long as they are representative of the edible portion of the standardized recipe.

Each laboratory has its own packing and shipping requirements, but in general, plan to ship the samples overnight or next day in the condition in which they must be to remain edible (e.g., refrigerated or frozen products should be shipped in a refrigerated or frozen state, respectively).

Most labs have a set price for an analysis of the nutrients included in a Nutrition Facts labeling package, and some also offer additional testing services for labeling of food allergens, gluten-free products, nutrient content claims, and additional voluntary nutrients (e.g., B vitamins, selenium, vitamin C). Ask whether the laboratory can deliver both a compliant Nutrition Facts label and a Certificate of Analysis (COA),

> ## *Quick Tip*
> "When sending in samples for laboratory analysis, be extra clear with direction. Provide details in the analysis request form with clear instructions of what you want (or don't want) the lab to do. For example, a lab once removed the skin from fish, even when the sample preparation instruction did not specify this."
> —Sarah Hendren, MS, RDN, Regulatory Affairs Scientist for Frito Lay North America

if that is what is required (see sample). Most laboratory analyses provide a COA of unrounded data for 100 grams of a product for total calories, total fat, saturated fat, *trans* fat, cholesterol, sodium, total carbohydrates, dietary fiber, total sugars, protein, vitamin D, calcium, iron, and potassium as well as ash and moisture results.

No laboratory-based analytical method exists to determine which sugars in a food are natural and which are added. A laboratory report will provide only the total amount of sugars in the food. Some laboratories offer services to assist with determining the added sugar content. This is often performed by a nutrition professional using nutrition analysis software.

Limitations of Laboratory Analysis

Several variables in a laboratory analysis can influence accuracy of the results. These include the variations in raw ingredients; the stability of nutrients during transport and storage; adherence to obtaining a representative sample for analysis; staff competence; and quality control (how the machines are maintained, serviced, and calibrated).

In addition, a laboratory analysis represents the nutrients found by one particular laboratory in one particular sample at one particular point in time. If the recipe changes, or if products or ingredients in the recipe change, the laboratory analysis will no longer be accurate. If food products and ingredients used in a recipe change frequently, a laboratory analysis might not be the best option.

Example of a Certificate of Analysis Report

A Certificate of Analysis (COA) communicates the results of a laboratory analysis for a food product or recipe.

Certificate of Analysis

NUTRITIONAL ANALYSIS

Serving Size: 100.0 g

Household Measure: 100 g

Analytes	Units	Results Per 100g	Amount Per Serving	Test Date	Test Location
Calories		1509.0	1510	05/31/2021	
Total Fat	g	162.59	163	05/31/2021	
Monounsaturated Fat	g	2.03	2.03	05/31/2021	
Polyunsaturated Fat	g	5.39	5.39	05/31/2021	
Saturated Fat	g	149.01	149	05/31/2021	
Trans Fat	g	0.02	0.02	05/31/2021	
Cholesterol	mg	<0.8	<0.8	05/31/2021	
Sodium	mg	432	432	05/31/2021	
Potassium	mg	109	109	05/31/2021	
Total Carbohydrate	g	<0.25	<0.25	05/31/2021	
Dietary Fiber‡	g	3.82	3.82	05/31/2021	
Sugars‡‡	g	4.59	4.59	05/31/2021	
Fructose	g	0.80		05/31/2021	
Glucose	g	0.49		05/31/2021	
Lactose	g	<0.25		05/31/2021	
Maltose	g	3.30		05/31/2021	
Sucrose	g	<0.25		05/31/2021	
Protein (F=6.38)	g	11.42	11.4	05/31/2021	
Calcium	mg	97.4	97.4	05/31/2021	
Iron	mg	2.50	2.50	05/31/2021	
Moisture	g	30.32	30.3	05/31/2021	
Ash	g	1.59	1.59	05/31/2021	
Vitamin D2	mcg	<0.75	<0.75	05/31/2021	
Vitamin D3	mcg	<0.55	<0.55	05/31/2021	
Total Vitamin D	mcg	<0.55	<0.55	05/31/2021	

‡ This Total Dietary Fiber measurement may include polysaccharides not currently recognized as dietary fiber by FDA. Clients must review their formulas and ingredients to determine fibers not currently recognized as fiber. Clients may need to consult with their fiber manufacturers to determine the regulatory status of their fiber.

‡‡ The reported Total Sugars value is the sum of all naturally occurring and added sugars. Quantifying added sugars must be separately performed using food formulas, production records, and ingredient specifications.

Sample report provided courtesy of Mérieux NutriSciences

SELECTING A LABORATORY FOR CHEMICAL ANALYSIS

Use the list below as a starting point when researching options for accredited laboratories. The cost typically ranges anywhere from $600 to $1,200 or more per item. Expect additional cost for added sugar software analysis, verification of nutrient content claims, and allergen testing and statements.

Analytical Food Laboratories (AFL): afltexas.com/lab-analyses/nutritional-analysis

EMSL Food Testing Lab: foodtestinglab.com/food-nutritional-analysis

Eurofins: eurofinsus.com/food-testing/services/testing-services

Food Safety Net Services: fsns.com/services/chemistry-testing/nutritional-labeling

Medallion Labs: medallionlabs.com/our-services/nutritional-labeling-testing

Merieux NutriSciences: merieuxnutrisciences.com/na/labeling-regulatory-services

Michelson Laboratories, Inc: michelsonlab.com

Q Laboratories: qlaboratories.com/food-chemistry

Nutrition Analysis Method: Software Analysis

The alternative to laboratory analysis is using nutrition analysis software to calculate the nutrient content of a recipe. The software must contain up-to-date data from the USDA and international food databases, as well as data from food manufacturers and restaurants. When used by skilled professionals, software offers the advantage of quickly and easily analyzing the nutritional content of recipes at a relatively affordable price. No physical food samples are needed for software analysis calculation: it is performed using information provided by the written recipe.

When to Use Software for Nutrition Analysis

Nutrition analysis software is an important tool for analyzing recipes for websites, blogs, print and digital publications, and cookbooks. It can also be used during product development, for recipes printed on food label packages, and for restaurant and foodservice menu labeling. Using software has many advantages: ease of use, flexibility, speed, and reduced cost. For example, adding or subtracting an ingredient in a software database when a recipe changes is much easier and more cost-effective than sending new food samples to a lab.

Quick Tip

"Nutrition analysis is its own specialty. It is not a data entry job. Yes, it requires data entry, but to perform it correctly and professionally, you must understand food composition, nutrition, and cooking."
—Karen Duester, MS, RD, President, Food Consulting Company

Learning to Perform a Nutrition Analysis

Recipe developers and testers should understand the basics of nutrition analysis—in particular, they should know what ingredient and product information is necessary to perform an accurate analysis. Even if your analyses are performed by other food or nutrition professionals, learning the basics allows you to better manage the process and can enable you to assist the publisher, foodservice company, or food manufacturer in choosing a reputable software application or hiring the appropriate professional to perform the work.

No matter who performs the nutrition analysis, professional best practices must be followed. Mislabeled and miscalculated recipes can cause problems in many forms, including brand negativity (repercussions of noncompliance or wrong information), a loss of the consumer's trust, and potential endangerment of consumer health with inaccurate nutrition information and nutrient claims.

Quick Tip

"For recipes that require FDA compliance and the focus is on accuracy, evaluate nutrient analysis software programs based on this parameter." —Chris Eakin, Director of Sales, ESHA Research

Quick Tip

"It is not the software that does the work, it's the person using the software that really matters. An analysis will only be as good as the food and nutrition knowledge of the person using it." —Cheryl Dolven, MS, RDN, co-author of *Recipe Nutrient Analysis*

NUTRITION ANALYSIS: FINDING A QUALIFIED EXPERT

A registered dietitian nutritionist (RDN) with culinary and regulatory expertise has the educational background and professional experience necessary to perform and manage the nutrition analysis for consumer recipes, food products, and restaurant menu labeling.

The Academy of Nutrition and Dietetics offers a Find an Expert resource page (eatright.org/find-an-expert); choose "nutrient analysis" as the expertise search option, and the site will bring up a variety of qualified professionals. The Academy's Food and Culinary Professional practice group (fcpdpg.org) and food labeling professional groups on LinkedIn are good resources as well.

A qualified professional should:

- understand how cooking and handling food affects nutrient content and make necessary professional judgments during the analysis (e.g., choosing the correct database ingredient item), know when an appropriate ingredient substitution needs to be made, or adjust the nutrients in a specific database item.

- stay current on the complexities of and research related to recipe nutrition analysis, food labeling, and software choices.

- understand the FDA guidelines and rules for food product and restaurant menu labeling (including regulatory compliance for the Nutrition Facts label) and verify nutrient content claims, health claims, and food allergen statements.

- be able to identify the nutrient benefits of a food item or recipe and translate them into FDA-compliant labeling claims or messaging for a food product's marketing department.

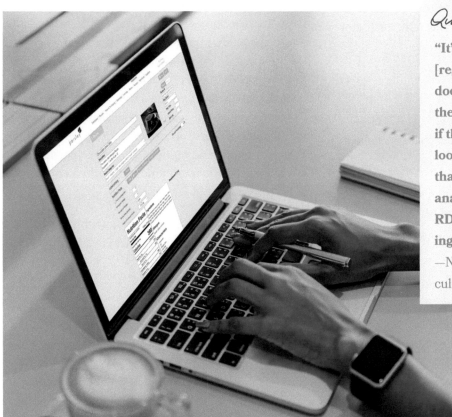

> ## Quick Tip
>
> "It's helpful if an RDN [registered dietitian nutritionist] does the nutrition analysis since they have the ability to evaluate if the final nutrient numbers look right. It's their judgment that you want. Also, since an analysis is just an estimate, the RDN knows to be consistent with ingredient database choices."
> —Nancy Macklin, MS, RDN, LDN, culinary nutrition consultant

Best Practices for Analyzing Recipes Using Nutrition Analysis Software

Nutrition analysis of a recipe using software may appear to be straightforward, but it's actually quite complex. The accuracy of the results is dependent on the recipe analyst's ability to correctly interpret and assess the recipe, choose accurate ingredient data from the database, and estimate an accurate yield if the written recipe does not include this information. Complicated preparation and cooking techniques can also affect the accuracy of the analysis.

The recipe analyst must attempt to obtain all the recipe details, stay current with nutrient analysis research, and follow best practices to ensure as much accuracy as possible. The more precise the recipe information is, the more accurate the nutrient estimates will be, which increases the likelihood of meeting the FDA's 80-20 compliance standard, a benchmark for menu labeling and consumer recipe analysis (see page 289 for more information).

Follow these general **best practices** when analyzing a recipe using a software application; each step will be discussed in more detail.

Step 1: Review the recipe.

Step 2: Compile a precise list of recipe ingredients and measurements.

Step 3: Review the preparation and cooking methods.

Step 4: Determine the correct edible portion for each ingredient.

Step 5: Evaluate recipe yield and servings.

Step 6: Enter the ingredient information into the software program.

Step 7: Review nutrition analysis results.

Step 8: Communicate nutrition information.

Step 1: Review the Recipe

The first step in a software nutrition analysis is to carefully review the recipe, whether it is a standardized recipe used at a foodservice establishment or a consumer recipe written for a publication. This step also includes obtaining and reviewing all subrecipes within the recipe in order to ensure that the analyst has all information necessary to perform an accurate and complete nutrition analysis. For example, a salad recipe may contain a subrecipe for a dressing.

The style and details of recipes written in a standardized recipe format or a consumer format can vary. It's most accurate to perform the nutrition analysis using detailed information that includes the gram weight of each ingredient, single serving size, and total yield. See Standardized Recipes on page 19 for more on standardized quantity recipes.

Step 2: Compile a Precise List of Recipe Ingredients and Measurements

Detailed ingredient descriptions and precise measurements are necessary to ensure an accurate analysis. If the written recipe does not provide this level of detail, the recipe analyst must obtain it. The ideal way to get this information is to work alongside the developer and take notes, but if that's not feasible, call or send recipe questions to the chef, recipe developer, or recipe tester. This critical step will help you choose ingredients from the database more accurately during the analysis. While carefully reading through the recipe, ask these key questions as you examine each ingredient item:

- Is this ingredient information clear as it is written?

- Is there sufficient detail, such as the ingredient's type, brand, form, and preparation?

OBTAIN PRECISE INGREDIENT INFORMATION

The following summarizes the type of ingredient and measurement information needed for an accurate nutrition analysis. (Refer to Chapter 7 for more guidance on recipe ingredients.)

Ingredient description

Is there a specific brand, or is generic acceptable?

Is the ingredient fresh, dried, dehydrated, frozen, canned, cooked, or nutrient altered?

Is product clarification needed? If so, ask for pictures of the label, Nutrition Facts panel, and ingredient statement.

Examples:

- **Tomatoes:** Are they fresh or canned; whole, diced, crushed, or peeled; no salt added?
- **Corn:** Is it fresh, canned, or frozen; with salt or no salt added?
- **Canned fruit:** Is it packed in syrup or water; with sugar or no added sugar?
- **Spinach:** Is it whole or chopped leaf; regular or baby; with or without stems?
- **Milk:** Is it whole, 2%, 1%, or nonfat?
- **Butter:** Is it salted or unsalted?
- **Breadcrumbs:** Are they fresh or dried?

Ingredient preparation

How is the ingredient prepared? Peeled, sliced, seeded, chopped, julienned, diced, minced, grated, pureed, trimmed, etc.?

Examples:

- **Potatoes:** Is it with skin or peeled?
- **Broccoli:** Is it florets only or stems and florets?
- **Cheese:** Is it sliced or shredded?
- **Meats:** Is it whole, cubed, or pounded thin?

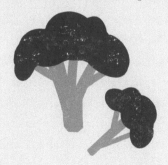

Weight measurement

Obtain the weight measurement for each ingredient. Weight may be in metric measurements (kilograms, grams), or US customary measurements (pounds, ounces), or both.

For retail, food manufacturing, and food service operations obtain current specifications and technical data sheets for all processed ingredients to include 100-gram, unrounded nutrient data.

Examples:

- 16 ounces (454 grams) boneless and skinless chicken thighs
- 1 cup (227 grams) unsalted butter
- ½ cup (100 grams) granulated sugar
- 1 medium head (910 grams) cauliflower, about 6 cups cauliflower florets

Package size

For packaged products, obtain both a volume amount and a weight measurement. If an ingredient in a recipe is given in can sizing (e.g., #3 can), refer to a resource that lists weights and volumes for each can size.

Size of produce

If an ingredient is listed as small, medium, or large, know if that information is adequate and, if not, when to obtain the weight. For example, "1 small apple" will likely be included in a database, while "1 large head broccoli" may not. Obtaining the weight is always best.

To taste, optional, and garnish

If an ingredient includes the terms "to taste," "optional," or "for garnish," provide written guidelines on how to account for these amounts in the nutrient analysis.

Use Weight Measurements Whenever Possible

Using weight instead of volume measurements for ingredients will provide a more accurate nutrition analysis. Weight is a measure of the heaviness of an ingredient, while volume measurements provide the space or capacity the ingredient takes up in a measuring spoon or cup. Volume measurements vary due to the different sizes and shapes of ingredients and how they are measured. Many consumer recipes are written in volume measurements (e.g., cups, teaspoons, tablespoons). While these measurements are useful for home cooks, they can increase the variability and inaccuracy of the final nutrient analysis.

Best practices If the recipe includes both the weight and volume measurements of ingredients, use the weight measurement for a more accurate nutrition analysis. Be aware of the variability of volume and weight measurements, even with the same type of food item. For example, note the differences in weight for 1 cup of cheddar cheese in various forms:

Volume of cheddar cheese	Weight
1 cup, shredded	113 grams (4 ounces)
1 cup, cubed	132 grams (5 ounces)
1 cup, melted	244 grams (9 ounces)

Quick Tip

"Work with the recipe developer in advance to create a common understanding of what information is needed for an accurate analysis. Ask them to weigh, not just measure, ingredients during their development. This advance communication will increase the likelihood that you get the details you need and will increase their efficiency and decrease any potential later frustration." —Cheryl Dolven, MS, RDN, coauthor of *Recipe Nutrient Analysis*

UNDERSTANDING OUNCES VERSUS FLUID OUNCES

It is important to be aware of potential confusion about ounces and fluid ounces. If a recipe lists an ingredient amount in ounces (weight) or in fluid ounces (volume), understand that these are two very different measurements.

- *Ounce weight* is a unit to measure solid (e.g., flour) and semisolid (e.g., sour cream) ingredient weights.
- *Fluid ounce* is a liquid volume measurement (e.g., for milk, oil, sauce, dressing, soup, and other liquid ingredients).

There is only one scenario where weight ounces and fluid ounces are the same: 8 fluid ounces of water weighs 8 ounces. This is the exception. All other liquids with differences in density will vary. For example, 1 cup honey (8 *fluid* ounces) weighs 12 ounces, rather than 8 ounces.

Having a conversion table with approximate volume-to-weight values on hand can be quite helpful; consider also keeping a chart that provides weight and volume amounts for various types of commonly used ingredients. See the appendix Common Ingredient Equivalencies and Conversions on page 349.

Quick Tip

"Be as specific as possible when listing ingredients. For example, what size can is used, and include any instructions with it. Listing an ingredient as 1 can of corn or 1 can of tuna will require answering the follow-up question of what size can, and is it drained or is the liquid included?" —Laura Ali, MS, RDN, culinary consultant and former senior manager of nutrition and regulatory affairs at Starkist

Step 3: Review the Preparation and Cooking Methods

The next step is reviewing the recipe directions to ensure they clearly describe exactly what needs to be done to prepare the recipe. The preparation and cooking methods used will affect the final nutrient values and recipe yield. Read the recipe directions carefully to ensure the following:

- preparation and cooking directions are clear and complete, and they include detailed information on equipment, pan sizes, time, and temperature of baking or cooking

- recipe yield is compatible with the portion size and number of servings

Calculating the nutrient values of a recipe and accounting for the effects of the recipe's preparation and cooking methods is straightforward in some cases, particularly if the recipe does not involve cooking. Yet some preparation and cooking techniques make calculating the nutrient values more complex and difficult to analyze. For example, foods cut into small pieces are subject to more nutrient loss or gain compared to whole foods or those cut into larger pieces; more fat is lost as meat is cooked for a longer period of time; and covering (or not) of food during cooking results in a difference in evaporation and moisture loss. These factors require a thorough understanding of the culinary technique being used and how it can change the caloric and nutrient content of the food.

Evaluating which food item is the best database choice comes from understanding these factors, and others, and deciding if a manual nutrient adjustment in a database item is necessary for accuracy.

Quick Tip

"An alternative way to adjust for moisture loss is to use the cooked weight of the product and apply it to a comparable cooked product in the USDA database." —Maria Caranfa, RDN, global nutrition strategist

Step 4: Determine the Correct Edible Portion for Each Ingredient

A recipe's nutrition analysis must convey the nutrient value of the food *after* preparation in the form that it will be consumed, which is also known as the *edible portion*. A recipe analyst's knowledge and experience will enable them to choose the database ingredient in the correct form to be entered for nutrition analysis. If the recipe's raw ingredients are analyzed in their raw state, despite the fact that they will be cooked when the recipe is prepared, the nutrition analysis will not be accurate. This requires an understanding of the following nutrition analysis terms:

As purchased (AP) is the ingredient amount in its purchased state—the raw form, prior to any preparation or cooking. Recipes typically list ingredients and amounts in their AP form in the ingredient list. For example, a recipe for a main-dish salad may list a store-bought cooked rotisserie chicken as an AP ingredient.

Yield percentage is the percentage of usable and edible food left after accounting for any trimming, draining, or cooking losses (also known as the yield factor). For example, according to the USDA Table of Cooking Yields for Meat and Poultry, a cooked whole rotisserie chicken's yield percentage is 45%. A yield percentage may represent just the trim yield (how much is left over after raw food is trimmed) or the cooked yield (how much food is produced after cooking).

Edible portion (EP) is the edible amount of food that is left after removing waste and, for some foods, after cooking. For example, if a cooked whole rotisserie chicken weighs 3 pounds, the weight of the shredded meat after the carcass is disposed of is 1.35 pounds (45% of 3 pounds), which is the EP. The EP is the amount of the ingredient left after the following:

- removal of all inedible portions (e.g., bones, stems, seeds, skins, drained juice or brine)
- all waste is trimmed or removed (e.g., fat from meat)
- accounting for cooking yield and weight changes from moisture loss (e.g., shrinkage, evaporation); water absorption (e.g., boiling); fat absorption or loss; or gains or losses in sodium content during preparation and cooking

Obtaining Correct Ingredient Information

A cook following a recipe thinks of the ingredients in their AP form. A recipe analyst, on the other hand, must choose the closest possible ingredient in the nutrient database in the form that it will be consumed (the EP), which could be raw or cooked. Software databases cannot possibly include every food item in an edible portion form, so consider obtaining this information through one of the following methods:

1. Ask the recipe developer, chef, or recipe tester if they can provide both the AP and EP measurements. Ideally, the recipe developer or recipe tester should weigh the recipe's raw and cooked ingredient yields whenever possible and provide this information to the recipe analyst, who can use them when inputting and choosing database ingredients. This is particularly important for meat, poultry, and fish.
2. Consult a reference book of ingredient yields. Use a yield percentage factor to calculate the EP of an ingredient based on a purchased weight (see formulas).
3. Create a "cheat sheet" based on other recipes analyzed (or your own kitchen measurements) by documenting an ingredient's EP after preparation (e.g., peeling, butchering) and/or cooking (e.g., loss or gain in ingredient weight). The corresponding yield percentage can then be calculated and used for future recipe analyses (see formulas that follow).

Raw (Uncooked) Ingredients

When analyzing recipes that do not involve cooking, the analyst must account for the loss and waste involved in the preparation of ingredients (e.g., trimming leaves or stalks, peeling, removing bones or skin) and choose accordingly from the database. In this scenario, the analyst has two options:

- If the software program offers this option, select the raw AP ingredient, enter the amount, and let the software calculate the EP yield.
- Select the ingredient and enter the EP amount after preparation (trimming, peeling, removing bones, etc.) into the software. This EP can also be calculated using a yield percentage for the ingredient (see Raw Ingredients: Determining Edible Portion and Yield Percentage).

RECOMMENDED RESOURCES FOR INGREDIENT YIELD INFORMATION

The Book of Yields: Accuracy in Food Costing and Purchasing, 8th Edition, by Francis T. Lynch. 2010. John Wiley & Sons.

Food for Fifty, 14th Edition, by Mary Molt. 2017. Pearson.

USDA's Food Buying Guide for Child Nutrition Programs: *fns.usda.gov/tn/food-buying-guide -for-child-nutrition-programs*

USDA Table of Cooking Yields for Meat and Poultry: *ars.usda.gov/ARSUserFiles /80400525/Data/retn/USDA_CookingYields _MeatPoultry.pdf*

USDA Table of Nutrient Retention Factors: *ars.usda.gov/ARSUserFiles/80400525/Data /retn/retn06.pdf*

USDA Food Yields Summarized by Different Stages of Preparation: *ars.usda.gov/ARSUser Files/80400530/pdf/ah102.pdf*

Quick Tip

"Culinary acumen and relationship building with recipe creators is key to understanding a recipe, applying correct nutrition analysis techniques, and getting the necessary information required for complete and accurate nutrition analysis. When faced with ambiguity in a recipe, always ask questions."
—Maria Caranfa, RDN, global nutrition strategist

Quick Tip

"In the absence of benchmarks—be consistent and create your own standards."
—Mindy Hermann, MBA, RDN, recipe developer and nutritional analysis consultant

RAW INGREDIENTS: DETERMINING EDIBLE PORTION AND YIELD PERCENTAGE

A recipe developer should follow these steps to determine the edible portion (EP) weight of a raw ingredient so this information can be entered for nutrition analysis of a recipe.

1. Record the original weight of the ingredient as listed in the recipe's ingredient list. This is the raw as purchased (AP) weight.

2. Using this amount, process (or prepare) the ingredient according to the recipe directions. Weigh and record the amount of waste.

3. Subtract the amount of waste from the AP weight to determine the EP weight:

   AP weight − waste = EP weight

Another option is to calculate the EP using the AP weight and a yield percentage for that specific food.

   AP weight × yield % = EP weight

Yield percentages can be found in various sources (see Recommended Resources for Ingredient Yield Information on page 260) but may not be available for all foods. It's helpful to know how to calculate a yield percentage so this can be recorded in your nutrition analysis "cheat sheet" to use for future analyses:

   (EP weight ÷ AP weight) × 100 = yield %

Examples of calculating raw edible portion* and yield percentage

AP weight	Waste or trim weight	EP weight	Calculated yield %
5½ pounds (2.5 kilograms or 2,500 grams) whole beef tenderloin	750 grams tenderloin trim (fat, sinew, etc.)	1,750 grams raw beef tenderloin	70% yield
1 (19-ounce/539 grams) can cannellini beans	300 milliliters liquid (194 grams)	345 grams cannellini beans	64% yield
3 large heads broccoli, about 4 pounds	1½ pounds	2½ pounds broccoli florets	62.5% yield
2 pounds shrimp, with shells and tails	0.4 pounds (shells, tails)	1.6 pounds raw peeled shrimp	80% yield

* A raw edible portion for meat, poultry, and fish can be entered with software that has the ability to convert to cooked yields.

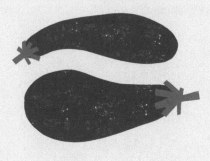

MEAT, POULTRY, AND FISH: DETERMINING YIELD PERCENTAGE AND COOKED YIELD

Some nutrition analysis software programs will automatically convert raw as purchased (AP) or raw edible portion (EP) data (e.g., trimmed, deboned) to cooked yield data for different types of meat, poultry, and fish using a known cooked yield percentage. However, even the most complete databases and yield reference books will not include a corresponding cooked yield for every ingredient. According to the USDA, the most accurate way to calculate the yield percentage for cooked meat, poultry, and fish is:

1. Record the following weights:

   - raw weight before cooking
   - cooked weight after the ingredient is cooked and is still hot, with a very brief resting period

2. Calculate the yield percentage:

   (weight of cooked sample while hot ÷ weight of raw sample in recipe) × 100 = cooked yield %

If a recipe for analysis does not include a cooked yield weight, the recipe analyst can select a known yield percentage for a specific type of meat, poultry, or fish (this will vary based on the cooking method). See Recommended Resources for Ingredient Yield Information on page 260. The cooked yield, which is the weight entered for nutrition analysis, can be calculated from the raw weight using this formula:

   raw weight × yield % = cooked yield weight

Sample calculations for cooked yield and cooked yield percentage

Example 1: Calculate the *cooked yield* for 2 pounds ground sirloin or ground chuck cooked in a skillet. According to USDA's Table of Cooking Yields for Meat and Poultry, ground chuck cooked in a pan has a 62% cooked yield (12.6% fat loss) and ground sirloin has about a 69% cooked yield (1.4% fat loss).

   - 32 ounces raw ground sirloin (cooked in skillet) × 69% = about 22 ounces cooked yield
   - 32 ounces raw ground chuck × 62% = about 20 ounces cooked yield

Example 2: Using the raw weight and cooked weight (22.4 ounces), calculate the *cooked yield percentage* of 2 pounds of salmon, skin removed and roasted or grilled.

   - 22.4 ounces cooked weight ÷ 32 ounces raw weight × 100 = 70% cooked yield percentage

Use this 70% yield percentage for future recipes that provide the AP amount to convert to an EP cooked amount.

Examples of cooked yield percentages and cooked yield for meat, poultry, fish

AP amount	Yield percentage (cooked and waste removed)	Cooked yield (EP) amount
2 pounds shrimp	65%	1.3 pounds cooked peeled shrimp
1½ pounds lobster	26%	0.4 pounds or 6.4 ounces cooked lobster meat
2 pounds boneless, skinless chicken breast	75%	1.5 pounds cooked
2 pounds flank steak, fat trimmed to 0%	81%	1.62 pounds cooked

Cooked Ingredients

Recipes that involve cooking are more complicated because ingredients change as they are cooked based on preparation techniques, cooking times, and temperature; as a result, so do their nutritional values. For this reason, recipe analysts must enter or choose ingredients in the database carefully to ensure that the analysis will be representative of the recipe as it is prepared and consumed. The databases of more robust nutrition analysis software programs contain nutrient data for raw AP amounts and corresponding cooked EP amounts, but even the best databases don't contain this information for every type of preparation and cooking method for every possible ingredient. The analyst has two options:

- If the software program offers this option, select the ingredient, enter the AP raw amount, and let the software calculate the EP cooked yield.
- Select the cooked ingredient and enter the cooked weight. This can be obtained from the recipe developer, your own kitchen measurement, or by using a yield percentage to calculate a cooked amount (EP) using the raw (AP) amount.

Cooked Yields for Meat, Poultry, and Fish

Determining a cooked yield for meat, poultry, or fish depends on several factors, including the cut, the amount of fat (the percentage [%] lean), whether the skin is included (for poultry), and whether the bone is included. Varying preparation and cooking methods also affect the cooked yield. For example, the final cooked weight of a roast or steak will vary depending on if a dry or moist heat cooking method is used. A rare steak will have a different cooked yield weight than a well-done steak; with a roast, the amount of fat and moisture lost increases with higher heat roasting.

For meats with differing amounts of fat, fat loss can vary even with the same cooking method (in particular, ground beef's open structure causes significant variance). The fat content of higher-fat ground beef can be significantly reduced once it's cooked, while the change in fat content of very lean ground beef after cooking is negligible. When a cooked yield weight is not provided to the recipe analyst, this must be calculated (see Meat, Poultry, and Fish: Determining Yield Percentage and Cooked Yield on page 262).

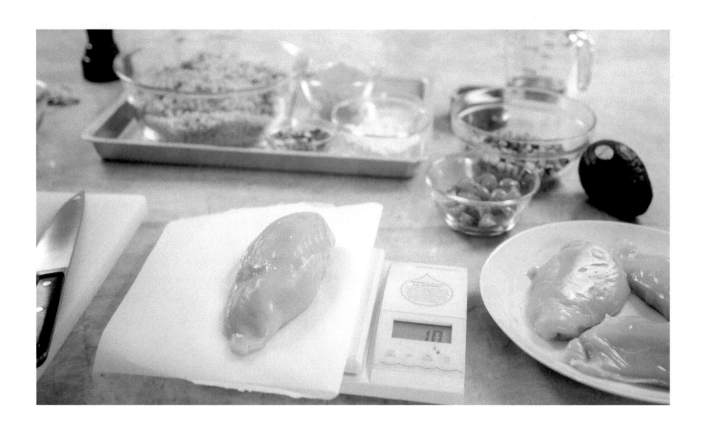

Step 5: Evaluate Recipe Yield and Servings

In the culinary world, the term *yield* has a dual meaning: the amount of usable ingredient remaining after it is prepared (peeled, butchered, cooked, etc.), as well as the recipe's total yield, including the number of servings and serving size. The recipe analyst's responsibilities include making sure the recipe's total yield and number of servings/serving size make sense.

A recipe's total yield can be listed in a variety of ways. For example, a tomato soup recipe's yield could be represented as 1 gallon or 4 liters; a muffin recipe may yield 24 muffins; and a tuna noodle casserole recipe may yield 1 (2-quart) casserole. A complete recipe yield should include the following:

- total yield in weight or volume
- number of servings in weight or volume
- individual serving size in weight or volume

Always check the total recipe yield and individual serving size to see that it makes sense before starting the analysis.

Examples:

Blueberry Muffins

Yield: 24 muffins

Serving size 1 muffin

Analyze with 24 servings for the nutrition analysis.

Tomato Soup

Yield: 1-gallon soup (16 cups)

Number of servings: 8 servings

Serving size: 1½ cups

Cannot analyze since the yield and serving size do not match: 1.5 cups × 8 servings = 12 cups. The recipe states a yield of 16 cups.

If you are working with a recipe and encounter a discrepancy like this, check with the recipe developer or chef for clarification or to confirm whether you should make your own assumptions and corrections during the nutrition analysis. If you make changes to the recipe serving size or yield, be sure to note them carefully.

In the soup example, the discrepancy can be corrected in either of two ways: 1) Perform the analysis for 8 (2-cup) servings and note the serving size change to 2 cups; or 2) Perform the analysis for 10 (1½-cup) servings and note the total servings change to "around 10 servings."

Pan size When analyzing recipes that include only a pan size, ensure that the serving size makes sense.

Example:

Mac and Cheese

Yield: 1 (2-quart) baking dish

Number of servings: 10

Analyze as a side or main dish?

Two quarts is equivalent to 8 cups, so each of the 10 servings would be about ⅔ cup. While that would be an adequate serving size for a side dish, it is small for a main dish serving size. In this example, the recipe analyst may choose to use their professional expertise to provide nutrition information for 10 side-dish servings (about ⅔ cup per portion) and also for 6 main-dish servings (about 1⅓ cups per portion).

Step 6: Enter the Ingredient Information into the Software Program

Once the recipe's details (e.g., clear ingredient measurements and weights, cooking methods, recipe yield, number of servings, and serving size) have been collected, you are ready to begin entering information into the nutrition analysis software. Be aware that even with detailed information, nutrition analysis discrepancies can occur. The cause could be the software's database, human error, or both.

To minimize the potential for discrepancies, obtain all the recipe details prior to performing the analysis, use an application with a robust database that is updated regularly (see Choosing A Nutrition Analysis Software Application on page 284) *and* learn the full functionality of the software. Using the application correctly will require training and good professional judgment. Consider the following steps for entering ingredients:

- Add new ingredients and subrecipes (sometimes referred to as user-added ingredients) to the database.

- Add missing nutrient data for an existing database ingredient.

- Search and choose the best "as consumed" ingredient options in the database for the recipe (e.g., raw, cooked, USDA generic, alternate brand).

- Adjust nutrient values if necessary, based on moisture or nutrient loss or gain due to the recipe's preparation or cooking methods.

- Be careful when choosing all ingredients, including those that seem straightforward and simple. (Software training courses are available such as through ESHA Research.)

Quick Tip

"Supplier nutrient data should be used, if available, especially for proprietary or custom ingredients. Ingredient suppliers should provide unrounded nutrient values per 100 g, as well as the source of their data." —Rachel Huber, MPH, RD, foodservice and restaurant dietitian

Quick Tip

"It is essential to evaluate the accuracy of supplier data (i.e., the data you use to generate the nutrition analysis). Never assume supplier data is always correct. Double check the values, ask for nutritional information in 100-g unrounded form, the source of their data, and the date the information was created. Always question the accuracy and validity of the input data as that will substantiate the accuracy of your final analysis." —Sarah Hendren, MS, RDN, Regulatory Affairs Scientist for Frito Lay North America

Add New Ingredients to the Database

Before starting the recipe analysis, add any new or brand-specific ingredients to the database that are used in the recipe but not found in the database. The most direct source for obtaining missing data is the food manufacturer or its supplier. Request the unrounded nutrient values for 100 grams of the food product. Distributors, growers, chefs, or restaurants might be able to provide this information as well.

Once nutrient values per 100-grams and per individual serving (the amount eaten by the consumer) are added to the database, label the new ingredient clearly with information that includes the supplier, restaurant, or unique product name and manufacturing item number so that it can be easily retrieved.

If the nutrition information on the product's label is the only data available, add that information to the database, as it's better than omitting the ingredient from the analysis. However, Nutrition Facts panels display rounded values for calories and nutrients per serving, so they will not accurately represent the nutrient information for a recipe calculation that uses more than one serving in the recipe. For example, consider a salad dressing that contains 6.4 grams total fat in its 16-ounce bottle. The serving size is only 2 tablespoons, and the Nutrition Facts panel rounds the fat content to 0 grams per serving. If the recipe that is being analyzed uses the entire 16-ounce bottle (454 grams/6.4 grams total fat), the recipe analysis will not accurately reflect the grams of fat from the salad dressing.

EXAMPLE: INGREDIENT SELECTION FOR BONELESS AND SKINLESS CHICKEN BREASTS

Depending on which software is used for the analysis, an ingredient search in its database may pull up only a single choice or dozens of choices (if the software has a robust database). Recipe analysts must use their own professional expertise and judgment to make the right choices. Many variables affect the likelihood of a database containing an appropriate choice, including the quality of the database, the type of ingredient, and the amount and type of processing the ingredient undergoes in the recipe.

The following example shows the ESHA database options for boneless and skinless chicken breasts, a commonly used ingredient. Skill is required to pick the best choice from the software's database, especially since it has many similar chicken breast options. In this example, the ESHA database provides 66 choices for boneless and skinless chicken breasts. The recipe analyst should search among these choices and select the best option.

ESHA Database Choices for Boneless and Skinless Chicken Breasts

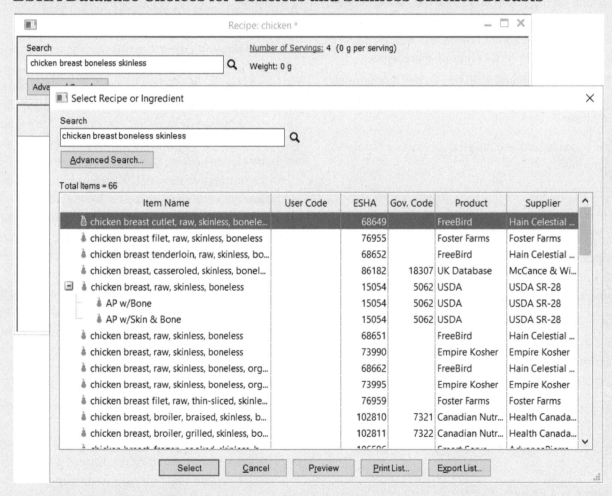

Image provided by the ESHA Research Nutrient Database, ©(2021) ESHA Research, Inc.

BOX CONTINUES >

Once a database choice is selected, the analyst should enter the correct ingredient amount for the recipe. For example, if a recipe calls for 1½ pounds boneless and skinless chicken breast, the analyst should select "AP [as purchased] boneless" and enter "1.5 pounds" as the amount. The database will use the US Department of Agriculture's loss and retention factors to calculate the correct cooked amounts. Thus, the software will convert the raw AP amount to the cooked edible portion (EP) amount. In this example, choosing "1.5 pounds chicken breast, roasted, skinless" would be incorrect, since that value represents 1½ pounds of cooked, rather than raw, chicken.

The example that follows shows the nutritional differences that exist among similar forms of the same type of chicken. Since not all software programs are capable of calculating cooked weight, obtain a cooked ingredient weight from the recipe developer or calculate the cooked yield using a yield percentage (see page 262).

Nutrient Differences in Various Forms of Chicken Breasts

Item Name	Quantity	Measure	Wgt (g)	Cals (kcal)	FatCals (kcal)	SatCals (kcal)	Prot (g)	Carb (g)	T
Chicken Example									
chicken breast, roasted, skinless	1.5 Pound		680.39	1122.64	218.61	61.85	211.06	0	
chicken breast, roasted, skinless (AP Raw w/Bone)	1.5 Pound		358.22	591.07	115.10	32.56	111.12	0	
chicken breast, roasted, skinless (AP Raw w/Bone & Skin)	1.5 Pound		318.42	525.40	102.31	28.94	98.77	0	
chicken breast, roasted, skinless (AP Raw-Boneless)	1.5 Pound		442.25	729.72	142.10	40.20	137.19	0	
Total									

Spreadsheet: Chicken Example *

Image provided by the ESHA Research Nutrient Database, ©(2021) ESHA Research, Inc.

Add Missing Nutrient Data to the Database

Sometimes, certain fields for an existing ingredient in a database are empty (e.g., added sugars) or missing a component (e.g., omega-3 fatty acids, whole grains) that is needed for a recipe analysis report. Some applications have the ability to add nutrient fields as long as the nutrient has a number tied to it. If possible, contact the ingredient supplier for the unrounded amount per 100 grams and add it to the database or, if the work in question is a consumer recipe analysis, call or email the ingredient manufacturer to obtain the needed missing nutrient data.

Add Subrecipes to the Database

Many recipes—especially those developed for and by restaurants—contain subrecipes. A subrecipe is a finished dish listed as an ingredient in the main recipe (e.g., marinara sauce, salsa, pesto). A subrecipe must first be calculated and added to the database as a new and separate recipe. Once a subrecipe has been entered into the database, it is available for use as an ingredient in the main recipe calculation.

Subrecipes present a challenge to recipe analysts in terms of determining the total yield and then the amount needed in the main recipe. Here the recipe analyst's expertise is of fundamental importance.

In the following Pasta with Pesto example, the subrecipe must first be entered into the database as a separate recipe before the nutrition analysis for the main recipe can be calculated. Because the main recipe and subrecipe include accurate ingredient measurements and the subrecipe has a total yield and calls for a specific amount in the main recipe, the calculation is straightforward.

Main Recipe: Pasta with Pesto

Yield: 4 servings

1 pound spaghetti
1 pint grape tomatoes
1 yellow pepper, thinly sliced
1 cup (240 grams) Pesto Sauce

Subrecipe: Pesto Sauce

Yield: 2 cups (480 grams)

2 cups fresh basil leaves, stems removed
2 tablespoons pine nuts
2 large garlic cloves
½ cup extra-virgin olive oil
½ cup (about 1 ounce) grated Parmesan cheese

In other cases, information may be missing. In the Quinoa Bowl with Creamy Cilantro Dressing example, the main recipe is missing a total yield and serving size. The subrecipe does not include exact ingredient measurements, a total yield, or the amount needed in the main recipe.

Main Recipe: Quinoa Bowl with Creamy Cilantro Dressing

Yield: 4 servings

¾ pound boneless, skinless chicken breast
2 cups cooked quinoa
1 (15-ounce) can sweet corn, drained
3 ounces (about ½ cup) cotija cheese
4 green onions, chopped
¼ cup extra-virgin olive oil
2 tablespoons fresh lime juice
¾ teaspoon kosher salt
¾ teaspoon freshly ground black pepper
1 avocado, peeled and cubed
Creamy Cilantro Dressing, for serving

Subrecipe: Creamy Cilantro Dressing

Yield: unknown
Serving size: unknown

4 garlic cloves, minced
4 jalapeño peppers, seeded
5 tablespoons fresh lime juice
Kosher salt, to taste
½ cup canola oil
1 cup packed fresh cilantro leaves

The main recipe cannot be analyzed properly unless the cilantro dressing's total yield and the amount used in the main recipe is provided. In this example, Creamy Cilantro Dressing should be added as a new recipe or ingredient in the database. As for the next step, there are a few options for gathering the missing information:

- Ask the recipe developer or chef to provide the missing information. For the main recipe (quinoa bowl), obtain the total yield and serving size. For the subrecipe (creamy cilantro dressing), find out amount of salt used in the recipe, the total dressing yield, serving size, and amount needed for the main recipe.

- If necessary, test the recipe to determine the missing information needed for analysis.

- Research similar recipes to estimate an individual serving size for the quinoa bowl and the dressing. Estimate the amount of salt needed and total dressing yield by using your own culinary expertise, and be sure to document it. For example, if you estimate 1 teaspoon salt in the dressing, 1 cup for the total yield of the dressing, and 2 tablespoons of the dressing per serving in the main recipe (total ½ cup), include that information in the note section of the analysis.

Quick Tip

"When calculating a recipe for a restaurant group, be sure to use supplier product nutrition information and do not just choose a generic brand from the database. You want the nutrition information to represent what you're actually serving to the consumer."
—Maria Caranfa, RDN, global nutrition strategist

Search the Database and Choose the Best Ingredient Option

Searching for and choosing specific ingredients or food items from an application's database is sometimes straightforward, but often, even the simplest ingredients have multiple database entries, which can lead to confusion. Each choice that is made should be intentional and careful, ensuring that the ingredient selected best represents the ingredient and cooking method shown in the recipe.

If a specific brand of ingredient is called for in the recipe, be sure to choose it in the database; otherwise, choose a USDA generic version unless an agreed-upon ingredient standard has been predetermined. In addition to the guidelines presented in Step 4 on page 259 for determining the correct edible portion for each ingredient, other tips include the following:

- Search for foods using a variety of names until you find the desired result. For example, if the recipe includes scallions, consider trying other names in your search, including "green onion," "spring onion," or even just "onion." Knowing other search terms for an ingredient, such as chickpeas or garbanzo beans as alternates for ceci beans, makes it easier to find the correct ingredient.

- If the recipe includes ingredients that will not be cooked, choose the best option in the database for the raw EP of the ingredient.

- If the recipe is cooked, select the best option in the database for the raw AP amount and its corresponding cooked EP amount.

- Choose a cooked form of an ingredient if there is not an option in the database that converts AP to a cooked EP.

ADDED SUGARS DATA

If added sugars data is missing for an ingredient, the added sugars field in a database will be blank. Recipe analysts should manually add added sugar information to this data field. When there is only one type of sugar in a food, calculating the value and adding it to the database is straightforward. However, when there is a combination of naturally occurring and added sugars in a food, such as in an ingredient like barbecue sauce or ketchup, it is best to contact the manufacturer or ingredient supplier to obtain this information. Many companies rely on ingredient suppliers to provide a formula that allows them to calculate the percentage of added sugars.

Keep in mind that a laboratory analysis can only test for total sugars because a chemical test does not exist to distinguish added sugars from naturally occurring sugars found in foods like milk, fruit, and vegetables. Added sugars may include sugar, brown sugar, corn syrup, agave syrup, malt syrup, maple syrup, molasses, honey, and concentrated fruit and vegetable juices.

Step 7: Review Nutrient Analysis Results

Once a recipe's ingredients have been evaluated and entered into the database, the next step is to examine the final nutrient values and evaluate the numbers to ensure they make sense. Some professionals refer to this as the reality check. Viewing the analysis in a spreadsheet format makes it easier to identify food items or ingredients with missing nutrient data. If a nutrient result shows up as 0, the food item does not contain that nutrient; a blank field reveals that reliable data has not yet been collected.

If an ingredient does contain a blank field instead of a nutrient value, contact the manufacturer or grower to obtain the information or try a different database to find the missing data. If necessary, you can always use your professional judgment to estimate the missing value based on that of a comparable product.

Use Nutrition Knowledge

Look closely at the nutrient data for each ingredient to catch errors and to judge the accuracy. Use the 4-4-9 formula to make sure the calories add up correctly: 4 calories per gram of carbohydrate and protein, and 9 calories per gram of fat. Use your knowledge of ingredients, nutrition, and culinary techniques to quickly verify other nutrition data. And be sure to document your nutrition analysis process in the recipe note section in the nutrition analysis software. Apply the same logic when inputting user-added ingredients to the database. If any information you add to the database is incorrect, future nutrition analyses involving the same ingredient(s) will be wrong as well.

Step 8: Communicate Nutrition Information

Robust nutrition analysis software applications allow users to customize the nutrients and nutrient components that are analyzed. For example, some databases include as many as 180 nutrients. For ease of use, these applications group a variety of nutrients into lists, so recipe analysts can choose which they wish to analyze (e.g., mandatory food label nutrients, carbohydrate only, fat only). In many cases, the reports can be printed or exported, for example, as a spreadsheet, a pie chart, or a Nutrition Facts label. Most recipes are analyzed for nutrients found on the Nutrition Facts label or nutrients that have a *Daily Value* (DV)—the recommended amount of nutrients to consume or not to exceed in a day—associated with them. Software-based analyses can also report the mandatory and voluntary %DV for nutrients found on Nutrition Facts labels.

Understanding Daily Values

The %DV is how much of a nutrient in a single serving of an individual packaged food or recipe serving contributes to one's total daily diet. To determine whether a recipe serving is high or low in an individual nutrient, it's best to reference the %DV:

- 5% DV or less of a nutrient per serving is considered low.
- 20% DV or more of a nutrient per serving is considered high.

See page 35 for more on the DVs for specific nutrients.

Communicate Nutrition Information in Rounded Values

Nutrition analysis software applications can provide data in either unrounded or rounded numbers. Some publications share very precise recipe nutrition information (e.g., 352 calories, 3.69 grams fat, 451 milligrams sodium), which leaves consumers with the impression that the data is exact. That is hardly the case; in fact, all nutrient calculations are estimates. Variations in foods, recipe preparation techniques, and actual portion sizes all influence the results, as nutrient analysis is not an exact science. To avoid this impression, round the nutrition data for recipes. Rounded nutrition information for the example above would be 350 calories, 3.5 grams fat, and 450 milligrams sodium.

The FDA has mandated that rounding must be used on Nutrition Facts labels to make them easier to read. Likewise, in nutrition analyses, it's best to communicate rounded values for calories and nutrients, as shown in Rounding Regulations for Nutrition Facts Labels.

Quick Tip

"There is a reason the FDA has companies round the nutritional information on labels. Food varies and a recipe will never be exact, so providing a rounded number really is the best practice. Having done chemical analysis and built databases of products over time you would be amazed at how much food items can vary." —Laura Ali, MS, RDN, culinary consultant and former senior manager of nutrition and regulatory affairs at Starkist

Quick Tip

"Provide your clients with notes on how you analyzed the recipe—including the assumptions you made during the analysis. It's helpful for them in case they receive consumer questions." —Mindy Hermann, MBA, RDN, recipe developer and nutritional analysis consultant

ROUNDING REGULATIONS FOR NUTRITION FACTS LABELS

Nutrient	Round to and report
Number of servings	
Servings between 2 and 5	Nearest 0.5 serving (e.g., about 3.5 servings)
Calories	
Fewer than 5 calories	Zero
5 to 50 calories	Nearest 5-calorie increment
More than 50 calories	Nearest 10-calorie increment
Fat	
If less than 0.5 grams	Zero
0.5 grams to 5 grams	Nearest 0.5 grams
Greater than 5 grams	Nearest 1 gram
Cholesterol	
If less than 2 milligrams	Zero
2 to 5 grams	Less than 5 milligrams
If greater than 5 milligrams	Nearest 5 milligrams
Total carbohydrate, dietary fiber, sugars/added sugars	
If less than 0.5 grams	Zero
If less than 1 gram	Less than 1 gram
Greater than 1 gram	Nearest 1 gram
Protein	
If less than 0.5 grams	Zero
If less than 1 gram	Less than 1 gram
Greater than 1 gram	Nearest 1 gram
Sodium	
If less than 5 milligrams	Zero
Up to 140 milligrams	Nearest 5 milligrams
Greater than 140 milligrams	Nearest 10 milligrams
Iron	Nearest 0.1 milligrams
Calcium	Nearest 10 milligrams
Vitamin D	Nearest 0.1 micrograms
Potassium	Nearest 10 milligrams

Source: US Food and Drug Administration, Code of Federal Regulations Title 21 Food and Drugs,

CALCULATING CARBOHYDRATE CHOICES FOR DIABETES MEAL PLANS

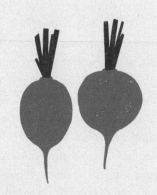

Carbohydrate counting is a tool for people with diabetes to help manage their blood glucose (or blood sugar). When including carbohydrate choices for people with diabetes as part of a recipe's nutrition information, keep in mind that no matter what food you're analyzing, one carbohydrate choice provides 15 grams of carbohydrate. Calculate the number of carbohydrate choices per serving by dividing the total carbohydrate amount per serving by 15.

Foods that contain carbohydrates:

- grains (e.g., breads, crackers, rice, hot and cold cereals, tortillas, and noodles)
- starchy vegetables (e.g., potatoes, peas, corn, winter squash, lentils, and beans)
- fruit and juices
- milk and yogurt
- sweets and desserts

Communicate Explanation of Nutrition Information to Readers

Nutrient calculations should always carry a disclaimer explaining that they are estimates based on calculations made using a specific database, software application, API, or website plug-in, along with the professional judgment of the person who performed the analysis. Because software analysis or an automated calculation of recipes can vary widely, consider including a disclaimer in your print and online publication or website that all nutrition values are estimates. Several examples for different settings are provided below.

Food Service/Restaurants

Nutrient information is approximate based on current product and recipe data in [name of database/software application] and supplier information. While we make every effort to obtain the most current nutrient ingredient data and allergen information, it's possible that a manufacturer may change their formulation without the recipe analyst's knowledge.

Nutritional information provided on this website about our menu items is based on standardized recipes, representative values provided by suppliers, analysis using industry-standard software, published resources, or testing conducted in accredited laboratories, and are expressed in values based on federal rounding and other applicable regulations. A number of factors may affect the actual nutrition values for each product and, as such, we cannot guarantee the complete accuracy of the nutritional information provided.

Print and Digital Publications

Nutritional values used in our calculations come from [name of database/software application/version number], USDA Agricultural Research Service Nutrient Data, USDA FoodData Central, or food manufacturers. If information for a nutrient in an ingredient is not available, it is listed as N/A.

The information shown is [name of API]'s estimate based on available ingredients and preparation. It should not be considered a substitute for a registered dietitian or nutrition professional's advice.

Nutrition information is provided as a general guideline to our readers. Various online calculators produce different results depending on the data source chosen, cooking techniques considered, and precision of ingredient measurements. Values are not calculated or reviewed by a nutrition professional.

Analyzing Complex Recipes

Many recipes are prepared in a way that makes them inherently complex to analyze. Some involve preparation or processing that needs special consideration; ideally, it would be best to send these to a laboratory for the most accurate chemical analysis. (In fact, if the complex recipe is being analyzed in order to create a Nutrition Facts label, it *should* be sent to a laboratory.) However, this isn't always realistic or affordable. In such situations, recipe analysts can follow best practice guidelines for nutrition analysis that have been assembled over many years of documented cooking and nutrient research and also consult veteran food professionals working in the field.

When no guidance or precedent is available, put your own expertise to use and carefully document how you arrive at each of the estimated nutrient values. Throughout the process, maintain ongoing communication with the recipe developer or chef so you can quickly get answers to questions you encounter while performing the analysis. In nutrition analysis, consistency and substantiation of results are paramount.

This section covers the following challenging recipe analysis scenarios:

- deep-fat frying, panfrying, sautéing, and stir-frying
- breading, flouring, and batter coating
- sodium absorption from cooking water
- salting to taste
- marinating, brining, pickling, and fermenting
- stocks, broths, sauces, and strained foods
- alcohol

Deep-Fat Frying

Determining the amount of oil absorption by a food when it is deep-fat fried is a complex process, as many factors and variables can affect how much oil is absorbed. Calculating fat absorption by measuring the weight of the food before and after it is fried is not recommended because all foods absorb fat when they're fried, but they also lose water. It's difficult to discern how much of the weight change is due to fat absorption, moisture loss, or a combination of both.

Best Practices

- Use 10% of the ingredient's weight to determine the estimated amount of oil absorbed.

  For example, if a recipe calls for 2 pounds bone-in chicken breasts dipped in buttermilk, dredged in a flour mixture, and then deep-fried, calculate the fat absorption as follows:

  - 2 pounds (907 grams) bone-in chicken breasts + 190 grams dredging/flour mixture = 1,097 grams

  - 1,097 grams × 10% = 109.7 grams fat

  - 109.7 grams fat/oil should be used for the calculation (equivalent to about 8 tablespoons oil [14 grams fat per 1 tablespoon oil])

- Weigh the finished ingredient and find a comparable item in the database. Choose an item that represents an average: *do not* choose the worst-case or best-case scenario for the fat content of the food. Use the nutrient values of the comparable product (e.g., fat grams) as a reference point and adjust the fat grams in the analysis accordingly. Fast-food restaurant chain websites and USDA resources are good places to start for estimating the fat absorbed in fried foods. These benchmarks will reveal whether your calculation is in the range of comparable items. An alternative is to look up an uncooked item and compare it to a cooked version—e.g., frozen french fries (not fried) and frozen french fries (fried)—to gauge how much fat is absorbed by a fried item.

- Use the USDA Table of Cooking Yields for Meat and Poultry as a reference to calculate for percentage (%) gain or loss of fat in a variety of cooking methods, including deep-frying (see Nutrient Analysis Resources and Bibliography on page 294).

- If the analysis is for a home-cooked recipe, another option is to measure the weight of the oil used before cooking. After the ingredient has been cooked per the recipe instructions, remove any food particles and weigh the remaining oil. The difference represents *an estimate* of the amount of oil absorbed. This is the least optimal method.

FACTORS AFFECTING OIL ABSORPTION

Moisture content: In general, plant foods absorb greater amounts of fat than animal foods. Plant foods have a much higher water content, and the amount of oil uptake is directly proportional to the amount of moisture lost during frying.

Porosity: The initial porosity (air space) of a food affects its oil absorption. When raw food is placed in hot oil, the oil bubbles furiously due to the rapid release of steam from the surface of the food. This release of moisture from the food as steam creates a sponge-like tunnel network for oil absorption during frying. When a food is removed from oil, the film of hot oil that coats it is rapidly absorbed.

Surface area and food size: Foods with a greater surface-to-volume ratio absorb more oil. The smaller the food, the more oil it will absorb compared to thicker and larger pieces of food (e.g., a chicken breast versus a chicken tenderloin).

Oil type: There is no conclusive evidence as to whether the type of oil has a direct effect on oil absorption.

Prefrying and postfrying methods: Prefrying (e.g., par frying, blanching, microwaving, or baking), coating the surface of a food with batter or breading, and the postfrying cooling process can reduce surface permeability prior to frying; as a result, it can reduce oil absorption in some foods. Postfrying oil penetration occurs while the food is cooling; the flow of oil transfers from the surface of the food into the food during this time. Blotting the food after it is fried may help diminish some oil absorption. With some foods, if the frying process is done correctly, the hot fat forms a crisp crust on the food, preventing excess fat penetration into the food's core.

Frying oil temperature absorption and frying time: The influence of oil temperature on oil absorption is unclear. However, oil absorption has been shown to increase with longer frying times, especially for thinner foods.

Panfrying, Sautéing, and Stir-Frying

Panfrying, sautéing, and stir-frying are common techniques seen in many recipes. The same variables that affect fat absorption in deep-fat frying apply with these techniques as well. The only difference is that much more oil is used in deep-fat frying. For example, a deep-fried fish recipe may call for 6 cups oil, whereas a panfried fish recipe may use only ¾ cup.

Best Practices

- For sautéing and stir-frying, use all of the oil called for in the recipe and assume that 100% of the oil has been absorbed.

- For recipes that involve panfrying, calculate the amount of oil absorbed using 5% of the ingredient's weight, according to Karen Duester of Food labels.com. See the bone-in chicken breast example for calculating a 10% absorption on page 273.

- Weigh or measure the fat before and after panfrying to estimate how much fat was absorbed by the food (to increase the accuracy of your results, strain out any bits of food left in the oil once it cools).

Breading, Flouring, and Batter Coating

Many recipes—including those for breaded chicken cutlets, eggplant Parmesan, fried calamari, and beer-battered fish, to name a few—call for foods to be covered in a dry or wet coating before deep-frying, panfrying, or baking. Getting an accurate analysis for these types of foods can be quite difficult, since consumer recipes usually list a greater amount of dredging or coating ingredients than is truly needed for the recipe, and the amount of fat absorbed is an estimate. When you choose a best practice to follow, remain consistent for the length of the project.

Best Practices

- Weigh the amounts of flour, egg wash, breadcrumbs and/or batter before preparation and then again afterward to determine how much of the ingredients were actually used in the recipe.

- Create your own estimated average to calculate the amount of dredging and coating ingredients used in these types of recipes and use this average consistently. Some food professionals rely on 80% as a factor based on their kitchen measurements.

- Use all of the dredging and coating ingredients called for in the recipe in the analysis. This choice is best when the recipe is written with a small amount of dredging or coating ingredient in relation to the food product being fried. Your own kitchen experience helps in this situation.

- Refer to the best practices for deep-fat frying and panfrying for fat absorption (see pages 273 and 274) if the breaded product is also being fried.

ADJUSTING NUTRIENT VALUES IN A DATABASE

If the results of an analysis do not match expectations based on nutrient loss or gain from preparation and cooking practices, more advanced software applications allow users to override a final nutrient value after the analysis is complete. For example, adjusting the final amount of total fat should be made based on nutrition analysis assumptions and guidelines. If an override is made, keep precise notes in the saved recipe in the software to keep track of changes and the reason for the override.

Sodium Absorption from Cooking Water

Adding salt to the cooking water for grains, pasta, or vegetables helps enhance flavor, so most cooks follow this technique. If a recipe calls for salted cooking water and no salt is used in the analysis, the sodium content information will be inaccurate.

Some grain or pasta recipes call for a specific amount of salt in the ingredient list, but many recipes just list salt without a specified amount. Recipes that do not state an amount usually provide direction to either cook according to the package directions or state that the cooking water should be salted in the recipe directions. Thus, the first step when analyzing recipes is to read the recipe from start to finish and determine whether all of the water (and the salt) is absorbed or the cooking water is drained off.

For most grain recipes that use an absorption cooking method, the salt recommended for the cooking water ranges from ¼ to 1 teaspoon per cup of dry grain (e.g., rice, quinoa, millet, farro).

When it comes to pasta, Marcella Hazan, author of *The Essentials of Classic Italian Cooking*, suggests that at least 1½ tablespoons of salt per pound of pasta should be added to the cooking water (many recipes advise that pasta cooking water should be "as salty as the ocean"). Many cooks use between 1 to 3 tablespoons of salt per 4 quarts of water; in general, the saltier the water is, the saltier the pasta will be. A USDA study of the uptake of sodium into potatoes, pasta, and rice after adding salt to cooking water found that the amount of sodium absorbed is directly related to the amount of salt added to the cooking water.

How much of the salt is actually absorbed? A 2019 study published in *Food Chemistry* examined the sodium content of prepared pasta under different cooking conditions. Using laboratory analysis, the results for cooking 1 pound of spaghetti to al dente in 6 quarts of water with 1 tablespoon of salt showed a sodium absorption of 128 milligrams for 1 cup of cooked pasta (140 grams). To extrapolate this finding, if 1 tablespoon of table salt (6,975 milligrams sodium) is added to the cooking water, the amount of salt absorbed is *about* ½ teaspoon (1,024 milligrams sodium) per pound of pasta. Note that FoodData Central reports 162 milligrams of sodium per cup for spaghetti cooked in salted water (NDB 20321), but the amount of salt added to the water is not specified.

Cook's Illustrated laboratory tested 1 pound each of six different shapes of pasta (spaghetti, linguine, penne, rigatoni, campanelle, and orzo) cooked in 4 quarts water with 1 tablespoon salt to al dente. Their sodium absorption results were slightly lower; the amount absorbed was about ¼ teaspoon salt (580 milligrams) per pound of pasta. Each pasta shape absorbed about the same amount of sodium. The bottom line: the amount of sodium absorbed by pasta from salted water is relatively low but calculating a pasta recipe with 0 milligrams of added sodium from the salted water is inaccurate.

When blanching or boiling vegetables in salted water, much depends on how much salt is added to the water, how long the vegetable remains in the boiling water, the type of vegetable, and the vegetable's method of preparation (e.g., peeled or unpeeled). Given all the different variables and varieties of vegetables, there are no accurate overall best practices for vegetables.

Best Practices

Consider the audience and adjust your nutrition analysis guidelines accordingly. For example, if you are conducting a recipe analysis for sodium-sensitive populations, use a specific amount of salt in the calculation based on an assumption versus choosing to analyze the recipe without added salt.

For grains that use an absorption cooking method (e.g., rice, quinoa), do the following:

- Calculate the entire amount of salt called for in the recipe and assume total absorption of both the salt and the water if the recipe does not instruct to drain the water.

- If the recipe ingredient list does not include an amount of salt or states "cook according to package directions," create your own standard to follow and note how the sodium content is calculated, such as:
  - Calculate using the entire amount of salt the recipe developer or chef used.
  - Calculate using a "cooked with salt" database choice for the grain, if available.
  - Create your own standard of how much salt is used when calculating dry grains. Choose an amount (e.g., ½ teaspoon per 1 cup dry grains) and consistently document the amount used in calculations for dry grain recipes that absorb all the salt and water.
  - Clearly state whether the recipe was analyzed without salt added to the grain's cooking water.

For dishes that are drained (e.g., pasta):

- Calculate using a "cooked with salt" database choice, if available.

- Estimate *about* ½ teaspoon of table salt (or 1,024 milligrams of sodium) per pound of pasta for recipes that call for cooking in salted water.

- Create an ingredient subrecipe (e.g., 1 pound dry pasta with 4 quarts water and ½ teaspoon table salt), which will provide consistency among all pasta main recipes you analyze.

For vegetables cooked in boiling salted water, calculate using a "cooked with salt" database choice for the specific vegetable if available.

Salting to Taste

It is important to try and obtain an amount of salt, even if the recipe says "salt to taste" in the ingredient list or "season to taste" in the recipe directions. Omitting the salt may be an acceptable choice for some publishers, food companies, or restaurants, but in general, it can be misleading.

Best Practices

- Obtain an estimate of the typical amount of salt used or needed from the recipe developer or chef, or, if possible, watch as the recipe is prepared and note the exact amounts of salt used.

- Use your own culinary expertise to determine the right amount or prepare the recipe yourself to determine the amount of salt needed.

- Include notes about any assumptions made for the recipe analysis (e.g., "Recipe is calculated using [quantity] amount of [salt type] of salt" or "Recipe is calculated without salt").

Another approach for deciding the right amount of salt to use in recipes that call for salt to taste is to create your own set of culinary standards. For example, vinaigrettes are typically made with salt, so providing nutrition information that includes almost no sodium would be inaccurate. For vinaigrette recipes, you could estimate 1 teaspoon of kosher salt per each 1 cup of oil, and document that assumption in a note at the end of the recipe that states, "Recipe is calculated using 1 teaspoon of Morton kosher salt. Salt may be reduced or omitted if the sodium content needs to be lowered." Likewise, if a recipe is analyzed without salt, make sure it's noted so the information is not misleading (e.g., "Recipe calculated without salt because a specific amount was not provided").

Marinating, Brining, Pickling, and Fermenting

Recipes with marinades or brines, as well as recipes that involve pickling or fermentation, are challenging to analyze because the analysis must account for the nutrients absorbed by the food. If laboratory analysis is not an option, you can establish your own nutrition analysis assumptions based on such factors as the concentration or amount of fat, salt, sugar, or acid in the recipe; the length of time the food spends immersed in the liquid solution; and the type, cut, porosity, and surface area of the food, as all of these factors influence the rate of absorption. For example, foods like eggplant and mushrooms absorb more sodium than less porous foods, such as onions and peppers. The larger the surface area of a cut of meat is, the more solution will be absorbed by it; for example, a chicken breast cut up into 1-inch cubes will absorb more marinade than a whole chicken breast.

Marinades

Marinades require consideration of additional factors, such as the following:

- Is the marinade only being used to infuse flavor or tenderize the food before being discarded?

- Will the remaining marinade be used to baste the food during cooking? Or will it be boiled and made into a sauce?

- Is the length of the marinating time short (e.g., 30 minutes) or long (e.g., 24 hours)?

- How will the food be prepared? (If the food is broiled or grilled, some of the marinade will burn off.)

A close reading of the recipe directions will help you make better assumptions when calculating for the marinade.

Best Practices

- Document nutrition assumptions based on marinating time and type of food.

- Create a separate subrecipe for the marinade and use it as an ingredient in the main recipe.

- If you are also testing the recipe, measure or weigh the amount of marinade the recipe produces before adding the food to the marinade, and then measure or weigh the amount of marinade that's left over after the food is removed. The difference between these two numbers can be used as an estimate of how much marinade was absorbed by the food during the marinating process.

- If the marinade's weight measurements before and after the food is marinated are not provided, assume a rate of absorption of 6% to 10% and document the standard based on the marinating time. Follow these guidelines:
  - 6% absorption of total marinade in a recipe that requires 1.5 hours or less of marinating time
  - 10% absorption of total marinade in a recipe that require 2 hours or longer of marinating time

EXAMPLE OF SODIUM ABSORPTION FROM A MARINADE

Cooking Light magazine prepared samples for a laboratory analysis of an unmarinated grilled pork tenderloin and a pork tenderloin marinated in a mixture of reduced-sodium soy sauce, sesame oil, green onion, garlic, black pepper, and fresh ginger for 1½ hours, which were then grilled. The results:

- Unmarinated grilled pork: 54 milligrams sodium per 3-ounce serving
- Marinated grilled pork: 276 milligrams sodium per 3-ounce serving

While only 6% of the sodium in the marinade was absorbed by the pork, the marinated pork contained five times the amount of sodium compared to the unmarinated meat.

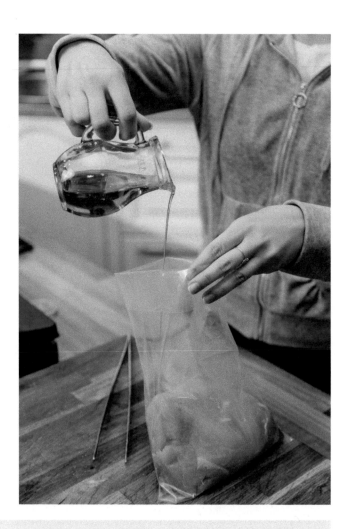

SODIUM IN BRINED POULTRY

Cooking Light magazine soaked three 12-pound turkeys in a brine solution containing ½ cup kosher salt (46,000 milligrams sodium) and sent the samples, along with a turkey that was not soaked in a brine, to a laboratory for analysis.

Results (per 4 ounces roasted turkey): About 0.6% to 1% of the total sodium from the brine was absorbed.

- No brine (sodium amounts found naturally in meat): white meat, 55 milligrams; dark meat, 90 milligrams
- 12-hour brine: white meat, 151 milligrams; dark meat, 235 milligrams
- 18-hour brine: white meat, 186 milligrams; dark meat, 254 milligrams
- 24-hour brine: white meat, 223 milligrams; dark meat, 260 milligrams

Cook's Illustrated magazine also sent cooked samples of boneless and skinless chicken breasts and boneless center-cut pork chops that were brined for 1 hour in 2 quarts of water with ¼ cup table salt to an independent laboratory for sodium analysis. The results: about 1% of the salt was absorbed into the food.

Food	Sodium absorbed	Salt equivalent
1 (6-ounce) boneless and skinless chicken breast	270 milligrams	Less than ⅛ teaspoon
1 (6-ounce) boneless center-cut pork chop	218 milligrams	Less than ⅛ teaspoon

* ¼ cup of table salt contains 28,320 milligrams of sodium

Brines

When a meat is brined, salt enters the meat's cells and alters the structure of the muscle fibers and proteins, ultimately swelling their water-holding capacity by about 10%. The result: juicier meat. Since most meats lose about 20% of their moisture during cooking, brining can cut the moisture loss of meat almost by half.

In most cases, the largest sodium increase occurs during the first 12 hours of brining time and then tapers off, according to a laboratory analysis performed by *Cooking Light* magazine. A test of brines performed by *Cook's Illustrated* magazine revealed that some meats absorb somewhat more or less than others and that lean muscle may absorb differently than fatty tissue (chicken absorbed significantly more brine per pound than pork, for example).

Best Practices

Document your nutrition assumptions based on the brining time and the type of food.

- Calculate using 1% total brine as a standard reference for the estimated amount of brine absorbed in the food. Document the following assumptions:
  - 1% total brine absorption if brining for 1 hour or less
  - 1% absorption if brining a very large food item (e.g., a turkey that's 12 pounds or heavier)

Adjusting Sodium Content of Canned Products

Draining and rinsing canned foods, such as beans, tomatoes, capers, artichokes, and roasted red peppers, can significantly decrease their sodium content. Draining alone can reduce the content by as much as 36%; draining and rinsing can reduce it by about 40%.

Best Practices

- Calculate a 30% reduction of sodium when canned products are drained.

- Calculate a 40% reduction of sodium when canned products are drained and *rinsed.*

- Use the weight of the drained canned product for the analysis, rather than the weight of the can or the can size. (The can's Nutrition Facts label serving size will indicate whether the weight given is for the drained weight; if the drained weight is not noted, the serving size weight will include the liquid.)

- Create a new food ingredient in the database saving as XYZ product, drained, sodium adjusted 30% or XYZ product, drained and rinsed, sodium adjusted 40%.

Example:

If the recipe calls for 1 (15-ounce/425-grams) can Brand XYZ black beans, drained and rinsed, first:

- Measure the drained, rinsed weight of canned beans. The drained weight of the beans is what should be entered into the database (in this case, 290 grams).
  - Net weight of beans with brine: 425 grams
  - Weight of brine: 135 grams
  - Weight drained and rinsed: 290 grams

- Choose USDA black beans or in this case, Brand XYZ black beans in the database and adjust the sodium in the database so it reflects the 40% reduction from draining and rinsing.
  - 1,350 milligrams sodium for the entire can
  - 1,350 milligrams sodium × 40% = 540 milligrams sodium
  - 1,350 milligrams − 540 milligrams = 810 milligrams sodium

- Adjust the sodium value in the database to 810 milligrams of sodium. Rename and save the new ingredient as "Canned black beans, drained and rinsed, sodium adjusted 40%."

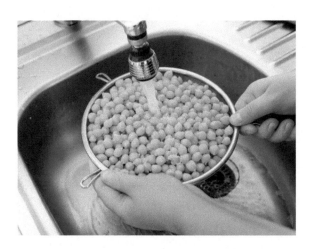

Stocks, Broths, Sauces, and Strained Foods

Analyzing stocks, broths, sauces, and strained recipes can present a challenge. When food cooks for a long time in a liquid, much of the liquid evaporates. Ingredients like vegetables, mirepoix (carrots, onion, and celery), meat, fish, and bones do infuse nutrients into cooking liquids, but these are often removed and discarded from the simmering liquid at the end of cooking.

The USDA's FoodData Central database does not include stocks, which further increases the challenge. Simply inputting recipe ingredients into the database for calculation without adjusting for losses or changes resulting from these preparation and cooking methods will affect the accuracy of the nutrient values. A laboratory analysis is the only accurate way to analyze the nutrients leached from ingredients that are strained out of a stock or broth, the heat-sensitive nutrient losses caused by long cooking times with sauces, and for the losses of fiber and other nutrients that arise from straining homemade baby food, sauces, and pureed soups.

Best Practices

Although these practices can improve the accuracy of software analyses, keep in mind that they will always be estimates.

Homemade broth or stock

- Add a laboratory-analyzed homemade stock or broth to the database of the software you use.

- Find a comparable low-sodium or reduced-sodium packaged broth or stock product in the database and assume its nutrient content is similar to the homemade version, as homemade broths and stocks usually contain significantly less sodium than purchased ones. Keep notes on which brand is used in the analysis.

Sauces

- If no ingredients are removed during or after the cooking process or before pureeing the sauce, conservatively calculate all ingredients in the recipe.

- Read the recipe instructions carefully and estimate how much fat is poured off or added to a sauce. Subtract this estimated amount of fat when making the calculation. For example, a recipe that includes sautéed meat might instruct the cook to pour off some of the fat before deglazing the pan to make the sauce.

- For larger sauce amounts, calculate the recipe using the final yield. Weigh or measure the liquid before and after the sauce is cooked. The final yield will provide an estimate of the moisture lost during cooking; while the volume is reduced, the calories are not. As for nutrients, some may increase and others (e.g., vitamin C) may degrade during the cooking process. This can only be measured by a laboratory analysis.

- Find a comparable product in the database that is assumed to have a similar nutrient content to the homemade version and compare the fiber and other nutrients in the analysis. Make fiber adjustments for the analysis referencing these products.

Alcohol

Alcohol retention after cooking ranges anywhere from 4% to 85%, according to a study conducted by the USDA's research division. The degree to which alcohol is retained depends on many factors, including the severity of the heat when alcohol is added during cooking; the ingredients in the recipe; the cooking method; and the type of cooking vessel. For example, the USDA demonstrated that more alcohol would evaporate if a recipe is cooked in a 12-inch pan than if it was cooked in a 10-inch pan because of the larger pan's greater surface area.

Best Practices

Using USDA's retention factors for alcohol in cooking, estimate the loss in calories from the alcohol that evaporates based on cooking time and subtract these calories from the calories provided by the alcohol (7 calories per gram of alcohol).

- Alcohol, flamed: 75% alcohol retained

- Alcohol, stirred, baked/simmered for 15 minutes: 40% alcohol retained

- Alcohol, stirred, baked/simmered for 30 minutes: 35% alcohol retained

- Alcohol, stirred, baked/simmered for 1 hour: 25% alcohol retained

- Alcohol, stirred, baked/simmered for 2 hours: 10% alcohol retained

- Alcohol, stirred, baked/simmered for 2½ hours: 5% alcohol retained

Example

A recipe calls for 1 cup white wine (198 calories) that cooks for about 15 minutes in a sauce: 198 calories × 40% alcohol retained = 79 calories

Adjust the wine calorie amount in the database to 79 calories.

Moisture Loss or Gain

A food's water content can increase or decrease when it's cooked. Ideally, these differences should be accounted for in a nutrition analysis if both the beginning and final weights of the recipe are known. Moisture loss impacts the nutrition analysis of many foods, and some software applications are capable of calculating moisture adjustments in recipes.

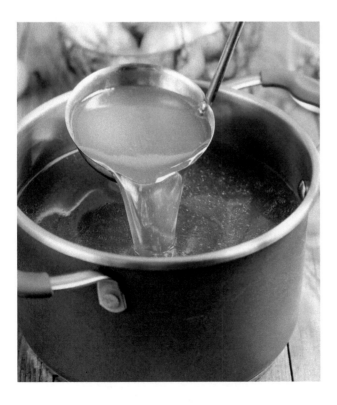

Creating a Nutrition Analysis Assumptions Document

Consistency is critical when analyzing recipes. For that reason, it's wise to create a document containing your project, publication, or company nutrition analysis assumptions and best practices. Maintaining nutrition analysis consistency across all recipes in a project is key. Additions or edits to this document should be made as new information comes to light and science evolves. Make sure to save each document version with a new date.

A nutrition analysis assumptions document (see example below) acts as a set of instructions for the recipe analyst. When creating a working document like this one, add or change as needed depending on your specific project or publication or when new ingredient information and evolving science is available. When adding a commonly used ingredient to this document, choose a brand that represents a generic or average amount of calories, sodium, sugar, and fat.

Example: Nutrition Analysis Assumptions Document

When the ingredient list includes alternative ingredients	Analyze with the first ingredient listed in the recipe when more than one option is given (e.g., "1 cup chicken broth or water").
When the recipe includes optional ingredients or garnishes	Do not include optional ingredients and garnishes in nutrition analyses.
When a range of ingredients and servings is provided in the recipe	Ingredient: Analyze using the *larger* amount listed in the recipe. For example, if "3 to 4 apples" is listed in the ingredient list, use 4 apples for the analysis. Servings: Analyze with the *smaller* number when a range is given. For example, if "4 to 6 servings" is listed as the number of servings, use 4 servings for the analysis. When both a weight and a conventional measurement (e.g., "1 cup") are provided in the ingredient list, use the weight, as it is always the most accurate measurement.
When cooking spray or a fat is used to grease pans	Do not include the cooking spray or fat in the analysis.
When a salt type or amount is not specified in the recipe	Use iodized table salt unless specified otherwise. If kosher salt is specified, use Morton kosher salt (480 milligrams sodium per ¼ teaspoon) instead of Diamond Crystal kosher salt (280 milligrams sodium per ¼ teaspoon). When a dash of salt is specified use ⅛ teaspoon; for a pinch of salt use 1/16 teaspoon.
When the amount of salt or other seasonings is listed to taste, do one of the following and document it	Ask the recipe tester, recipe developer, or chef to measure and specify the actual amount used in the recipe. Use your own culinary knowledge to estimate the amount of salt needed to enhance the dish's flavor. Calculate using this amount in the analysis and document it. Use a standard quantity of salt and black pepper in your analyses (e.g., for entrées, ¼ teaspoon salt and ⅛ teaspoon black pepper; for side dishes, ⅛ teaspoon salt and 1/16 teaspoon black pepper). Add a clear statement regarding how "to taste" entries are analyzed. Example: "Salt is calculated only if a recipe lists a specific amount. When recipes state unquantified amounts of salt (e.g., salt to taste, season to taste, add salt to cooking water), the salt is not included in the recipe analysis."

When the recipe includes a packaged food	Use the unmodified or full-fat version of the product unless a modified product is specified (e.g., low-fat, no-salt-added).
When the recipe includes pasta	Choose the version cooked in salted water, if available. If an appropriate choice is not available in the software's database, add ½ teaspoon of table salt per pound of pasta to the recipe analysis.
When the recipe includes canned vegetable and beans	Use a salted version unless otherwise specified. Estimate a 30% reduction in sodium content for drained and a 40% reduction for drained and rinsed canned products. Create a new database food item that reflects this change in sodium values.
When the recipe includes cheese	Use ounces or grams rather than cups for shredded cheese amounts. Weight is more precise for nutrient values on shredded cheese, since freshly grated cheese in cup measurements can vary.
When the recipe includes butter	Analyze using salted butter in savory recipes unless instructed otherwise. Analyze using unsalted butter in baking recipes unless instructed otherwise.
When the recipe includes milk	Analyze using whole milk unless otherwise specified (e.g., nonfat, 1%, or 2% milk).
When the recipe includes Dijon mustard	Analyze using [insert specific brand name] brand of Dijon mustard if no specific brand is recommended.
When the recipe includes jarred marinara sauce	Analyze using [insert specific brand name] brand of marinara sauce if no specific brand is recommended.
When the recipe includes soy sauce	Analyze using [insert specific brand name] for naturally brewed soy sauce and [insert specific brand name] for naturally brewed, reduced-sodium soy sauce, if no specific brand is recommended.
When the recipe includes chicken broth or stock, do one of the following and document it	Analyze using regular salted canned broth unless otherwise specified. Decide which brand to use for recipe analysis and document it. Analyze using US Department of Agriculture (USDA) estimates for reduced-sodium or low-sodium broth or stock when this type is specified. Analyze using low-sodium canned broth or stock for recipes using homemade broth or stock or use the USDA Food and Nutrient Database for Dietary Studies product identified as "chicken broth prepared from recipe."
When the recipe includes a cooked whole rotisserie chicken	Use 45% as the yield percentage if the weight of the whole cooked chicken is known.
When the recipe includes chicken breasts	Use 6 ounces for 1 raw boneless, skinless chicken breast if the weight is unspecified. Use 8 ounces for 1 raw boneless chicken breast with skin if the weight is unspecified. Use 10 ounces for 1 raw bone-in chicken breast with skin if the weight is unspecified.
When the recipe includes frozen shrimp	Analyze using USDA's 518717 brand of frozen shrimp (1 pound large raw shrimp contains 2,567 milligrams sodium). Different brands and types of frozen shrimp vary in sodium content based on the amount of brine used to wash and soak them.
When the recipe includes meat	In general, meat shrinks by about 25% when it is cooked; therefore, it has a 75% yield percentage. For example, 1 pound (16 ounces) raw boneless and skinless chicken breast will yield about 12 ounces cooked chicken.
When the recipe has missing ingredient and product information	Use 100-grams unrounded nutritional information from supplier or food company instead of the Nutrition Facts label for missing information.

Choosing a Nutrition Analysis Software Application

Nutrition analysis of recipes has come a long way since the labor-intensive process of manually looking up each ingredient, adding the data to a spreadsheet, and calculating the nutrient values by hand. It is now a highly efficient computerized process. When it comes to selecting recipe analysis software, choices range from free online options to sophisticated and expensive software applications. Food professionals face an increasingly difficult task of determining which API, software, or app is best for their recipe analyses. Following are some questions to consider when evaluating and selecting different recipe analysis software applications:

- What is your reason for analyzing recipes?
- What do you know about the application's database?
- What features do you need?
- What type of computer will you use?
- What is your budget?

What Is Your Reason for Analyzing Recipes?

If you are a nutrition professional for whom calculating nutrition values is routine practice, select a more advanced software application. In return, your analyses will be more accurate and you'll have access to a larger database, a comprehensive data management system, and the ability to create FDA-compliant labels. This may include professionals who do any of the following:

- work for a food manufacturer, restaurant group, or foodservice company and may be involved in creating nutrition information and Nutrition Facts labels that comply with FDA regulations

- analyze recipes that are health- or nutrition-focused or recipes that make specific nutrient content claims (e.g., recipes for people with diabetes or heart disease or allergen-specific recipes)

- analyze recipes for print or digital publications, such as cookbooks, newspapers, magazines, or food company websites

If you work for a publication with a high volume of recipes, a nutrition analysis API might be a good choice, as it can quickly calculate rough estimates of nutrition information. If you are a recipe developer looking to estimate your recipes' nutrition information during development or a food blogger or content creator with a desire to manage various recipe, diet, and fitness needs, you'll likely have more flexibility in choosing the software, website plug-in, or app that is right for you.

What Do You Know about the Application's Database?

Recipe analysis software applications, APIs, and apps are only as good as the data they rely on. Evaluating where the data comes from and how often the database is updated is a key step in evaluating the software.

Where Does the Data Come From?

A quality recipe analysis software application gathers data from many reputable sources to ensure accuracy. These sources include the latest USDA National Nutrient Database for Standard Reference Legacy Release (abbreviated as SR Legacy); the USDA Food and Nutrient Database for Dietary Studies (abbreviated as FNDDS); the USDA Global Branded Food Products Database (abbreviated as Branded Foods); and data supplied directly by food manufacturers and restaurants. If you are interested in learning more about food and ingredient databases, consider attending the biannual National Nutrient Databank Conference (see Nutrient Analysis Resources and Bibliography on page 294 for more information).

Nutrition analysis software applications and APIs should be transparent about the quality of their data on foods and ingredients, including providing the source of the data for each entry, no matter whether it comes from a government source, a food council or association, a food manufacturer or restaurant, or a professional research article. **All data in a recipe analysis database should be supported by documentation.**

Crowd-sourced data can be useful at times, but it is unreliable and shouldn't be used for professional recipe analyses. Databases containing information submitted by consumers, whether they enter the data themselves or provide pictures of foods or scanned labels, have little to no oversight or verification. As a result, they often include inaccurate data, incorrect product details and descriptions, and duplicate items—sometimes with different nutrient values for the same food item. And remember that information from Nutrition Facts labels feature rounded calorie and nutrient values, which are not necessarily accurate for nutrition analysis.

How Often Is the Database Updated?

Quality recipe analysis databases are updated with the latest food and ingredient data on an ongoing basis. After all, hundreds of new food products are introduced every month, and packaged foods that are no longer on the market should be removed from the database during updates as well. Ask representatives of the software manufacturer or developer if the company has procedures in place to ensure that the values in the ingredient composition database are reviewed and updated as needed and also on a regular basis (ideally, updates should occur at least once or, better yet, several times per year).

How Extensive and Complete Is the Database?

A robust database includes a wide variety of foods and ingredients—everything from raw foods to name-brand items. The database should also provide all of the nutrient data needed to produce an accurate calculation, as missing data leads to inaccurate recipe analyses.

Can You Add Ingredients to the Database?

Since an analysis should be as close as possible to the actual recipe, the software should allow you to enter your own ingredients if necessary, and the ingredients you enter should be visible only to you.

Is the Database Easy to Search?

The database should have a consistent and functional naming convention, as disparate naming conventions needlessly complicate searches.

What Features Do You Need?

Different recipe analysis software applications offer different features, so it's important to determine early on what features you need for your business. The main functions offered by nutrition analysis software applications include:

- recipe analysis, which includes recipe management; the ability to save new ingredients and rename existing ones; the ability to enter overrides for specific nutrients; generation of nutrient analysis reports; generation of carbohydrate choices; generation of allergen statements; generation of ingredient statements; identification of nutrient content claims; and export of regulation-compliant domestic or international food labels

- diet and fitness needs, which may include management of client or patient diet and recipe records and nutrition need assessments

- menu planning and management, which includes menu creation and analysis as well as management of food costs, scaling, inventory, and purchasing

- platform interfacing, which includes an application's capability of publishing directly to a website or to interface with other business features, mobile apps, point of service systems, and more

Some applications are focused on only one of these functions, while others offer some or all of them. Also, consider the training and customer support services provided by the software manufacturer. Any application you choose should be user friendly, but additional software training tools can be a valuable asset that helps you maximize the accuracy of your analyses and minimize frustration. In fact, whether an application offers easy-to-access technical support may be a deciding factor when choosing an application. Some manufacturers provide both technical support and customer service via phone, chat, or email.

What Type of Computer Will You Use?

Will you need software that's designed for a Windows or a Mac computer, an online or cloud-based application, or an API?

Desktop Version (Windows or Mac)

Most nutrition analysis software applications are designed for Windows-based computers, but Mac owners can successfully use Windows-based applications by installing licensed software that can run Windows applications on a Mac. If you purchase a desktop version of a nutrition analysis software application, you will install it on your machine and perform your own updates.

Cloud-Based/Online

Some software applications do not reside on local computers. Instead, these applications are used entirely online by logging in with a username and password, and updates are handled by the manufacturer.

Application Program Interface

You or your company can build third-party proprietary software using a nutrient data API or a nutrition analysis API, a tool that allows programmers to add recipe analysis functionality to recipe text.

What Is Your Budget?

Investing in a nutrition analysis software application will cost much less than a laboratory nutrition analysis, but it's still an expense, and there may be ongoing expenses to maintain and update the software. Free or low-cost nutrition analysis software applications exist, but they may use questionable or unsubstantiated data and may not be routinely updated. Most are not capable of accounting for nutrient changes during cooking and have limited capacity for adding or changing information.

The cost of nutrition analysis software applications varies depending on their features. There are also many different cost models, including monthly subscription plans, single- or multiple-user server licenses for desktop applications with renewal fees for updates and ongoing support, cloud-based or online subscriptions, and API licensing fees. Each

category has options to choose from, making software an accessible and affordable option for most professionals. Free sites are fine for quickly looking up an estimate for an ingredient's nutrient information, but a high-quality, professional analysis requires investment in a reputable software application.

If you consider using a free application (other than the USDA FoodData Central), remember that nutrition analysis APIs, software applications, and apps are typically developed by individuals who are skilled in writing code; no food, nutrition, or food regulatory knowledge is needed.

Nutrition Analysis Software Options

Contact laboratories or colleagues who work with food and beverage companies to ask for their recommendations for the best professional software applications for nutrient analysis. Some of these applications enable users to easily create Nutrition Facts labels.

If you are looking for basic nutrient information about an ingredient or food when developing recipes, FoodData Central (fdc.nal.usda.gov) is a great first stop: a well-respected and extensive database that is free to use. FoodData Central contains five different databases or "data types," as USDA refers to them, and provides source date information, so you know when the nutrient data was most recently updated. FoodData Central also offers a free API that is available to software and app developers.

Quick Tip

"When evaluating nutrient analysis software, ask the company or developer where their nutrition data comes from and how they verify the information's accuracy. Find out how often they update the data and if you, the user, are able to update or add missing nutrient information or ingredients. It's helpful if the software is cloud-based so that updates are quick and easily backed up. And make sure there is support and training for the program." —Laura Ali, MS, RDN, culinary consultant and former senior manager of nutrition and regulatory affairs at Starkist

RECIPE NUTRITION ANALYSIS SOFTWARE AND DATABASES*

This list of software applications, apps, APIs, and plug-ins is not exhaustive and is subject to change as new options become available.

Software applications for nutrition professionals

Below are software applications recommended for nutrition professionals who want to analyze menus, foods, and recipes with higher accuracy, larger databases, ongoing updates, more capabilities, and comprehensive data management.

Axxya Nutritionist Pro	nutritionistpro.com
EGS Calcmenu (food service and restaurants)	eg-software.com
ESHA Research	

Food Processor
   Genesis R & D Food Formulation
      & Labeling Software
	esha.com/products/food-processor
	esha.com/products/genesis-rd-food-labeling-software

LabelCalc (for food manufacturing food labeling) and MenuCalc (food service and restaurants)	labelcalc.com menucalc.com
NutriBase Professional	nutribase.com
Nutrihand Pro	nutrihand.com
Nutritics	nutritics.com
Nutritionix	nutritionix.com/business/interactive-nutrition-tools
Parsley (for foodservice and restaurants)	parsleysoftware.com
USDA list of approved applications for school food service	fns.usda.gov/tn/usda-approved-nutrient-analysis-software

Database APIs

Database application program interfaces (APIs) are recommended for developers who wish to incorporate nutrient data into their applications or websites for the purpose of syncing data between two systems. For example, website plug-ins integrate with a nutrition database API to automatically calculate recipe nutrition analysis based on ingredients entered. APIs have different functionalities—some offer real-time integration and can calculate nutritional information for recipes automatically using a proprietary algorithm.

Edamam	developer.edamam.com
ESHA Research Genesis	esha.com/products/genesis-api
FoodData Central	fdc.nal.usda.gov/api-guide.html
Google Fit	developers.google.com/fit
Nutritics	nutritics.com/p/api
Nutritionix	nutritionix.com/business/api
Spoonacular	spoonacular.com/food-api

BOX CONTINUES >

Recipe website plug-ins for WordPress

Delicious Recipes	wpdelicious.com
Nutrifox	nutrifox.com
Recipe Card Blocks	wordpress.org/plugins/recipe-card-blocks-by-wpzoom
Recipe Maker	wordpress.org/plugins/wp-recipe-maker
Tasty Recipes	wptasty.com/tasty-recipes

Multiuse software

Software recommended for health professionals that includes diet and fitness capabilities along with recipe analysis

Cronometer	cronometer.com
ESHA Research ESHATrak App	esha.com/products/eshatrak-online-nutrition-app
My Food Record	myfoodrecord.com
MyNetDiary	mynetdiary.com
ReciPal	recipal.com
That Clean Life	thatcleanlife.com
Whisk (recipe analysis only)	whisk.com

* This list is not comprehensive and reflects products available at the time of writing. Crowd-sourced apps are not recommended for use with ingredient data and recipe analysis.

Quick Tip

"Be mindful if using free databases when calculating nutrition analysis, as user input data can lead to inaccurate nutrition calculations. Regardless of what database or software you use, nutrition analysis is only as good as the person performing the analysis. Your experience, culinary knowledge, understanding of nutrient loss and retention, and evaluating the final outcome are essential tools to your success.

—Sarah Hendren, MS, RDN, Regulatory Affairs Scientist for Frito Lay North America

Quick Tip

"Commercially available databases vary in completeness, accuracy, and inclusion of branded items and must be kept up to date especially with branded consumer packaged goods. And they must have the option for entering new products into the database. I have entered the nutritionals from supplier specification sheets for thousands of specific products based on 100-gram nutrient data provided. I ask suppliers for an update often since it is best practice to use the actual product in the analysis, not just a generic product." —Wendy Hess, MS, RD, nutrition analysis consultant

Using Federal Guidelines for Reporting Nutrition Information for Recipes

The FDA has not issued rules or guidelines for analyzing consumer recipes and reporting this nutrition information. Professionals should follow best practices for recipe nutrition analysis, which includes using the 80-20 rule as a benchmark and following the FDA's regulations for making nutrient content and health claims (see pages 36 through 38) and providing allergen statements (see Chapter 5).

FDA Labeling Compliance Standards: The 80-20 Rule

Food Products and Nonalcoholic Beverages

The FDA set compliance standard 21 CFR 101.9 (g) for labeling of packaged food and nonalcoholic beverages in order to evaluate the accuracy of nutrition label information against a standard for compliance purposes. The compliance standard, which allows manufacturers the flexibility to account for natural variances in their products, is referred to as the 80-20 rule. It stipulates that for any nutrient whose consumption is encouraged (i.e., "beneficial nutrients"), the actual nutrient level in the food must be 80% or more of the declared label value. For any nutrient that should be avoided in excess (i.e., "nutrients to limit"), the actual level in the food must not be greater than 20% above the amount declared on the food label. To calculate the percentage, use the formula:

(actual value ÷ label value) × 100 = XYZ%

These allowable variances are designed to ensure that beneficial nutrients are not overstated and nutrients that should be limited are not understated. If nutrient values vary outside of this rule, then the product is considered out of compliance.

Beneficial nutrients (80% or more) The nutrient content of vitamin D, vitamin C, calcium, iron, potassium, total carbohydrate, protein, dietary fiber, polyunsaturated fat, and monounsaturated fat must be present at 80% or more of the value declared on the label.

For example, consider a product whose label states that it contains 260 milligrams of calcium per serving. A laboratory analysis finds that the product contains 240 milligrams calcium. The ratio between the laboratory (actual) and declared value is $(240 \div 260) \times 100 = 92\%$. The actual calcium value exceeds 80% of the declared value, and as a result, the product is FDA compliant.

Nutrients to limit (not in excess of 20%) The nutrient content of calories, total sugars, added sugars, total fat, saturated fat, *trans* fat, cholesterol, and sodium cannot exceed 20% of the value declared on the label.

For example, consider a product whose label states that it contains 6 grams total fat per serving. A laboratory analysis finds that the product contains 8 grams total fat per serving. The ratio between the laboratory (actual) and declared value is $(8 \div 6) \times 100 = 133\%$. The actual fat value is 33% above the declared value, which exceeds the 20% limit, and as a result, the product is not FDA compliant.

Food manufacturers are responsible for assuring the validity of the stated nutrient values found on their product labels via a laboratory nutrition analysis, calculations from nutrition analysis software, or a combination of both methods. No matter which method or combination of methods is used, each manufacturer must have rigorous controls in place to conduct and document its accurate nutrition analysis to meet the 80-20 rule standard. If they fail to maintain these standards, their products are at risk of being considered mislabeled. If a manufacturer makes a nutrient claim (e.g., low sodium) on a product, a laboratory analysis is recommended to substantiate the claim.

Alcoholic Beverages

Most alcoholic beverages (distilled spirits, wines that are 7% to 24% alcohol by volume, and malted beverages) are regulated by the Alcohol and Tobacco Tax and Trade Bureau (TTB). Nutrition labeling is optional for these products. Other alcoholic beverages, including hard seltzers and low- and no-alcohol wine and spirits, fall under the jurisdiction of the FDA and must follow all nutrition labeling requirements.

Restaurant Menus

FDA has recognized that the 80-20 rule for menu labeling regulations is unrealistic for foodservice operations. Restaurant foods differ from packaged foods due to the wide range of human, environmental, and ingredient-related variables in a restaurant setting. As a result, the FDA uses a "reasonable basis" standard for compliance in restaurant menu labeling. While adhering to the 80-20 rule is not required for restaurants, it's a good benchmark to follow for recipe analysis. To comply with this reasonable basis standard, a recipe analyst should use a standardized recipe and follow the same best practices for analyzing packaged food products.

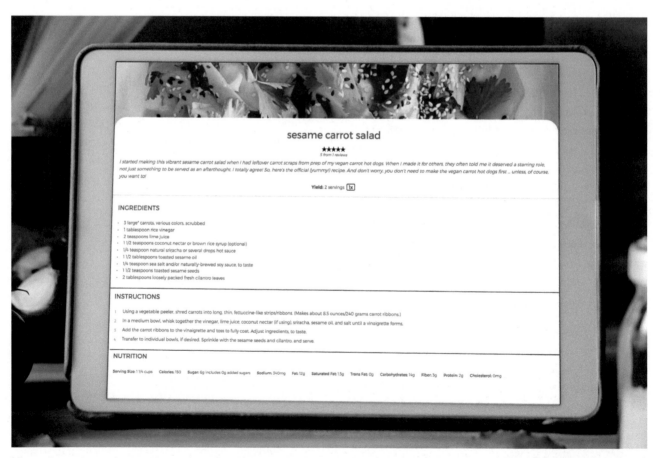

Most online recipes today provide nutrition information for consumers. Recipe courtesy of Jackie Newgent, RDN, CDN (jackienewgent.com).

Food product labels

Food labeling practices originally emerged as a consumer safety precaution following a series of foodborne-illness outbreaks in the 1850s. Nutrition information on labels was left to the discretion of manufacturers until 1990, when the US Food and Drug Administration (FDA) mandated that all food product labels must include standardized nutrition information and consistent health claims.

The FDA's Nutrition Labeling and Education Act (NLEA) of 1990 states that nutrition information is required to be listed on all packaged retail foods. Food manufacturers must comply with the labeling regulations of the NLEA for their food product labels and must stay current with any changing legal requirements.

NLEA helps ensure proper labeling by food manufacturers. Compliance with the Act requires inclusion of a Nutrition Facts label, ingredient listings, allergen statements, and substantiation of health and nutrient content claims like "low sodium" on the product's packaging. The nutrients required to be listed on the Nutrition Facts label are calories, total fat, saturated fat, *trans* fat, cholesterol, sodium, total carbohydrate, dietary fiber, total sugars, added sugars, protein, vitamin D, calcium, iron, and potassium.

For additional food industry labeling guidance, review the FDA's Food Labeling Guide or Code of Federal Regulations–Title 21.

Nutrition Facts	
8 servings per container	
Serving size	**2/3 cup (55g)**
Amount per serving	
Calories	**230**
	% Daily Value*
Total Fat 8g	**10%**
Saturated Fat 1g	**5%**
Trans Fat 0g	
Cholesterol 0mg	**0%**
Sodium 160mg	**7%**
Total Carbohydrate 37g	**13%**
Dietary Fiber 4g	**14%**
Total Sugars 12g	
Includes 10g Added Sugars	**20%**
Protein 3g	
Vitamin D 2mcg	10%
Calcium 260mg	20%
Iron 8mg	45%
Potassium 240mg	6%

* The % Daily Value (DV) tells you how much a nutrient in a serving of food contributes to a daily diet. 2,000 calories a day is used for general nutrition advice.

Restaurant menu labeling

A provision in the FDA's Patient Protection and Affordable Care Act (ACA) of 2010, *Food Labeling: Nutrition Labeling of Standard Menu Items in Restaurants and Similar Retail Food Establishments*, requires restaurants and similar retail food establishments with more than twenty locations doing business under the same name to provide consumers with calorie and other nutrition information for standard menu items. The rationale behind the menu labeling law is to help Americans make informed choices for better health. The final rule was published in 2014 and went into effect on May 7, 2018.

Recipe Analysis Checklist and Worksheet

A recipe analysis checklist can be used to ensure that you have complete and correct information before beginning the nutrition analysis. After receiving a hard copy or digital version of the recipe for nutrition analysis, review it closely using the questions shown in the sample checklist as a guide. As you review, make note of any additional information you will need from the recipe developer, chef, or editor.

Another option is to use a recipe analysis worksheet, which can be completed by the recipe analyst or with the help of the recipe developer or chef to ensure that recipe information is clear and complete before performing the nutrition analysis. The worksheet can also be shared with a recipe developer to complete and submit with each recipe for nutrition analysis. This makes it clear what is needed for an accurate analysis, and it can save time on future projects. A recipe nutrition analysis worksheet can also serve as documentation of your process, which can be useful in case of questions or an audit where it may be necessary to show proof that the analysis was performed with best practices.

Recipe Information Needed for Nutrition Analysis

Checklist	Yes/No	Notes
Ingredients		
Are all ingredient names clear, including product type, brand, and form indicated (e.g., fresh, frozen, canned, Heinz ketchup versus store-brand ketchup)		
Does each ingredient indicate the preparation technique to be applied to the ingredient and size if necessary? (e.g., peeled, sliced, drained, cut into ½-inch cubes)?		
Is there a weight or volume listed for each ingredient?		
Directions		
Do the recipe directions clearly describe exactly what needs to be done to prepare the recipe?		
Are equipment and pan sizes indicated?		
Is the cooking temperature and time listed?		
Yield and serving size		
Is the total recipe yield indicated?		
Is number of total servings indicated?		
Is the individual serving size indicated?		
Is the individual serving size given in volume or weight measurements?		
Are the serving size and number of servings listed in the recipe correct based on the total yield?		

Recipe Analysis Worksheet

Recipe Name: _____

Recipe Yield: Total amount (weight/volume): _____ **Total servings per recipe:** _____ **Single serving size:** _____

Weight (grams/ounces): _____ **Household measurement** (e.g., 1 cookie, cups/tablespoons, fluid ounces, liters): _____

Recipe Ingredient* (brand name, if applicable)	Weight (AP)	Ingredient Description (package size and type: fresh, frozen; can, box, vacuum-packed, bottle; low-fat, reduced-sodium, enriched Cut of meat: raw or cooked, prime or choice; bone-in or boneless, etc.)	Preparation steps (minced, chopped, grated, stems removed)	Weight (EP)	Volume Measurement

Directions (step-by-step procedures for combining and cooking ingredients, cooking times and final cooking temperatures):

_____

_____

_____

_____

_____

_____

_____

_____

_____

_____

Baked, roasted, or fried (circle one)	Initial recipe weight before cooking: _____ grams	Final recipe weight after cooking: _____ grams	Weight loss during cooking: _____ grams
Fluids including sauces, soups, and cooked liquid ingredients	Initial amount recorded in volume/fluid ounces, or weight: _____	Final recorded in volume/fluid ounces, or weight: _____	Loss during cooking: _____
Marinade (yes/no)	Initial amount of marinade (weight and volume measurement): _____	Leftover amount of marinade (weight and volume measurement): _____	Amount of marinade used: _____

* Include ingredient information and product nutrition information specification sheet for 100 grams or photo of Nutrition Facts panel for specialty ingredients; include (or attach) nutrition analysis for a recipe's subrecipe.

Abbreviations: AP = as purchased; EP = edible portion.

Nutrient Analysis Resources and Bibliography

Books

The Book of Yields: Accuracy in Food Costing and Purchasing, 8th Edition, by Francis Talyn Lynch. 2010. John Wiley & Sons.

Food for Fifty, 14th Edition, by Mary Molt. 2017. Pearson.

Food Analysis, 5th Edition, by Suzanne Nielsen. 2017. Springer Publishing.

Recipe Nutrient Analysis: Best Practices for Calculation and Chemical Analysis by Catharine Powers and Cheryl L. Dolven. 2015. Culinary Nutrition Publishing.

Laboratory Analysis Resources

AOAC Standards and Scientific Methods:
aoac.org/scientific-solutions

ISO/IEC 17025, Testing and calibration laboratories:
iso.org/ISO-IEC-17025-testing-and-calibration-laboratories.html

FDA Food and Menu Label Resources

Code of Federal Regulations Title 21 [80/20 rule: 21 CFR 101.9(g)]:
accessdata.fda.gov/scripts/cdrh/cfdocs/cfcfr/cfrsearch.cfm?fr=101.9

FDA Issues Final Guidance Regarding the Declaration of Added Sugars on the Nutrition Facts Label for Honey, Maple Syrup, Other Single Ingredient Sugars, and Certain Cranberry Products:
fda.gov/food/cfsan-constituent-updates/fda-issues-final-guidance-regarding-declaration-added-sugars-nutrition-facts-label-honey-maple-syrup

FDA's Policy on Declaring Small Amounts of Nutrients and Dietary Ingredients on Nutrition Labels: Guidance for Industry:
fda.gov/media/98834/download

Guidance for Industry: Guide for Developing and Using Data Bases for Nutrition Labeling:
fda.gov/regulatory-information/search-fda-guidance-documents/guidance-industry-guide-developing-and-using-data-bases-nutrition-labeling

US Food & Drug Administration. Labeling & Nutrition Guidance Documents & Regulatory Information:
fda.gov/food/guidance-documents-regulatory-information-topic-food-and-dietary-supplements/labeling-nutrition-guidance-documents-regulatory-information#nutrition

Menu Labeling Requirements:
fda.gov/food/food-labeling-nutrition/menu-labeling-requirements

Menu Labeling: Supplemental Guidance for Industry. Published May 2018:
fda.gov/files/food/published/Menu-Labeling-Supplemental-Guidance-for-Industry-PDF.pdf

USDA Resources

Ingredient Yield: Food Buying Guide for Child Nutrition Programs:
fns.usda.gov/tn/food-buying-guide-for-child-nutrition-programs

Cooking Yield: USDA Table of Cooking Yields for Meat and Poultry:
data.nal.usda.gov/dataset/usda-table-cooking-yields-meat-and-poultry

Nutrient Retention: USDA Table of Nutrient Retention Factors, Release 6:
data.nal.usda.gov/dataset/usda-table-nutrient-retention-factors-release-6-2007

Nutrient Analysis in School Meal Programs: USDA Approved Nutrient Analysis Software Programs:
fns.usda.gov/tn/usda-approved-nutrient-analysis-software

Standardized Recipes: USDA Recipe Standardization Guide for School Nutrition Programs:
theicn.org/cicn/usda-recipe-standardization-guide-for-school-nutrition-programs

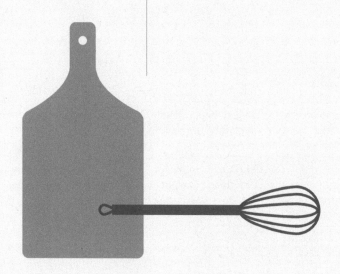

Complex Recipe Analysis Resources

Fat Analysis
Understanding Oil Absorption During Deep-Fat Frying by Pedro Bouchon. *Advances in Food and Nutrition Research.* 2009; 209-234.

Salted Water
Cooking parameters affect the sodium content of prepared pasta. LM Bianchi, KM Phillips, RC McGinty, et al. *Food Chemistry.* 2019;271:479-487. doi.org/10.1016/j.foodchem.2018.07.198

Cook's Illustrated. How much sodium does salted cooking water add to pasta?: cooksillustrated.com/how_tos/8903 -how-much-sodium-does-salted-cooking -water-add-to-pasta

USDA. Change in sodium content of potato, pasta and rice with different cooking methods: nal.usda.gov/fsrio/research-projects /change-sodium-content-potato-pasta-and -rice-different-cooking-methods

Marinades/Brines
Cook's Illustrated. How much sodium is in brined food? : cooksillustrated.com/how_tos/8474-how -much-sodium-is-in-brined-food

Sodium reduction in canned beans after draining, rinsing. RL Duyff, JR Mount, JB Jones. *J Culinary Sci Technol.* 2011;9(2):106-112. tandfonline.com/doi/full/10.1080/154280 52.2011.582405

Science of Brining.; edinformatics.com/math_science/science _of_cooking/brining.htm

Alcohol Retention
Alcohol retention in food preparation by J Augustin, E Augustin, RL Cutufelli, et al. *J Am Diet Assoc.* 1992;92(4):486-488.

USDA Table of Nutrient Retention Factors, Release 6: data.nal.usda.gov/dataset/usda-table -nutrient-retention-factors-release-6-2007

Nutrition Analysis and Labeling Regulatory Support

Food Consulting Company
Provides nutrition analysis and food label guidance and services to the food industry. The company writes a monthly newsletter and a LinkedIn group that is open to anyone who wants to share insights and ideas about nutrition, labeling, and regulatory compliance for the United States, Canada, Mexico, the United Kingdom, and the European Union. Food Label News Newsletter. foodlabels.com/food-label-news

Nutrient Databank Conference
The National Nutrient Databank Conference is held biannually to foster communication among nutrient database generators and users. Participation is open to researchers from academia, the food industry, government, and other interested parties. nutrientdataconf.org

Prime Label Consultants
Provides label training for regulatory and marketing professionals; hosts an annual food label conference bringing together government policymakers and industry experts in exchange of trends, ideas, and labeling best practices. primelabel.com/index.html

Nutrition Analysis and Labeling Networking Groups

ESHA Nutrition Labeling & Analysis Software Community: linkedin.com/groups/6936547

Food Label Community: linkedin.com/groups/3452458

Food & Nutrition Label; Dietary Supplement & Menu Labeling & Advertising: linkedin.com/groups/158141

Food Regulatory Affairs Professionals: linkedin.com/groups/163263

Regulatory Affairs Professionals Society (RAPS): linkedin.com/groups/110767

US FDA Nutrition and Labeling Laws Guidance: linkedin.com/groups/2482604

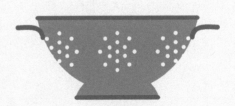

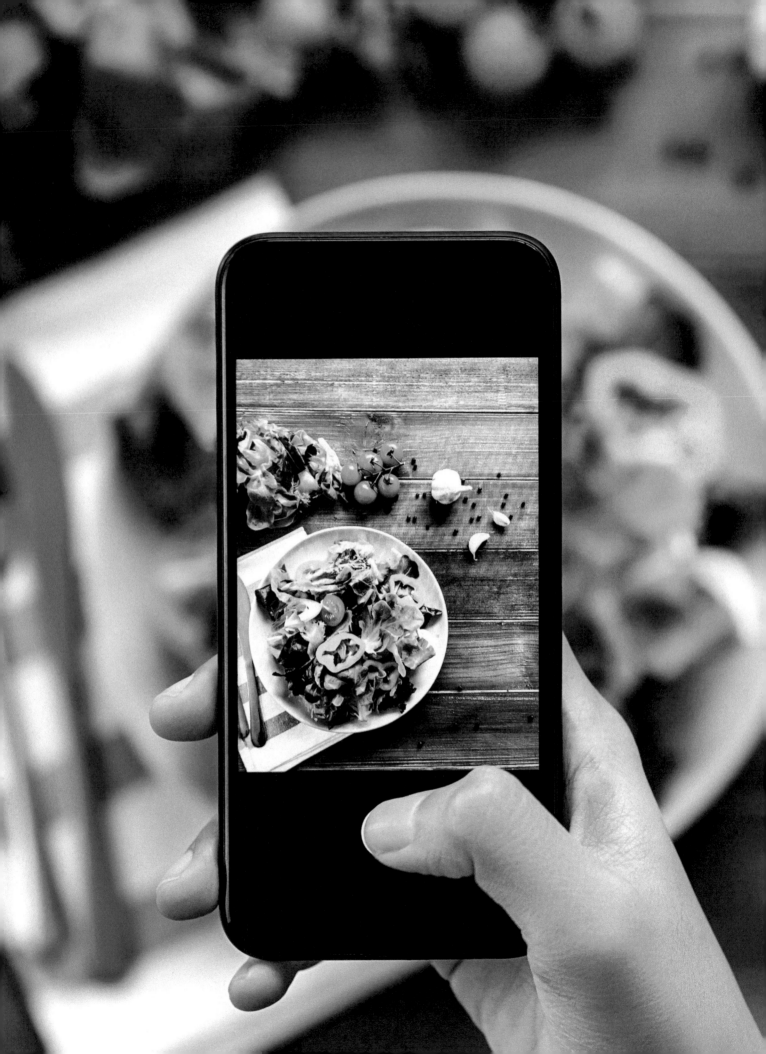

Chapter 10
Food Styling, Photography, and Videos

IN THIS CHAPTER, LEARN ABOUT:

- Food styling tips and tricks to make food look delicious

- Planning, shooting, and editing for food photography and food videos

- Equipment options for food photography and video

- How to use lighting and composition to elevate food photography and video

As digital technology has advanced, many recipe developers and recipe writers are expanding their skills to include food styling, food photography, and food videos. In this chapter, professional food stylists, photographers, and videographers who dedicate their careers to their craft share their wisdom and expertise so you can better understand the process behind the art of styling food, taking food photos, and recording food videos. Consider the following approaches for learning and practicing your skills:

Study the work of professionals. Follow different food stylists, photographers, and videographers on various platforms and publications. Determine qualities and approaches that you like. Imitation (the most sincere form of flattery) is a great first step in learning.

Assist a professional. Volunteer to work with someone you respect. Learn how they bring food and drink to life on set and in front of the camera—from preproduction to postproduction. As you learn, start your own experimentation based on what you observe. Sign up for live workshops at professional conferences, take online classes, or watch video tutorials produced by professionals. See Food Styling, Photography, and Video Resources and Bibliography on page 347.

See Food Styling, Photography, and Video Resources and Bibliography on page 347.

Quick Tip

"Getting good at food photography is like playing an instrument: practice makes you better." —Renée Comet, professional food photographer

Prioritize learning. Developing your skills as a food stylist, photographer, or videographer takes time, practice, and patience. Understanding how a food image or a video shoot comes together and the skills each member of the team provides is important—even if you're the *only* team member! Collaboration is the gateway to learning, whether you have the opportunity to work alongside great photographers and art directors or are working alone and asking other professionals to provide feedback.

Practice! While the information in this chapter is an excellent resource, the best way to learn is to jump in and start experimenting and practicing. The more experience you build, the more the strategies in this chapter will help you. Even if your first efforts are just for your own use, it's important to start somewhere and build a foundation you can improve upon.

PROFESSIONAL ROLES IN FOOD PHOTOGRAPHY AND VIDEO

The **recipe developer or writer** creates recipe(s) with visual interest in mind, provides inspirational or aspirational recipe content for readers, and keeps the overall vision in mind for the shoot.

The **prop stylist** chooses the props, fabrics, and tabletops for the shoot.

The **food stylist** makes food look good for the camera and knows a litany of tricks and techniques to create beautiful food. Food stylists often do the planning, grocery shopping, prep, and cooking for a shoot as well.

The **art director** communicates the look and feel—the overall vision—of the shoot.

The **photographer** plans, shoots, and edits images, ensuring the lighting, focus, and composition are right.

The **videographer** shoots and edits video footage and ensures the lighting, focus, and composition are right. Videographers often assume the responsibilities of a video producer for small productions or when shooting their own videos.

The **video producer** coordinates and manages the entire video production process, including setting the creative vision and strategy, writing the script, coordinating logistics and management for the shoot, directing on the day of the shoot, and working closely with the editor during postproduction to bring the vision and story to life.

Food Styling

Professional food stylists help create beautiful, interesting, and mouthwatering images of food by plating and arranging them to look their best; they are true artists with a creative eye. Food stylists know how to cook, but—more importantly—they can solve the problems that inevitably arise during a photo shoot quickly and with technical expertise. An amateur can create a food photo that looks like the recipe, but a professional food stylist can take one look at an image preview and know exactly what to change, not only to showcase the food but also to create a beautiful image.

Food styling is considered a niche career, but these days, all food professionals should know the basics of how to make food look good for the camera, whether they're using their skills as part of a team or for their own social media, blog, or e-newsletter. In a team setup, the photographer is the master of lighting and camera settings, and the stylist is the culinary expert who is responsible for the aesthetics. If you're doing it all on your own, you must first understand the fundamental techniques of photography (especially lighting) before moving on to food styling, and you must realize that the most important food styling "trick" is knowing how to cook.

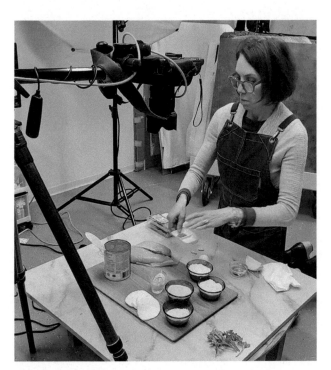

Food Stylist Lisa Cherkasky styling the ingredients for the photo shoot.

Prop Styling

Just as they do in the theater world, props help set the stage for a great food photo. Props are all of the items in food images other than the food—the surface or background, cookware, bakeware, plates, bowls, silverware, serving utensils, glasses, coffee mugs, teacups, table linens, napkins, and so on. The choice of props should support the message of the image—whether it's trying to convey a time of year, a location, a mood, or a celebration.

Traditionally, if the budget allows, a prop stylist on the shoot handles all the props. Sometimes, the photographer handles the props and the food stylist uses what is available, or the food stylist may do both the props and the styling. These days, many food professionals do the prop styling, food styling, and photo or video shooting themselves. Whether you're planning to hire a prop stylist or do the work yourself, consider assembling a collection of props, and think beyond kitchen and houseware stores when looking for props, such as online, or at thrift stores, garage sales, and flea markets.

Tips for Choosing Props

- Use props sparingly. Don't let props distract from the main focus of the images: the food.

- Choose a photo surface or background color that doesn't compete with the food and that reflects the emotions you are trying to convey. Some ideas for surfaces include marble, tiles, a chalkboard, a piece of slate, a cutting board, brown paper, parchment paper, linen, cheesecloth, and burlap.

- Gather image ideas from print or online publications to help plan the shoot. Present image ideas to the team and discuss (stakeholders may include the art director, photographer, food stylist, client, product manager, or account manager), or if you're doing it all yourself, put together a clear strategy to represent the look and feel of the shoot.

- If the photos are for a corporate client, review photos the client has used or published to get a sense of their brand and style, or ask for examples of images the client prefers to help create a vision that is also in line with their brand.

Quick Tip

"When using a prop stylist, try to schedule a call ahead of the shoot, preferably ahead of their shopping days. It's important that you are both on the same page. Ask questions like: 'Is this single serving or family sized?' 'Will this be shot in the dish it was cooked in?' It's best to have at least two [prepared recipes] of each dish—one for 'stand-in' on set and one to plate in the kitchen. Ideally, all the decisions on background, plate color, lighting, and camera angle are made before the hero food goes on set. We often use smaller plates, salad sized, for entrées. Some dinner plates are just too big, and you end up with a lot of dead space in your shot." —Mary Valentin, professional food stylist

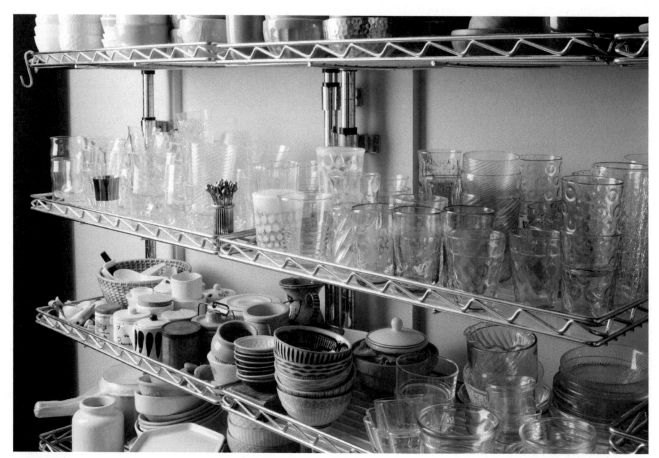

Professional photographer's prop closet. Photo credit: Renée Comet Photography

TIPS FOR CHOOSING DISHWARE, GLASSWARE, AND FLATWARE

The following are some general tips for choosing dishware, glassware, flatware, and other accessories when styling food for a shoot.

Color of dishware

Select dishware that frames the food well in a color or colors that complement those of the food:

- **White:** If you're starting out, several different sizes of matte white plates, bowls, and mugs are a must. Every type of food looks good on white but it is especially good with red foods (tomato sauce, red meat, beets). The shade of white makes a difference. For example, a bright white is sharp and pops whereas a warmer white is cozier, creating a calm and serene feeling.

- **Yellow:** Green foods (e.g., salads, pesto, green vegetables) look good on yellow plates. Yellow and green are both warm colors and next to each other on the color wheel (read more about the color wheel on the next page).

- **Blue:** Contrasting colors of yellow foods (e.g., eggs, corn, mango, yellow curries) look good on blue plates.

- **Black or brown:** Neutral or beige foods like chicken, cream sauces, and potatoes can work on black or brown plates.

Dishware finish

A matte finish on dishware makes food look great, while glossy dishware can create unwanted reflections.

Dishware size

Small bowls and plates give food an appearance of abundance and can accentuate smaller foods, (e.g., raspberries and blueberries).

Dishware depth

Use shallow bowls since deep bowls are more prone to shadows.

Glassware

Use low glassware (e.g., juice glasses) and wine glasses with a shorter stem as the size allows you to shoot from different camera angles when the focus is on the food.

Flatware

Flatware should be on the small size (e.g., a salad fork is less distracting or intrusive than a dinner fork), and a matte finish helps prevent unwanted reflections.

Additional considerations:

- **Mise en place shots:** Use clear small bowls or short plastic wine glasses.

- **Cutting boards:** Use different shapes and textures of cutting boards as an easy way to add interest in a shot.

- **Textured napkins and table linens:** These add interest, dimension, and contrast. White, off-white, or solid colors are a good place to start. Besides houseware stores, these can also be found at thrift stores and remnant bins at fabric stores.

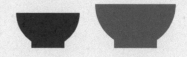

THE COLOR WHEEL

The **color wheel** is a diagram that organizes colors in a circular form into 12 basic hues:

- three primary colors (red, yellow, and blue)
- three secondary colors (purple, orange, and green), which are equal mixture of two primary colors
- six tertiary colors (red-orange, yellow-orange, yellow-green, blue-green, blue-violet, and red-violet), which are primary colors mixed with secondary colors

The color wheel can be a helpful resource when learning how different colors work together in food styling and photography. Don't be afraid to use color in your images, but be mindful that your choice of colors for props and the work surface can affect the color of the food. Most professionals find it easiest to start with a textured white background and a white plate, and let the food be the color in the image and the "star." As you begin to feel more comfortable with your skills, then begin experimenting with color.

Start by determining the main color of the food in the photo and choose a plate, work surface, props, or garnishes that are complementary in color—meaning that they are opposites, creating nice visual contrast—or analogous—meaning that the colors are similar and located next to each other on the color wheel, including the main color. If the food in the shot is a neutral color, select bright and colorful props, but remember, colors interact with each other. They'll look different depending on the other colors surrounding them. The practical takeaway is you don't have to be an expert in color theory—just know it exists. Learn by experimenting; choose a main color and then see what pairs well with it.

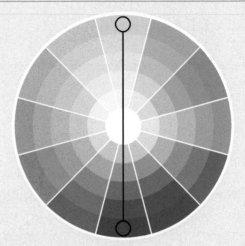

Complementary colors are opposite each other on the color wheel (e.g., blue/orange, red/green, purple/yellow).

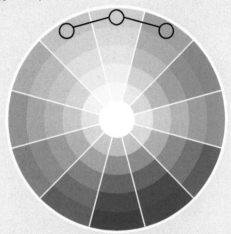

Analogous colors are colors next to each other on the color wheel (e.g., green and blue, yellow and green, orange and yellow, purple and blue).

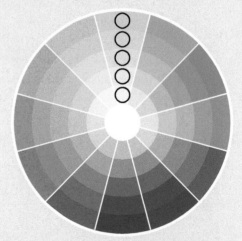

Monochromatic colors are varying shades of the same color (or hue).

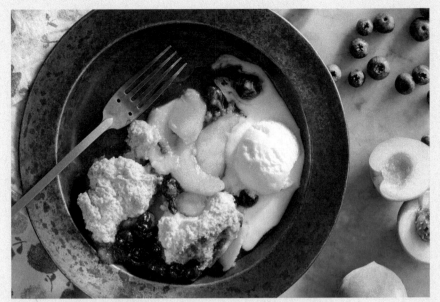

Example of complementary colors

This image shows colors opposite each other on the color wheel (orange/blue). A pewter plate makes the peach cobbler with ice cream pop. And the complementary colors of the yellow/orange peaches and blue/purple blueberries are an example of using complementary colors with the food and props.

Photo credit: Mark Boughton Photography

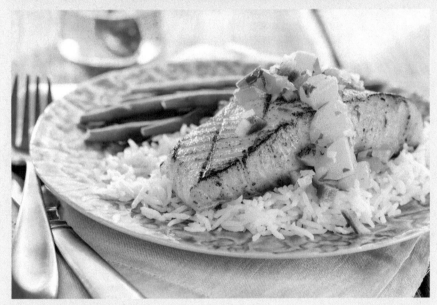

Example of analogous colors

This image shows the combination of colors next to each other on the color wheel (orange salmon, yellow mango garnish, and green asparagus). The blue plate is a complementary color choice to the main orange color of the salmon.

Photo courtesy of the National Honey Board

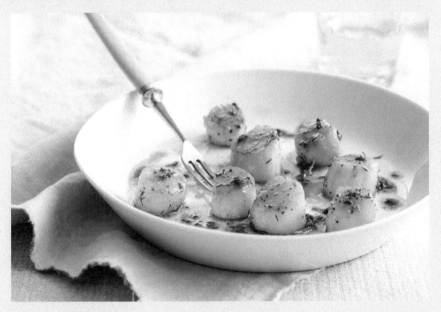

Example of monochromatic colors

This image shows varying shades of the same color for the plate, napkins, fork, and scallops (brown is a mixture of colors on the color wheel).

Photo credit: Mark Boughton Photography

HOW MUCH FOOD DO I NEED FOR A PHOTO SHOOT?

A commercial shoot performed in-studio with a team is quite different than playing the roles of both food stylist and photographer in your own home, but in both situations, you must have plenty of food on hand. For a commercial shoot, you might need as many as ten versions of some element that will be photographed—a product package, a baguette, or elements of a finished dish—to find the one that will ultimately be photographed.

When working with a client, whether online or in person, the shooting process may be slower, especially if changes are made along the way. This may also require having more food. So be sure to discuss the budget and amount of food you will have on hand to allow for changes. Obtaining more food during a photo shoot can add significant time and cost to the project.

If you're shooting at home or in a smaller setting, experts recommend you have at least two versions of each dish that is to be photographed—one to use while adjusting the lighting and composition of the image and the second for the final beauty shot.

Quick Tip

"Learn as much as you can about food, and really know how to cook. Take classes, do an apprenticeship, and travel, if possible. Knowing your craft makes you much more valuable to your clients—and to the reader."
— Denise Vivaldo, professional food stylist

Quick Tip

"Organization is key. Use a shopping list template to organize your grocery needs; it's especially good for shoots with multiple recipes and days. This list can also serve as a good reminder of what's in the pantry and [can] allow you to think through what garnishes, alternatives, and swaps might be needed. Also, be selective when grocery shopping and bag your own groceries, being careful to protect more delicate items like fresh berries and hamburger bun tops."
— Kathy Takemura, Cofounder, Culinary Garage

Quick Tip

"Wherever you go or whatever you do, you should always be on the lookout for small items—plates, dishes, silverware, and other props. You never want your food image to be all plate or dish. You always want your subject, the food, to be the hero. Small props allow your food to shine and when I say small, I mean mini. Some of the smallest props become some of your best and most used props." —Jeff Martin, professional food stylist and founder, Food Photo Affair

Quick Tip

"Matte white and pale colors look great with food. But instead of trendy, use a color that people may find unusual and do something unexpected and beautiful with it." —Lisa Cherkasky, professional food stylist, *Washington Post*

Quick Tip

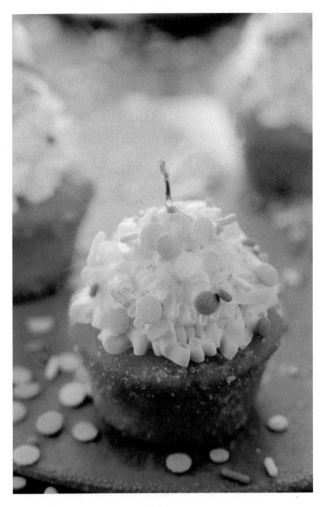

Placing item in the center makes it clear where the viewer's eyes should go. Photo credit: Nicole S. Young

Composing the Image

Defining the Inspiration and Mood

The first step to composing an image is to define the inspiration and mood of the scene: sketch it out on paper or talk it through with the team. Ask yourself, "What kind of story are we creating in this image? What is the goal?" Below are some examples of inspiration and mood in photography:

- a sense of place or in the moment look (e.g., bite taken out of a cookie, open wrapper, crumbs on the plate)
- mise en place shots (e.g., kitchen setup, organizational flow, efficiency, focus)
- setting (e.g., casual, elegant, vintage, minimalist, nostalgic)
- celebration (e.g., holiday, birthday)
- seasonal (i.e., time of year)
- aspirational (i.e., viewers can visually insert themselves into the image successfully)
- editorial (i.e., what the image is trying to sell, such as a slice of cheese or a deli sandwich)

Food stylist Lisa Cherkasky recommends a helpful preproduction team exercise to define the look and feel (or story) of an image: come up with a single adjective to describe it (e.g., trendy, homey, cozy, fun, simple, artisanal, homemade, sophisticated).

Selecting the Image Focal Point

When selecting the image focal point, you can choose a close-up of the food with one item as the focal point or develop a composition where other items in the image help support the focal point. Those who are just starting out often find it much easier to style

Quick Tip

"If you have unwanted reflections on silverware, hold a foam board to block the light causing the reflection, use some museum putty to hold the silverware in the exact place so you can control the reflection, or move the silverware so it doesn't catch any direct light. Alternatively, spray silverware with dulling spray to add a matte finish which will blur any reflections, including the reflection of the photographer taking the picture!" —Denise Vivaldo, professional food stylist

close-up shots, since there's little background and few props to worry about. To help support the focal point of the image:

- Place items in the image (e.g., other plates, silverware, props) so they direct the eye toward the focal point of the image. You effectively create lines of items directing where you want the viewer's eyes to go (these lines form diagonals toward the focal point).

- Isolate the subject, set additional items in the image off to the right or left so they don't compete with the focal point. Don't place another item right behind the subject, as this can create competition between the two items (e.g., if the image's focal point is the layers of a deli sandwich, don't place a can of cream soda right behind the plate; instead, place it off to the right a bit).

- Focus on the food and blur the background. If you're using a smartphone camera, you can do this automatically using the app's portrait mode setting; on a DSLR camera, use the aperture and focal length settings. The composition of the photo also plays a role by increasing the distance between the focal point of the food and the props in the background.

- Make sure that the light falls on or illuminates the focal point, creating the desired degree of contrast and focus.

Creating a Visual Weight Balance

To create an aesthetically pleasing image, you must closely examine the visual weight of all items in the image and decide how best to balance them. When you're setting up a shot, place empty dishware and props in the vertical or horizontal frame to see how they look, and then move them around until you feel that the composition is well balanced. You may find it helpful to use stand-in or "stunt" food while you set up the composition and lighting for the shot.

Remember that larger items carry more visual weight than smaller ones. This is true both when the image is viewed as a whole and also in terms of how the food arranged on the left and right side of a plate relate to each other. Objects with visible texture and vibrant color add more visual weight than smooth or solid objects. Elements positioned at the top of the image's frame will appear heavier. Negative space (i.e., areas of the photo that contain no objects at all) has visual weight in and of itself.

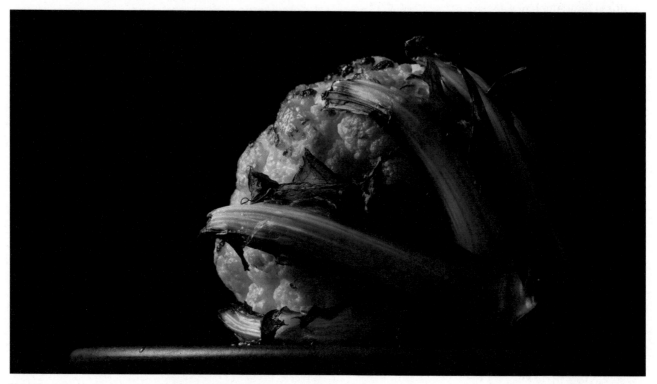

Use of negative space to create visual impact. Photo credit: Renée Comet Photography

Creating a Food Styling Kit

In creating a food styling kit, most food stylists find that they accumulate items over time and as they acquire more experience. To keep it organized, many professionals use cosmetic bags or tote organizer inserts inside a larger bin to keep everything in place.

Food Styling Kit Tools

Each item in a food styling kit serves one or more purposes. Use this as a guide to help build your own food styling kit.

Sharp knives A dull knife can ruin the edges of food.

Makeup sponges, makeup tip applicators, and microfiber glass cleaning cloth These come in handy when you need to wipe clean the edges of a bowl, plate, or glass (cotton swabs or cotton balls work as well, but they can leave fibers behind).

Paintbrushes A fine-tip paintbrush is great for adding realistic imperfections to foods, and a fan-type brush is good for sweeping unwanted crumbs off a plate.

Paper towels Spills are inevitable on food photo shoots, so have plenty on hand to wipe up messes.

Vodka or rubbing alcohol Easily clean off droplets of fat or frosting from edges of a bowl or plate with a makeup sponge, sponge-tip applicator, or a paintbrush dipped into some alcohol.

Tweezers Food styling requires moving items in very small increments. A pair of tweezers allows you to have much more control.

Scissors A pair of scissors will come in handy when you need to cut off imperfections or trim food to a desired size (bonsai or mini scissors work well for snipping in tight places).

Toothpicks and bamboo skewers Like tweezers, toothpicks and bamboo skewers are great for moving food around. They're also great for keeping an item in place.

Acrylic ice cubes These never-melting cubes can provide an excellent illusion of chill in a beverage or act as a food support when plating a dish.

Denture cream Denture cream (e.g., Poli-Grip) is a great way to glue food in place.

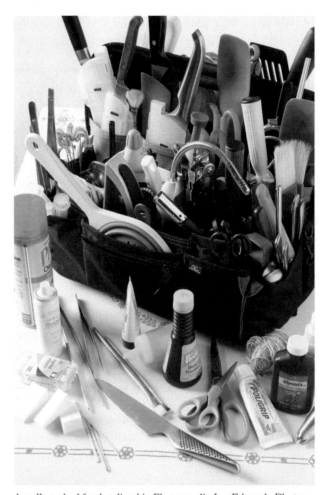

A well-stocked food styling kit. Photo credit: Jon Edwards Photography from *The Food Stylist's Handbook*, 2nd edition, by Denise Vivaldo and Cindie Flannigan. 2017. Skyhorse.

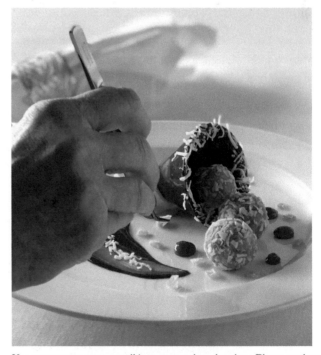

Use tweezers to move small items around on the plate. Photographer: Jon Edwards Photography; Food Stylist: Cindie Flannigan

Gorilla Glue or Zap-A-Gap These glues are invaluable to fill a crack in a piece of meat or a tortilla wrap.

Museum putty This tool will hold flatware in place so it doesn't have undesired reflections from the light and can hold up food at a desired angle.

Vegetable shortening or instant mashed potatoes Either option makes a great food support.

Ramekins or clear plastic cups in a variety of sizes These are handy for holding garnishes on set and can also be used as a food support.

Krylon dulling spray or matte finish spray These are great for spraying on shiny flatware or cookware to remove reflections. In a pinch, hairspray works, too.

Kitchen Bouquet, Marmite, or cocktail bitters These make great coloring agents for food or drinks. Mixed with water or oil, they can be sprayed or brushed onto the surface of meat. Mixed with water, they can stand in for bourbon, white wine, tea, or coffee.

Light corn syrup or a nonfoaming cooking spray containing dimethyl silicone (e.g., Pam) A coating of either will add sheen and moistness to food.

Scotchgard Spray on a food item to create a water-resistant barrier and prevent it from becoming soggy.

Glycerin Mix glycerin with water in a spray bottle to spray long-lasting droplets on a glass or food item.

Spray bottle with water or can of water mister Many foods benefit from a fine mist of water before the photo is taken.

Empty fine spray bottles Keep several on hand to fill with water, a glycerin-water mixture, or a diluted coloring agent.

Squirt bottles, eyedroppers, and drizzle spoons Each of these will give you more control when working with small amounts of sauces, dressings, or liquid of any kind.

Garnish tools Keep an array of graters, zesters, vegetable peelers, melon ballers, and channel knives handy to prep a garnish at a moment's notice.

Kitchen torch A kitchen torch can easily and quickly brown the surface area of a food.

Quick Tip

"Scotchgard sprayed on pancakes, waffles, or bread will keep moisture from making it soggy. Spray on, let dry a few minutes, then add condiments, syrup, butter or whatever you like. It's all about extending the life of your food while it's in front of the camera. And for syrup, use the cheapest syrup (real maple syrup is too thin for photography and will soak right into your product), put it in the freezer for at least 40 minutes, then pour over your pancakes or waffles. You may need to wait a few minutes to get the consistency you need, but your pour will be slower and easier to control." —Cindie Flannigan, professional food stylist

Quick Tip

"When using uncooked tortillas, as for burritos, rub [them] with either Corn Huskers Lotion or Gold Bond Aloe Vera Lotion. They coat the tortillas and prevent them from cracking without leaving a greasy shine. Keep the middle of omelets, burritos, crepes, and wraps from collapsing by using cotton balls in the middle." —Cindie Flannigan, professional food stylist

Mini pencil torch Often used for craft projects, a butane mini pencil torch can quickly warm up congealed fat or cheese.

Heat gun A heat gun can provide focused heat to help melt cheese or brown french fries.

Disposable gloves Having a set of gloves is invaluable on any set, but they're particularly important if you're working with raw fish or meat and the set location has no running water.

SHOULD STYLED FOOD BE EDIBLE?

Which is more important: making food look good for the camera using all of the tricks of the trade or eating it after the shoot? Your answer to this question will drive your food styling decisions. Food stylist Lisa Cherkasky shares, "If styling decisions make the food inedible, why is this worse than fixing issues with a photo editing software program in postproduction? The goal is to try and get the best shot right away, versus relying on editing later. This saves the photographer time." Food photographer Huge Galdones adds, "It depends on what food is being shot and what it is used for. If you're selling a burger, I like to make the burger 100% edible. If the side dishes aren't the main hero, I don't mind compromising the integrity of these secondary elements."

GENERAL FOOD STYLING TIPS

Always be on the lookout for inspiration and ideas. Look at how similar foods are styled in print and online publications and follow content creators on social media platforms.

Sketch out the image ahead of time, taking note of *color*, *balance*, and *texture*.

Select the best-looking ingredients, regardless of what food you are styling. Remember to buy extra ingredients for garnishes and background propping.

Use stand-in food when setting up the shot to ensure the right shape, size, color, and contrast of food on the plate.

Do not crowd the plate. Keep it simple and natural; use less food than you would serve a guest.

Start with clean dishes and glassware, and handle them with care so they stay clean. (Keep Windex and a microfiber cleaning cloth on hand so you can quickly attend to any greasy spots on set.) You can always add a little messiness as you go, advises food stylist Cindie Flannigan, but it's very difficult and time-consuming to do it the other way around.

If the food isn't photogenic, consider focusing on the vessel instead.

When it comes to adding food and props to an image, keep odd numbers in mind. In general, having an *odd number of elements in a photo is best*.

Set each element of the dish individually in the bowl or plate, gently layering the elements so each looks good. The process of plating for photography is quite different than at a restaurant or at home.

Look for empty spaces when plating foods and fill in the holes. Empty areas tend to create deep shadows. Be sure you don't fill in all the holes, however, or the image will have no contrast.

Carefully consider the placement of background food, drinks, and props. To keep the attention on the main food without drawing attention to the background, never place items right behind the main food. Instead, move them slightly off to the right or left in the corner of the image.

Make food ahead when possible, leaving more time to focus on food styling on the day of the shoot. For example, cakes, quick breads, muffins, cookies, crème brûlée, and puddings can be made ahead—if they're not fresh, no one will know.

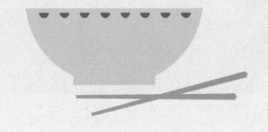

Food Styling Techniques

Following are some creative suggestions and techniques often used by professional food stylists.

Building a Support or False Bottom

- Clear glass stones or a small ramekin or bowl turned upside down in a larger bowl can support foods or create a false bottom (e.g., holding up noodles or a garnish in a soup). If the image is being used for advertising, it should represent what's being sold. Editorial photography is less restrictive.

- Mashed potatoes or vegetable shortening affixed to the bottom of a bowl or plate are an effective false bottom for room-temperature foods, including salad greens and cereal. Frozen wads of damp paper underneath a salad also give a salad height and keep the greens looking fresh.

- Museum putty is also great for holding food in place.

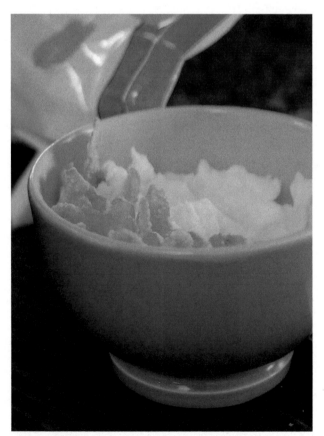

Create a false bottom using vegetable shortening so cereal will sit on top without sinking. Photo courtesy of the Denise Vivaldo Group. Food Stylist: Cindie Flannigan

Enhancing the Color and Shine of Foods

- To darken foods, use a kitchen torch or use Kitchen Bouquet, Worcestershire sauce, or soy sauce.

- To enhance a red color, try red food coloring, beet juice, paprika mixed with water, or maraschino cherry juice.

- To enhance shine, brush some light corn syrup (for pork, chicken, and fish) or dark corn syrup (for red meats) on the surface. You can also mix corn syrup into liquids to make them shine.

Creating Fresh-Looking Foods and Drinks

- Undercook the food so it stays visually appealing longer and doesn't dry out.

- Shoot the food at room temperature, as foods often shrink after refrigeration and expand when exposed to heat.

- A spray bottle filled with ¼ cup glycerin and ¾ cup water can be used to mist drinking glasses (be sure to place easily removable painter's tape around the rim of the glass to prevent drops from landing there) or to give the appearance of water droplets on fruits and vegetables. The glycerin helps hold the water droplets in place; water alone will evaporate much more quickly. Shake the bottle vigorously before spraying.

Quick Tip

"One of the most common problems is conveying temperature on set. There is nothing sadder than coagulated, cold-looking mac 'n' cheese. Use a good garment steamer to refresh cheesy, saucy recipes when you're ready for the final shot. It's always important to show a little shine somewhere to keep your food from looking dry. Fats are shiny and translucent when hot. Brush a little oil on the outside of cooked meats. Spray a little water on greens." —Mary Valentin, professional food stylist

Styling Tips for Specific Foods

Meat, Poultry, and Fish

- Get better grill marks by brushing the meat with a coating of either oil alone or dark corn syrup and then oil. Once the meat is placed in the grill pan or on the grill, do not move it until it naturally releases.

- Another option for grill marks is an electric charcoal starter or metal skewer that has been heated over a stovetop burner. The marks made this way aren't perfectly arranged, which creates a more natural and random look. Some food stylists choose to prepare steaks and chops in a sous vide and then add grill marks or searing and finishing details using a kitchen torch.

- Never cook meat, poultry, and fish all the way through, as it may end up looking dry and shriveled. Instead, brown the outer surface of meat or poultry skin with a kitchen torch for a more natural look.

- Fat is translucent when it is hot and turns white and hard when cold. Ideally, have a freshly cooked steak ready to put in once you're finished with lighting and composition (if not, the food might end up looking cold on the plate). Trim off any unwanted fat before styling; if needed, use coloring techniques (e.g., Kitchen Bouquet) to get the color just right.

- To darken meats in certain areas, paint on some Kitchen Bouquet, Vegemite thinned with water, or corn syrup and oil. If any unwanted marks make it into the shot, you can take care of them postproduction during editing.

- A light brush of oil will refresh meat and make it look juicy and hot. Be careful: too much will make it look greasy. Another option is to warm it up using a handheld steamer.

- Never place oil on the interior of meat. Instead, brush the cut surfaces with water to keep it looking juicy.

- Backlighting (light is facing the camera) can make meat look shinier, and sidelighting will highlight its texture.

- If a piece of cooked fish has a crack in it, fill it in with petroleum jelly (e.g., Vaseline) or white denture cream.

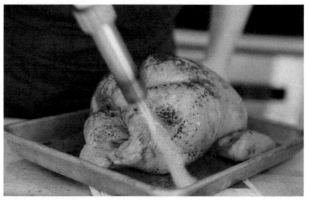

Create golden brown and tight skin by moving a kitchen torch over the skin. Photo credit: Jack Coyier. Food styling: Denise Vivaldo and Cindie Flannigan

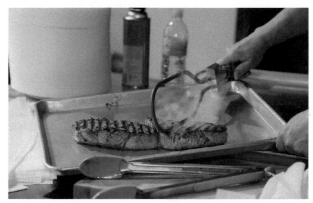

Creating grill marks using an electric charcoal starter. Photo credit: Diana Lundin. Food styling: Denise Vivaldo and Cindie Flannigan

Quick Tip

"When planning your shots, shoot the foods with a limited lifespan (i.e., most perishable) first and then move on to the ones that last longer. One trick to buy time is to understand and plan for what happens to food as it sits at room temperature. When roast beef is sliced hot, the juices will keep running out onto the plate. Instead, let it rest longer at room temperature before slicing so the juice stays in. The same goes for sauces; instead of a hot or cold sauce, let a sauce sit at room temperature and then either thin or thicken it as needed. Your goal is to stabilize the food so it looks the same for as long as possible. And of course, to save time, get the lighting and composition set with the stand-in and then plate the hero food." —Lisa Cherkasky, professional food stylist, *Washington Post*

Fruits and Vegetables

- Reserve the freshest and best-looking fruits and vegetables for garnish or props.

- Do not wash berries (e.g., raspberries, blueberries, blackberries), as they get mushy quickly. Spray strawberries with cold water to freshen them up.

- Buy bananas that are slightly firm. If a banana will be peeled, squeeze lemon juice over the exposed area or dip it in Fruit Fresh mixed with water.

- Wrap cut slices of citrus fruits (e.g., oranges, lemons, limes) in damp paper towels to keep them fresh.

- If apples are being used in a shot, consider using the Opal variety, as they do not oxidize when exposed to air.

- Prevent browning on sliced fruit or certain vegetables (potatoes and artichokes) by squeezing or rubbing lemon juice over the cut sides or by placing in a bowl filled with a mixture of 2 parts water to 1 part lemon juice. Alternatively, dip fruit in a solution of water and Fruit Fresh, an antibrowning powder. Pat it dry immediately afterward. Be careful to not use too much as it can cause the flesh of soft fruits to break down.

- If the photo will include an avocado, be sure to buy several firm avocados, as it's difficult to know whether the inside will look appealing. Keep them from turning brown by immersing them in or brushing them with vodka or Fruit Fresh mixed with water. If needed, give them a light spray of vodka on set.

- Add an acid, such as vinegar, to potatoes while they're cooking to keep them white.

- Retain the vibrant green color of vegetables by blanching them in boiling water with lots of salt and then briefly refreshing them in an ice bath. Wrap the blanched vegetables in damp paper towels and store them in a zippered bag in the refrigerator. If this process isn't possible, undercook the vegetables and add them to the plate right before you're ready to shoot.

- Sauté vegetables in oil rather than butter since the butter will harden into specks as it cools.

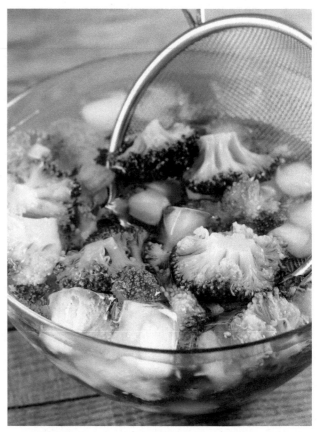

Retain the vibrant green color of vegetables by plunging them in an ice bath after quickly cooking in boiling water.

- If you're using tomatoes, cut them as close as possible to the time you will be shooting, and spray the cut surface with water or wrap it in a damp paper towel.

- Instead of washing mushrooms, just wipe off any specks of dirt and wrap them in paper towels to prevent moisture absorption.

- Mist vegetables with water to make them look appetizing and fresh. Alternatively, mist with a mixture of glycerin and water (usually a 1:1 ratio) if you need water droplets to hold for a longer period of time. Be aware that surfaces with glycerin cannot be wiped clean; it must be washed off.

- Consider using fresh vegetables as props or garnishes to add a pop of color in dishes like chili, where the color of the vegetables leaches out during the cooking process.

Salads

- Wash lettuce or any leafy green and wrap it in a damp paper towel. Store it inside a zippered bag in the refrigerator.

- Keep salads covered with damp paper towels until you're ready to shoot, and freshen them up the moment before you take the photo with a mist of water.

- Bring wilting greens and herbs back to life by dunking them in an ice bath or an ice bath with a little Fruit Fresh dissolved in it.

- Don't dress a salad until you're ready to shoot it because the leaves will wilt quickly. Use a dropper, a small spoon, or your fingertips to add dressing where it's needed to highlight a part of the salad or to drip it onto the plate.

- Build a salad on a foundation or platform so heavier ingredients don't fall to the bottom (a false bottom of vegetable shortening or cold mashed potatoes works well). Frozen wads of damp paper towels are also great for this purpose; keep a tray of them at the ready in the freezer. They provide height for the salad and the chill perks up the greens.

Pasta

- Undercook pasta so it retains a better consistency. Drain it, rinse it, and toss it with a very small amount of oil—be sure not to use too much, as it can make the pasta difficult to manage on set and can leave an odd, blotchy pattern on the pasta. Some food stylists rinse pasta only in cold water.

- Build a support for the pasta by adding a small amount of instant mashed potatoes, vegetable shortening, or damp paper towels to a serving plate or bowl and arrange a nice mound of pasta on top.

- Long pastas, like spaghetti, should be aligned with all the noodles facing the same direction, so you can take a small group of noodles and spiral them a bit. Keep them cool, damp, and tightly covered with plastic wrap.

- Loops and swirls of pasta should be loose and relaxed. It's tempting as a new stylist to create tight circles with pasta, but don't give in to temptation.

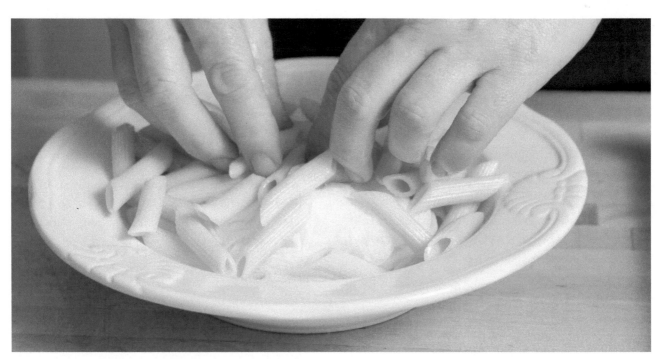

Add a support base of damp paper towels to keep pasta from flattening out. Photo credit: Jack Coyier. Food Stylist: Cindie Flannigan

Herbs

- To store fresh herbs, wrap them in a damp paper towel and place them in a zippered bag; store them in the refrigerator. Otherwise, place freshly cut herbs in a large glass of water, like flowers in a vase, and then place the whole glass in a plastic bag tied at the top, forming a mini-greenhouse. You can easily grab what you need and close it back up. For basil, keep it at room temperature on the counter top, as it can turn black if it's over-chilled.

- Perk up wilted herbs by shocking (briefly dipping) them in ice water.

- If possible, pick fresh herbs just before shooting.

Soups and Stews

- When shooting soups or stews, use shallow bowls, and shoot the photos from a high angle. Avoid the temptation to overpromise by making a soup look like it has more ingredients than it really contains.

- If needed, build a support or false bottom. Whole raw potatoes are great if you're shooting the soup in the pot; if you're shooting servings in bowls, use thick slices of potato. If you need to lift certain ingredients to the surface, use toothpicks.

Drinks

- To achieve a natural-looking condensation effect on a glass, use a 50-50 mixture of glycerin and water combined in a fine-mist spray bottle. Since you only want to create condensation where the drink actually touches the glass, first cover the rim or top section of the glass with painter's tape. Spray the glass with Krylon Crystal Clear Glaze, and then mist the glass with the glycerin mixture. Pour the liquid up to where the tape is placed on the glass.

- If the beverage should appear carbonated, insert a straw at the back of the glass and pour some salt, sugar, or crushed Alka Seltzer into the straw.

- To generate significant head in a glass of beer, shake some salt into the glass and stir.

- To give the appearance of bubbles in coffee when it is first poured, add a little coffee (or whatever brown liquid you're using to simulate coffee) and

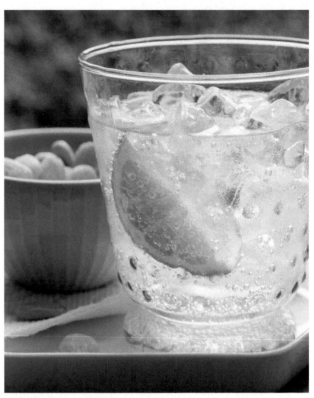

Capturing carbonation in a beverage. Photo credit: Renée Comet Photography

> ### Quick Tip
>
> "A cold syrup or sauce holds up longer than room temperature ones. I put syrups and some sauces in the freezer for a short time and always keep them really cold. The colder they are, the slower they will move."
>
> —Jeff Martin, professional food stylist and founder of Food Photo Affair

a drop of clear dish soap to a measuring cup. Mix well to create bubbles. Using a spoon, scoop out the bubbles and place them around the edges of the mug of coffee.

Miscellaneous

- **Cereal** Cereal often benefits from supporting material, such as vegetable shortening or mashed potatoes. Fill two thirds of the bowl with the support material so the cereal doesn't sink.

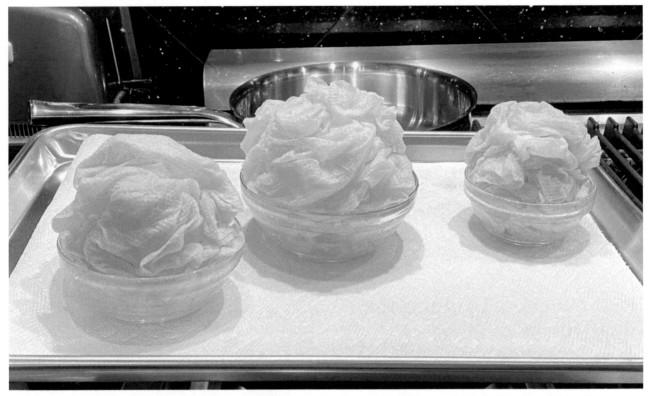

Peach ice cream stand-in to help set up composition and lighting for the photographer. Photo credit: Cindie Flannigan, food stylist

- **Thickened dairy products** Drain sour cream or yogurt through paper towels or a coffee filter to thicken it. Keep the thickened product in the refrigerator until the last possible minute and then put the dollop on the food right before shooting—or try thawed Cool Whip.

- **Ice cream** Freeze scoops of ice cream on a pre-chilled small metal tray lined with parchment or wax paper for at least 2 hours (or overnight). Set up the shot first and do all the styling using stand-ins for the ice cream (e.g., wads of damp paper towels molded to the correct scoop size); take the ice cream out of the freezer only when you're ready to shoot. Place a cooler on its side, place dry ice in the bottom, and store the ice cream inside the cooler while you style the shot.

- **Baked goods** Freeze pies, cakes, brownies, and bars before you cut them to get the cleanest slices.

- **Garnishes** Read through a recipe and note which ingredients are possible options for props or garnishes. Purchase extras of these, and only use ingredients that are in the dish. For example, if the dish you're shooting is pasta with butter, pancetta, and sage, be sure that you only use sage as a garnish or prop and not basil. The garnish is meant to highlight the dish, so consider matching the color of the plate to the garnish (for example, place a slice of chocolate cake with strawberries on a red plate).

Quick Tip

"Make fake ice cream by slowly beating 2 pounds powdered sugar into 1 cup vegetable shortening and 2 teaspoons cornstarch with the paddle attachment of a stand mixer until your mixture is the texture of Play-Doh. Add food coloring sparingly to get the desired color. Fake ice cream can be scooped just like regular ice cream. After using, wash off any sauces or ingredients in cold water, place in a resealable bag, and freeze." —Cindie Flannigan, professional food stylist

Food Photography

There are three distinct stages in the photography process. The amount of time spent in each stage will vary depending on the size and type of the project. Even small projects, like a series of images for social media posts, can cycle through these stages.

1. **Preproduction:** Planning the photo shoot, including the style elements and shot list
2. **Production:** Executing a photo shoot, including the work area, equipment, lighting, photo composition
3. **Postproduction:** Editing the piece for final presentation

Preproduction: Planning the Photo Shoot

Planning the photo shoot can begin once the recipes are developed and tested. Ideally, take your own quick photos, or ask the recipe tester to take photos during recipe development or testing of both the process and the finished dishes. These photos will serve as a helpful reference when planning the photo shoot.

The planning stage allows you, or you and the team, to think through and determine the overall goals, style, look, and mood for the project as a whole and to consider each recipe that will be shot in those contexts. This may include taking time to make decisions about colors and textures (e.g., surfaces, ingredients, garnishes, props), lighting, and camera angles. If the project is for a client, present two to three "inspiration photos" to elicit feedback about the client's preferences and get concrete direction for the shoot. Many professionals find it helpful to sketch out the pictures they plan to take before the shoot begins.

Once you've selected the styling elements for your photos, you can assemble a shot list. The shot list enables you to simplify the number of backgrounds and set changes you'll need to make and serves as a plan to ensure that you get all the photos you will need on the day(s) of the shoot (set changes eat up a lot of time). Prioritize this shot list so what must get done gets done; nice-to-have shots should only be made if time allows.

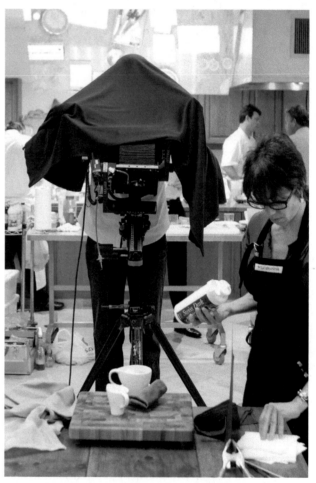

A studio food shoot with photographer Renée Comet and food stylist Lisa Cherkasky. Photo credit: Isaac Oboka

Taking time to plan carefully, including creating and finalizing a preproduction document, allows you to be more productive and effective during the photo shoot. You'll save time, money, and energy during the shoot, and you'll be sure to have the photos you need.

Production: The Photo Shoot

The photo shoot involves setting up a work area and making decisions on the equipment, lighting, and photo composition. The equipment needed for a photo shoot will depend on your skill level and reasons for the shoot. General descriptions and suggestions for work areas, equipment, and other helpful tools are provided to help get you started.

Work Area

Professional photographers often have studios, but some need little more than a designated area and a worktable or two. Any table can be used, but generally photographers find it useful to have one table that is rather low, making it useful for overhead shots (sometimes in conjunction with a sturdy step stool), and a second that is tall, for eye-level shots. Adjustable-height desks work well, too. It's also handy to have a rolling cart or a table on wheels if the shoot space has several natural lighting options to choose from.

A movable tabletop (also known as a photo surface) placed on top of the worktable can quickly change the look and feel of the photo. Numerous online sources offer backgrounds and surfaces to purchase that vary color and texture for a range of prices (see Food Styling, Photography, and Video Resources and Bibliography on page 347). Many photographers find that they have a variety of options on hand already to change the photo surface, such as a large, weathered cutting board, a marble cheese board, parchment paper, or tablecloths or large pieces of fabric.

Camera

All cameras, whether a high-end digital single-lens reflex (DSLR) camera or smartphone camera, are capable of taking excellent photos. So why choose one over the other? Simply put, a smartphone camera makes photography decisions for the photographer, while a DSLR camera allows the photographer to make adjustments independently.

A smartphone's native camera app is perfect for those who are just starting out and easing into the practice of adjusting the brightness, contrast, color, cropping, and other elements in their photos. For those who seek more creative control on photos taken with a smartphone, download onto your phone a photo editing and camera app like Adobe Lightroom

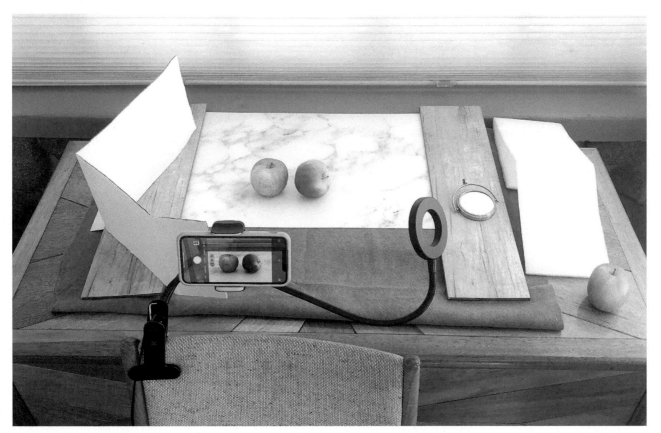

iPhone food shoot using a marble photo surface. Photo credit: Cindie Flannigan

Quick Tip

"A lot of professional photographers work on location and must make the space work for them. Ultimately, the photographer must find a way to light a 2 foot by 2 foot surface. Sometimes being nimble is equally as valuable as having all the right photography gear in hand." —Huge Galdones, professional food photographer

and use their in-app camera. These photo apps allow users to capture and modify photos and also perform postproduction editing, organizing, and storing of photos right on the phone (these apps can be used on a computer to manipulate photos taken with a DSLR cameras as well).

If you choose to use a DSLR camera, take the time to learn about the camera's different modes and settings (e.g., ISO, aperture, and shutter speed) and how to control the overall brightness or darkness of your photos (the exposure). Many food photography books explain how to use the manual settings on a camera to get the best possible results with food (see Food Styling, Photography, and Video Resources and Bibliography on page 347).

Lenses

Cameras and lenses are expensive, so consider renting a specific type of lens to experiment with it before investing in one. Following are a few different types of lenses and how they can be used in food photography:

- **50 mm f/1.8 prime lens** (sometimes called the "nifty fifty") is a good initial upgrade from the standard lens that comes with a camera. This lens allows for a narrower depth of field (i.e., subject is in focus, while the background is blurred) and is good for overhead shots.
- **24-70 mm f/2.8 macro lens** is a very versatile zoom lens that's good for close-up and portrait-style shots. (Any type of macro lens is good for these situations, including a 35 mm f/2.8, a 50 mm f/2.8 or a 100 mm f/2.8.)
- **100 mm f/2.8 macro lens** or 70-200 mm lens provides more working space between the food and the camera so the food can be styled without jostling the camera.

Tripod

A tripod prevents the camera from moving and allows for hands-free photos, which is critical for food photography. With a tripod, you can set up shots in advance and focus on creating and adjusting the photo's composition without disrupting the flow of the shoot. The photographer and food stylist can work together more effectively using a tripod, since each can preview the image from the same point of view with the camera in the exact same position. Tripods are available in lightweight tabletop or larger and heavier floor versions; some include a tripod head (the accessory that actually holds the camera), but heads can also be purchased separately. The tripod you choose should be sturdy, with a head that is easy to work with.

Tethering Tools

Tethered photography is the process of connecting a DSLR or smartphone camera to a laptop or computer monitor using an extra long USB cable and tethering software, such as Capture One or Adobe Lightroom. (A wireless option is available but often provides a less stable connection.) Tethered shooting allows the photographer to view a larger image of the photo on the monitor. Seeing the photo on the large screen makes it easier to reference and allows the photographer and

Quick Tip

"When using a smartphone, learn how to use the AE/AF lock—auto exposure and auto focus—once you have it set where you want it. Auto exposure adjusts the brightness of the image, and auto focus adjusts the sharpness. This can be helpful when taking images in low or changing light, when the background is busy, or when the focal point will be off-center. Just be sure not to change the distance between the camera and your subject—and also to unlock it when done. To lock, tap the camera screen to focus and hold on the focal point until you see an AE/AF Lock banner on the screen. Tap this to lock exposure and focus, then take the photo. Tap anywhere on the screen to unlock." —Huge Galdones, professional food photographer

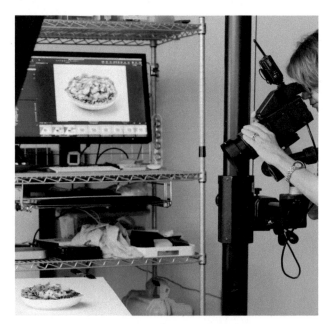
Tethered shooting allows photographer Renée Comet to view her image live on a computer monitor. Photo credit: Steven Redfearn

food stylist to be more intentional about what to keep or change with the shot and food styling. It also permits the photographer to shoot remotely, without touching the camera, and facilitates the workflow by immediately transferring photos to your computer for editing.

Lights

Many professional photographers will share that lighting is the most important element in the creation of quality photos. Learning how to use the light, whether it's natural or artificial, is key to creating beautiful food photos. Lighting affects every aspect of a photograph: the drama, depth, dimension, contrast, shadow, brightness, and darkness. Too much or too little light, color temperature of the light, or tiny movements of light sources can drastically change a photo's look and feel. (See Three-Point Lighting for Video Production on page 337.) Each photographer has their own technique for lighting, so selection of lighting design will always be a matter of personal preference.

Some photographers believe natural light is best—especially since it's free. Use it if you can, especially while you're learning. Lighting photos with artificial sources requires the purchase of equipment and another level of learning, but having alternate light sources does provide much more flexibility in terms of the photography schedule throughout the day. Following are lighting tools that can be helpful, whether shooting with natural or artificial light.

A diffusion panel is a light modification tool that softens the source of the light, reducing the effects of glare and harsh shadows. The best choice for situations where light is streaming in from a window is to place a *collapsible diffusion panel* (a translucent material stretched over a circular or rectangular frame that comes in a variety of sizes) between the window and the food. Alternatively, hang a piece of sheer white fabric over the window or tape paper that is somewhat sheer (e.g., parchment paper) over the window. A light modifier called a *softbox* or a *photography umbrella* can be used to diffuse and soften light coming from studio lights or the flash of the camera.

UNDERSTANDING BASIC PHOTOGRAPHY TERMS

Exposure: the overall brightness or darkness of a photo

ISO: the setting that will brighten or darken a photo by controlling the amount of light the camera lets in. It is the speed at which the camera's sensor registers information

Aperture: the hole in the camera's lens that lets light in and controls the photo's depth of field (i.e., whether the photo has a blurred background or the entire photograph is in sharp focus)

Shutter speed: the length of time the camera's shutter remains open to expose the camera's sensor to light

When the shutter speed is slow, the shutter remains open for a longer period of time and gathers more light; when it's fast, the shutter opens and closes quickly, allowing less light to get in. The aperture and shutter speed all affect a photo's exposure

White balance: the adjustment of colors in a photograph to make the image look more natural; makes sure that objects that appear white in person also appear white in the photo

The correct white balance depends on the color temperature—its relative coolness or warmth—of the light. If this is not done, food can have blue, orange, or green color casts. While adjustments to white balance can be made in postproduction, it's best to optimize the white balance (even if it only involves using an automatic white balance setting) at the time you take the photo.

A reflector or bounce card is a light modification tool that provides a surface to reflect or bounce light. Reflectors are available in different colors at photo and video equipment stores or online, or you can create your own homemade versions. The color of the reflector will affect the color of the light on the food: a white reflector softens and brightens food; silver also brightens food and adds contrast; gold adds warmth; and black reflectors (or black foam board) absorb light and block unwanted reflections. A black reflector can also be used to reduce the amount of light in the photo and can create desired shadows and depth.

It's best to start with a traditional white reflector. Its primary purpose is to reflect more light on to the subject of the photograph and to fix shadows by filling in the light. To create a homemade version, start with a large piece of white foam board (available at craft stores). Cut the rectangular board in half and then tape it back together so it can stand up as a reflector. You can prop the board up near the food or use *photography clamps* to hold it in place, if necessary.

Quick Tip

"Understanding color temperature, measured in degrees of Kelvin, is foundational to using light correctly. Lighting affects all the colors in a scene. Use this simple rule: pick either daylight or artificial light and stay consistent with it." —Michael Sutz, professional filmmaker, Twelve Plus Media

Quick Tip

"LED light technology continues to evolve—both in the quality of the light and its affordability. These lights require very little wattage and can be run on battery and can be softened by bouncing their light into a bounce card, a ceiling, or any other reflective surface. They can also be fitted with a variety of softboxes." —Michael Sutz, professional filmmaker, Twelve Plus Media

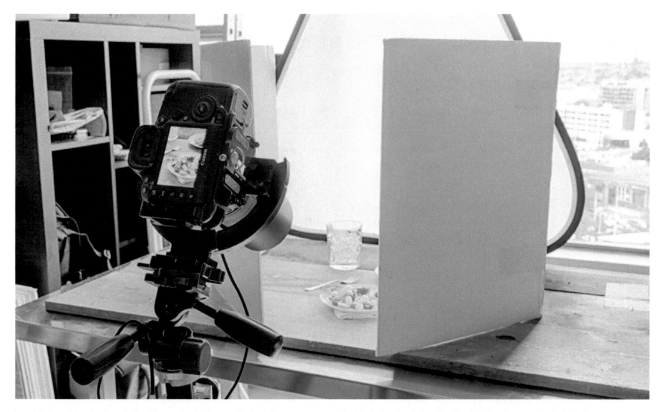

Backlight with window light: The light source is facing the camera and behind the food (food is backlit by the window). A diffusion panel is placed between light source (window) and the food to soften the light, and a white foam board (bounce card) is placed opposite the light source and acts as a reflector to bounce light from the light source onto the food. Photo credit: Nicole S. Young

GENERAL LIGHTING TIPS

One of the most critical aspects of getting lighting right with food photography is establishing where the light will be coming from—the direction of the light on the food. There are three options: front, back, or side lighting. With front lighting, the light source is behind the camera. Professional photographers do not recommend front lighting for food, as it tends to flatten food and cast unwanted shadows.

Back lighting: The light source is facing the camera so that food is backlit by the light/window, which adds texture and depth to food. This method works well to highlight the top of shiny foods, such as a grilled steak. The highlights help to bring the food alive.

Side lighting: The light source is at a 90-degree angle from the camera. Side lighting adds depth, shadow, and a feeling of texture to the photograph. It is particularly good for foods with reflective surfaces, such as soups and beverages.

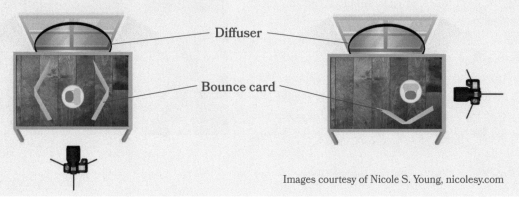

Images courtesy of Nicole S. Young, nicolesy.com

Natural light (produced by the sun)

If shooting outside, select a shady area. Indirect daylight gives food a bright and even glow. If shooting indoors, set up a table near a window (windows that face north or south window light are best since the sun never shines in directly). To soften the light, use a diffusion panel or hang a white sheet or thin white paper over the window. Most photographers do not recommend shooting in direct sunlight because the light is too harsh, creating dark shadows with less discernible texture and shape.

Only use a single source of light. If using natural light coming in from a window, turn off any overhead lights. Multiple light sources can cast different color tints on food, which makes adjusting the white balance difficult while editing.

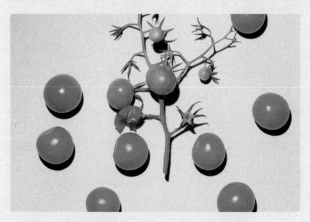 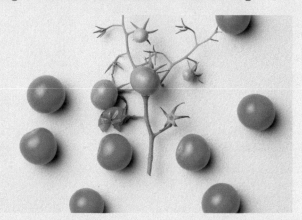

Hard light (left): strong, sharply defined shadows and contrast. Soft light (right): diffused light that is bright and balanced with minimal shadows. Photo credit: Renée Comet Photography

Artificial light

If you need to shoot at night or do not have access to good natural window light during the day, purchase a softbox, a relatively inexpensive and flexible box that fits over a light source (either LED or fluorescent) to help mimic the light of soft daylight. In general, the larger the softbox is, the softer and more diffused the light will be. The softbox can be purchased alone or as part of a lighting kit. Table-top lights, light tents, or light sheds (large shooting enclosures) are other options.

Many photographers recommend placing a softbox light slightly off center and to angle the light down toward the food. Placing a reflector or a piece of white foam board directly opposite the light will help create a brighter image by filling in shadows. Many books and tutorials on using artificial light are available (see Food Styling, Photography, and Video Resources and Bibliography on page 347).

The closer the light source is to the food or the scene, the softer the light will be; if the light is placed further away, the light will be harsher, creating more shadows and contrast.

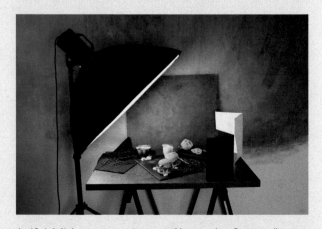

Artificial light set up using a softbox and reflectors (bounce cards).

Photo Composition

The elements of a photograph's *composition* include arrangement of all the food and props in the image; the choice of lighting; the distance at which the photo is taken; and the camera angle. The relationship among these various elements creates an image's composition.

Professional photographers recommend following the rule of thirds as a starting point in understanding how to create a well-balanced image. Once you learn this technique, experts suggest that you break away from it and instead use your own creative eye when composing an image.

The Rule of Thirds

According to the photography rule of thirds, a prospective image is divided into nine parts using two equidistant horizontal lines and two equidistant vertical lines, like a tic-tac-toe grid. (Smartphone camera apps conveniently provide such a grid.) Once the image is divided into thirds, both horizontally and vertically, the *focal point* of the food (the specific part of the food that needs to be highlighted) should be placed at the intersection of those dividing lines or along the lines themselves. Sometimes an image's focal point is obvious, but sometimes, you must decide what part of the image would be best to highlight (e.g., a specific part of a sandwich, pizza, or stew).

Support the Focal Point

Once the focal point of the image has been selected, the other items in the image should be arranged to support it and direct where you want the viewer's eye to go. This includes the lighting and any other items in the image (e.g., props), which can be arranged in lines to draw the viewer's eyes where you want them.

Closely examine the preview of the image in the camera's viewer or on a monitor and decide which elements should be changed or moved to better highlight

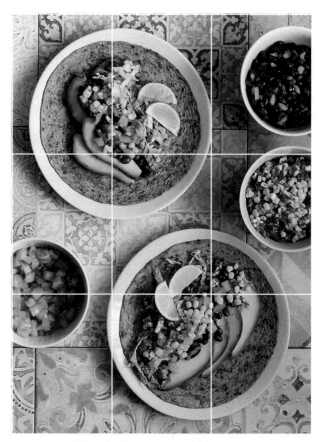

Use the rule of thirds guideline by placing food along gridlines or at a point where they intersect.

the focal point and keep the image balanced. Keep in mind that larger items, as well as items that have texture, patterns, or bold colors, will carry more visual weight. *Negative space*, or empty areas in the image, can be equally powerful. See page 306 for an example of a photo using negative space.

The Camera Angle

The choice of camera angle is certain to make a difference in a photo's composition. Which angle is best for a particular image depends on the food, how it's styled, and the perspective from which you want the viewer to see the food.

- **Flat-lay shot** (also known as an *overhead or 90-degree angle shot*): This shot gives a bird's eye view that is good for table scenes with multiple components and for foods that are flat, like pizzas, cinnamon rolls, or charcuterie platters.

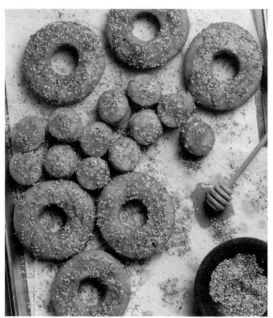

Overhead shot. Photo credit: Renée Comet Photography

Quick Tip

"If you plan on using a text overlay in the final image, such as for a cookbook cover, blog post, food advertisement, or product package, take a picture with negative space where you want the text to fit. And if there are many items in the photo, make sure the focal point of the image is not covered by the text. An alternative is live viewing the text overlay by importing a text PNG into a photo editing software [application], like Capture One. This enables you to shoot the food and view the image and text overlay live on your computer screen or monitor." —Todd Pierson, professional food photographer

- **Angled shot** (25, 45, or 75 degrees): Generally speaking, the flatter the food is, the larger the angle should be, and the taller the food and props are, the smaller the angle should be. A 75-degree angle mirrors the angle a person sees when sitting down to eat. This angle works well for soups or to capture the depth of a full plate of food.

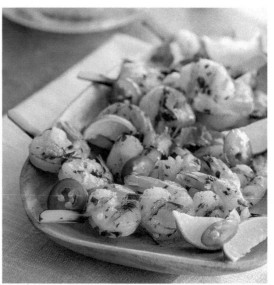

45 degree angle shot. Photo courtesy of the National Honey Board

- **Eye-level shot:** Use this shot for food and drinks that are tall and have more detail on the side or inside than the top, like sandwiches, burgers, and smoothies. Shooting eye-level can be quite effective to avoid showing drips on the plate; food stylists often refer to this as the "heroic" angle.

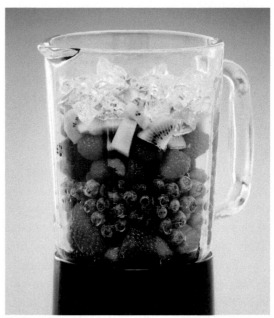

Eye-level shot. Photo credit: Nicole S. Young

The Depth of Field

A photograph's *depth of field* is the space that is in focus.

- **Large depth of field** has the majority of its elements in focus.
- **Narrow or shallow depth of field** has a specific point of focus and keeps the foreground or background out of focus. The advantage of this is to help the viewer's eye prioritize what's most important in the frame.

Smartphone camera apps offer a portrait mode setting that establishes the depth of field, but if you use portrait mode, be sure that you are not accidentally blurring elements that you intend to keep in focus. On a DSLR camera, use the aperture and focal length settings to adjust depth of field.

The Zoom Feature

Before you consider using the camera's *zoom feature* (either in or out), think about the content and mood you want to convey. Some photographers recommend that those who are just starting out should stick to shooting close-up photos so the focus of the image stays on the food and less on the props and background. Instead of using a zoom feature, get closer to your subject.

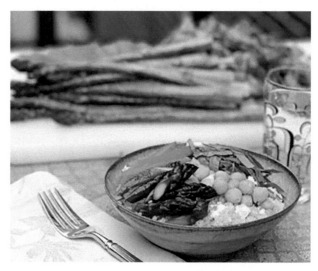

Shallow depth of field: foreground in focus, while the background is blurred. Photo credit: Raeanne Sarazen

Quick Tip

"Clients may want their packaging in the shot. Make sure to have the correct/approved packaging and learn the details of how visible the packaging must be. For example, can the package be blurred or can part of the package be cropped out?" —Dawn Jackson Blatner, RDN, author of *The Flexitarian Diet* and *Superfood Swap*

SHOOTING HORIZONTAL VERSUS VERTICAL

Deciding whether to shoot in horizontal or vertical orientation will depend on where and how the image will be used. For example, will the photo be included in a banner ad on Facebook (horizontal) or in a Pinterest post (vertical)? If both orientations are needed, the shoot will take more time and steps will be added to both the food styling and photography processes.

Horizontal images are wide and short, and vertical ones are narrow and tall. An image's orientation may force you to change or move props, and probably the lighting as well. Meanwhile, as the set is being rebuilt, the prepared food is losing its freshness. Professionals suggest building extra time and food prep into the schedules for shoots that require both horizontal and vertical versions of images; it's important to figure this into the strategy and add the extra time into the estimate for the client.

In some cases, you can build a set that can work both horizontally and vertically, depending on the image's final crop (this is a particularly good strategy for very perishable foods). The edges of the crop are part of the image's composition, so don't ignore them. In fact, the closer you can compose the image to its final cropped format, the stronger the image's composition will be. If an image will be needed in multiple formats and crops, be sure to preview all the crops while the image is being shot; it's always better to just nudge a few things around and take another shot.

The Editing Process

After food images are captured, the editing process workflow begins. This includes downloading, organizing, editing, storing, and sharing files. Selecting the right photo editing software is a highly personal choice. If budget is a concern, free photo editing apps are designed to edit images on a smartphone. Research the features and review ratings from users to find one that is right for you. Examples include Snapseed, VSCO, Adobe Photoshop Express, Adobe Lightroom Photo Editor, Foodie, LiveCollage, and PhotoGrid.

Professional photo editing programs can be expensive and are usually obtained through a monthly subscription. Options include Adobe Photoshop, Adobe Lightroom, and Capture One Pro. These programs offer a higher level of control in editing, so it may be worth the investment if photography is a skill set you wish to develop further.

See Food Styling, Photography, and Video Resources and Bibliography on page 347 for more information on photo editing apps and programs.

Raw and JPEG Formats

Most professional photographers save their photographs in raw format versus JPEG because raw format permits greater flexibility in editing. Images shot and saved in a raw format contain all of the image data collected by the camera's sensor, which means that editing of color, contrast, and light exposure will be easier to make. Saving images in a JPEG format compresses the data and thus limits the ability to edit the image. The downside of raw images is that the file sizes are much larger.

Editing Techniques

Editing photos takes practice. While trial and error is a worthwhile way to learn, taking a course in or referring to professional resources for photo editing can be helpful. Some techniques that are worthwhile to learn include fixing white balance; cropping; and adjusting contrast, brightness, and saturation. While photo editing software may not be able to correct flaws in composition, lighting, and styling, it can bring out a food's best traits to evoke a mouthwatering response.

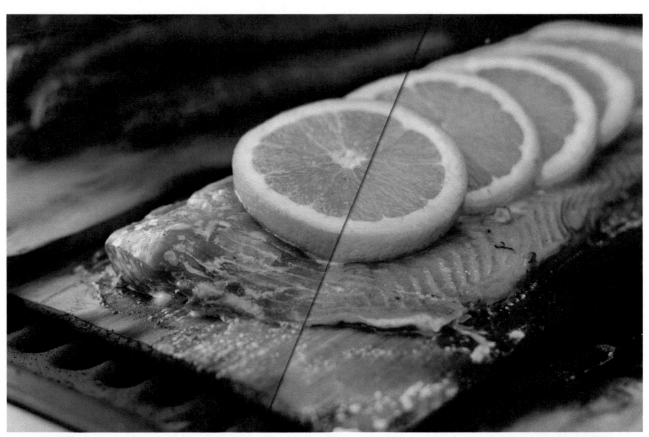

The raw image was first edited in Adobe Lightroom Classic to enhance the brightness, contrast, and overall color. Then, the photo was brought into Photoshop, where some minor touch-up work was done to remove blemishes, and additional tonal and color enhancements were made. Photo credit: Nicole S. Young

UNDERSTANDING IMAGE RESOLUTION AND SIZE

In photography, resolution refers to the level of detail of an image. It's typically measured in pixels, which is essentially the number of tiny squares that make up a digital image. A higher resolution and higher number of pixels means more image detail and a larger file size.

Megapixels (MP): This is the unit used to specify the number of horizontal and vertical pixels in a digital image. For example, an image with dimensions of 4032 × 3024 means there are 4,032 pixels across (width) and 3,024 pixels from top to bottom (height); $4,032 \times 3,024 = 12,192,768$ or 12 MP. Most smartphones capture optimum resolution at 8 to 12 MP for print and digital, with the main difference being in how large the image can be enlarged or printed without losing quality.

DPI (dots per inch) versus PPI (pixels per inch): Although DPI and PPI are often used interchangeably to describe resolution, PPI indicates the density of pixels in digital images while DPI indicates the density of ink dots that make up a printed image.

Kilobyte (KB) and megabyte (MB): These are the units that describe the digital file size. Generally, an image of higher resolution is a larger file size. A file size in MB is a larger (and usually higher quality) photo than one in KB.

For print publications: 300 DPI (or 300 PPI) is considered a high-resolution image, appropriate for cookbooks and other print materials. A smartphone image's default resolution is 72 DPI. Depending on the file size and the desired dimensions of the print image, it may need to be converted from 72 to 300 DPI to prevent it from appearing pixelated.

For online or digital publishing: 72 DPI and a file size between 20 to 200 KB are ideal. Graphic designers and web editors will want a 2 MB or greater file size so they can manipulate it. Photos taken on a smartphone are likely around 2 MB in size.

PHOTOGRAPHY AND COPYRIGHT

Photographers own the copyright to their works, according to the US Copyright Act. While it may be tempting to right-click and save an image you see on the internet or screen shot another person's image and use it without permission—especially when you need an image for your website or cookbook—you cannot legally do so. You must first obtain permission before using an image created by another person. Contact the owner and negotiate whether payment is required. Get the permission agreement in writing.

Some photographers allow free use of their photos on social media with proper acknowledgment and tagging—especially since the nature of social media is so fleeting—but others require a payment. That is why it's always wise to check first. In certain situations, you do not need to obtain permission, such as images that are in the public domain (owned by the US government), instances where the copyright owner has stated that the images can be used without permission, and some images with a Creative Commons (CC) license.* In addition, the Copyright Act's Fair Use provision provides some exceptions for using copyright-protected images in certain circumstances. To learn more about fair use, visit: copyright.gov/fair-use.

* There are six different types of Creative Commons licenses and a public domain dedication. These licenses give creators a standard way to grant public permission for reuse. Several of the types of licenses are free for anyone to use, but some restrict editing and others are only available for noncommercial use. Read more about each type of license at creativecommons.org/about/cclicenses.

Food Videos

A food video can be produced by a team of professionals—a producer, a videographer, a lighting expert (known as a gaffer), a sound technician, a prop stylist, a food stylist, a make-up artist, a wardrobe stylist, a host, and many assistants—or it can be just a solo professional. Similar to photography, an experienced video professional is a creative storyteller with knowledge and expertise in preproduction, shooting, and editing.

These days, food content is frequently presented via video, so adding video knowledge to your skill set can be invaluable. Watching cooking videos in different formats is a good place to start. Make notes about what you like. Draw inspiration from existing videos, and then imitate them. Watching a food video is easy, but creating one is considerably more labor intensive than you likely think.

Whether creating video content for a social media platform or a full-length food documentary, all types of film production go through three stages. The amount of time spent in each stage will vary depending on the project, but following this multistep process will help give structure to your workflow:

1. **Preproduction:** Creating a creative brief, script, shot list, storyboard, food and prop shopping list, as well as the food preparation
2. **Production:** Shooting the video
3. **Postproduction:** Editing the video

Preproduction: Planning the Video

The preproduction stage is important and time intensive. The more time you spend in this planning stage, the smoother the other phases will likely go—and the better and more engaging the video will be. While the preproduction stage for every video doesn't require the same amount of time and thoroughness, every video does need some type of plan or checklist. In general, the preproduction stage begins with the drafting of a short creative brief describing the overall project.

The Creative Brief

A creative brief informs the writing of the script, shot list, and storyboard. It may be often long and detailed,

including information on timeline, budget, competition, and more, but length can vary based on the project. At a minimum, a creative brief (or a simplified version of one) should answer certain key questions, or if it's a more complex video, it can involve writing the script and creating a shot list and storyboard (see Sample Creative Brief for a Video on page 345). A creative brief should answer several key questions:

Who is the audience? Whether you're producing a 20-second or 30-minute video, you must determine who your audience is and on what platform or platforms they will consume the video content. Invest time in getting a thorough understanding of who the viewers are and what their interests include; an idea of how much food and cooking knowledge they already have; and the problems they may want to solve.

This "pain point" or problem could be anything from a need for inspiration (quick entertainment) to a need for a descriptive how-to tutorial on a technique (e.g., stuffing a Thanksgiving turkey). If you know your audience well, you're in a better position to figure out the right tone of voice to use, the best video style, the most ideal visuals, and so on. (See page 7 for detail on developing content for a specific audience.)

What is the goal of the video? In other words, what will this video accomplish? The goal may be something general (e.g., marketing, education, training) or specific (e.g., to build a social media audience, sell a cookbook, develop a reputation as an expert, increase website traffic, or increase subscriptions to an e-newsletter).

What is the topic and recipe to be featured? The choice of topic and recipe depend on the video's target audience. Research what your audience is searching for online most frequently and seek inspiration from fresh and current trends. When you're deciding on the recipe, simplicity is important. The recipe should be approachable, with simple steps, and it should be visually engaging—both in terms of its ingredients and the final dish itself.

What are the key takeaways? These are what you want the audience to remember from the video. Making note of these short pieces of information will help you as you craft the messaging for the script and clarify what should be visually prioritized to reinforce the takeaways. Your key takeaways may include elements of brand messaging that your client believes are most important.

The Video Script, Shot List, and Storyboard

The preproduction work effort also involves the creation of an organizational process to shoot the video. Traditionally, this process includes writing a script and creating a shot list and storyboard, but any combination or variation of these elements is acceptable—including an abbreviated version of any of them. Video professionals document their process in many different ways; much depends on what you find works best for you, your team, and the project.

As a first step, many professionals find it helpful to write out step-by-step what will happen during the video shoot; they sit down with the recipe and think through the video from start to finish. It not only helps organize their thoughts, but it also provides a sense of direction for the video. This process could include the following:

- Decide whether the video will be "hands and pans" or if it will feature a host—or a mix of the two.

- Divide up the recipe into steps based on the video's time limitations and noting what steps aren't critical and what can be prepped, chopped, or put into mise en place ahead.

- Think about the dialog in general and note where you might want to use voice-overs.

- Determine which techniques you will demo on camera and where you will need a swap-out (e.g., if a dish needs to simmer for 20 minutes, you could simmer another version of the dish in advance and bring out the cooked version so the shoot isn't held up).

- Decide whether a final swap-out "beauty dish" needs to be prepared ahead so you can cut to the finished dish during the video without having to wait for it to cook.

- Note where key takeaways and subtopics fit.

- Determine which cookware, bowls, and utensils are needed.

- Make lists of ingredients, equipment, props, and swap-outs.

The Script

With video, if you don't capture the attention of viewers in the first few seconds, you risk losing them altogether. Good storytelling, through a well-written script, can help engage your audience from the beginning to the end of the video, minimizing the likelihood of viewers scrolling away to something they find more entertaining.

Not all videos have scripts—some are off-the-cuff and totally unscripted, but either way your scripted or unscripted video should follow this basic structure.

The hook (beginning) Tell the audience what you are going to do.

The content (middle) Do it (build trust, fix the audience's problem, key takeaways).

Call to action (end) Tell the audience what you did (in the form of a summary; ask for a call to action).

The Hook

Grab the audience's attention by telling them what will happen in the video and what they will learn by watching it. Consider adding a visual hook, such as taking a bite of the finished dish or showing a food action (e.g., pouring, sprinkling). Examples of effective hooks include:

- "Do you struggle cooking for guests with food allergies? If so, I have five delicious allergy-friendly menus for you."

- "What should you make for the vegetarians at your Thanksgiving table? I'll show you a dish everyone will love."

- "Today, I'm going to reveal my three secrets for making the best chocolate chip cookies."

The Content

This section of the script should translate the main messages or key takeaways into a story that resonates with the audience. During this stage, the host builds trust with the audience while helping them solve a problem. The more engaging, energetic, natural, and authentic the host or talent is, the more viewers will want to watch, regardless of the content. Helpful script-writing tips include:

- Write the script in chunks. Divide it into short sentences or very short paragraphs, with breaks in content.

- Note which lines the talent should deliver on camera and which lines should be delivered in the form of a voice-over, where the viewer can hear the talent speaking, but instead of seeing the talent's face, they view relevant video footage, photos, or graphics.

- Build your narrative around your audience's known pain points—this will help them engage.

- Keep key takeaways to two or three points.

- Be as succinct and clear as possible (especially true for social media videos). If what you want to say can be said in 10 seconds or less, don't spend several minutes on it instead.

- Write the script like you speak, using a conversational tone.

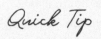

- Show, don't tell. Video is an inherently visual medium. Many videos are viewed on mobile devices with the sound off, so think through the visual elements of your story. Can the viewer understand your video just by watching it? Try to construct a story that's told primarily through images. This will help you write voice-over or narration text that communicates only the most critical information.

- Engage your audience emotionally. They'll remember the story and how it made them feel more than any facts you share.

Think about the other aspects of video storytelling: colors, composition, sounds of cooking, and background music. These critical elements help communicate with an audience on an emotional level and will bring the story to life.

The Call to Action

End the video with a summary of what you did and then finish up with a call to action. Tell them specifically what to do next: buy a book, visit website, sign up for a newsletter, come back next week, or swipe for the recipe link. Reinforce this call to action with a text overlay so that the audience clearly knows where to go next even if the sound is off. For example, "If you enjoyed this video, come back next Saturday for more tips on creating easy and healthy desserts. In the meantime, visit my website!"

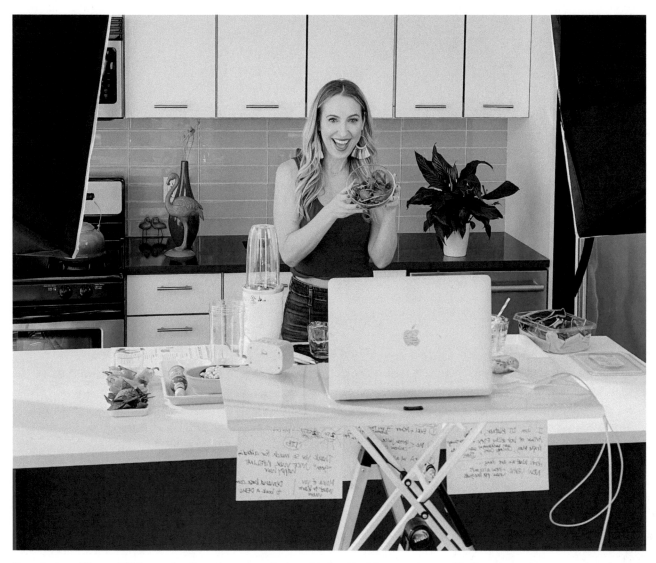

Dawn Jackson Blatner, RDN, records a live video using a laptop with the video's key messages and bullet points written on paper and taped under the lens of a laptop camera.

Quick Tip

"Once you have done all the scriptwriting and rehearsing and you are thoroughly prepared, let it all go and make it your mission to relax, have fun, and genuinely engage with your audience during the shoot itself. Don't stress about getting every single point across perfectly. It's much more important to the quality and impact of the video that you are at ease and enjoying yourself." —Ellie Krieger, MS, RDN, host of Food Network and PBS cooking shows and best-selling cookbook author

Quick Tip

"The expectation of video quality depends on the medium you are making the video for. Social media videos are far less produced than hosted videos, so it's fine to be raw. Imperfection is preferable. So when you're starting out, don't overthink it. Just make stuff and you'll get better." — Michael Grady, Executive Director of Programming, Dotdash Meredith

Practice

The host or talent should rehearse the script to test the video's length. Once the timing is set, practice in front of the camera. As you watch your practice sessions with the sound both off and on, pay close attention to facial expressions and critique yourself. This may seem counterintuitive, given the advice to keep it natural, but it's not. Practicing also ensures that you get the messaging down pat.

While rehearsing, walk through the video. Touch the items, note what you will do with each ingredient, and practice your message points. Make sure you are talking *and* doing at the same time.

For live videos, practice by doing a mini shoot and releasing it right away. Watch it, critique it, and take what you learn from it to make improvements next time, or record a rehearsal, watch it, and critique it before you go live.

Delivering the Script

Try to let your true personality come through. The most compelling videos are told in an authentic, genuine voice.

A **teleprompter** ensures that none of the message points will be left out, but practice is key. You want to look natural, like you're having a conversation, and avoid having your eyes dart back and forth. Using a teleprompter is an acquired skill that requires practice. Don't give up if your delivery seems unnatural the first few times.

Or, simply turn the script into several key messages for a more natural and conversational delivery. Then just focus on memorizing the hook, two or three sentences of the main message, and the call to action instead of trying to memorize everything.

And lastly, before you hit the record button, consider listening or dancing to music that gives you energy and makes you smile. Or use your own strategy to help avoid appearing flat in the video.

Quick Tip

"You don't necessarily need a teleprompter. A piece of paper with simple bullet points in large-enough-to-read font taped under the lens of a laptop camera or smartphone on a tripod can help jog your memory. Practice with your props. The food props themselves can help become cues [for] what to say. For example, when you touch the spinach to add in your recipe, it can be a reminder to share your talking points about storing greens." —Dawn Jackson Blatner, RDN, author of *The Flexitarian Diet* and *Superfood Swap*

Quick Tip

"If you are using a teleprompter, record your practice and watch the playback to see how you come across, and make adjustments as needed. You don't want to look like you are reading with your eyes moving across the screen; instead, try and look steadily at the camera lens."

—Ellie Krieger, MS, RDN, host of Food Network and PBS cooking shows and best-selling cookbook author

SAMPLE OPENING SCRIPT FOR A GLUTEN-FREE FOOD VIDEO

	Sound	Picture	Props
1	**Host:** Are you new to the gluten-free diet and unsure which ingredients and condiments contain gluten? In this video, I am going to take you through your fridge and pantry and show you what to keep and what to give away. Hi. I'm [Talent Name], a registered dietitian and mom of two kids with celiac disease.	Wide shot host direct-to-camera	
2	**Host:** Before we begin, let's talk about gluten. What is it, and where is it found? Gluten is a protein found in wheat, barley, and rye, which are key ingredients in foods such as bread, crackers, pasta, beer, and rye bread.	Graphics on screen: images of pasta with the word "wheat," glass of beer with the word "barley" and an image of rye bread with the word "rye."	
3	**Host:** Gluten is also found in many foods where you wouldn't expect it.	Wide shot of host on screen walking to refrigerator and opening refrigerator door.	Refrigerator door filled with condiments, including: soy sauce, hoisin sauce, salad dressings, and BBQ sauces
4	**Host:** Who would have thought that condiments like soy sauce and hoisin sauce contain gluten, and that some salad dressings and barbecue sauces may contain gluten, too? And there are surprises in the pantry, too, like malt vinegar and licorice. Some packaged products, like bouillon cubes and seasoning mixes, may contain gluten as well.	Medium shot: host pulls out soy sauce and BBQ sauce. Wide shot: host walks over to cabinet. Medium closeup: pulling out vinegar and seasoning mix.	
5	**Host:** The only way to know for sure whether a product contains gluten is to read the food label.	Split screen with host on left, soy sauce ingredient label on right. Wheat is circled/highlighted amidst bottle's ingredients.	
6	. . . .include 3 to 5 takeaways (or tips) . . . script ends with a summary and a call to action		

The Shot List and Storyboard

A shot list provides direction on what shots are needed for a particular scene and the order in which the videographer should shoot them. Sometimes, it makes sense to group similar shots together at one time (e.g., the video's opening and closing once the lighting is set up). Creating a shot list helps ensure you capture all the shots you need and optimizes the shoot. A shot list may include the following details:

- project title, description, location
- what's in the shot: including background, equipment, props, food, talent/host
- what actions take place
- shooting notes (e.g., wide shot, closeup, zoom, pan, camera angle); blend several styles to maintain visual interest
- brief dialogue or message points

For many videographers, the *storyboard*, or a visual representation of the video, is a foundational step. It provides a specific visual reference for how each shot should be framed. Similar to a comic book, the storyboard is a set of sketches or pictures representing each shot in sequence; it may include notes about what goes on in each shot, what's said in the script during that shot, and notes regarding the angle and composition of the shot. A storyboard (or a shot list, if that is your preference) helps give direction and clarifies what the video is trying to accomplish.

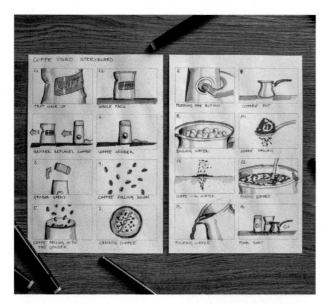

A storyboard is the visual representation of the individual shots planned for a video.

Spicy Sriracha Almonds

Preparation time: 5 minutes
Cooking time: 15 minutes
Yield: 8 servings (¼ cup per serving)

2 cups whole natural almonds
3 tablespoons sriracha sauce
1 tablespoon soy sauce
1 tablespoon olive oil
2 teaspoons crushed red pepper flakes
½ teaspoon kosher salt

Preheat oven to 350° F. Line a rimmed baking sheet with parchment paper. Spread the almonds in an even layer on the baking sheet. Roast 5 minutes. Remove from the oven and allow to cool while making the sriracha mixture.

In a medium bowl, whisk together the sriracha, soy sauce, oil, and red pepper flakes. Mix in almonds until coated evenly.

Return the almonds to the baking sheet and spread out in an even layer. Roast, stirring once halfway through, for 10 minutes.

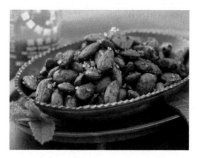

Remove the sheet pan from the oven. Sprinkle almonds with the salt; stir. Allow almonds to cool completely before storing in an airtight container.

Courtesy of Almond Board of California.

Shot	Notes
First scene: prep (overhead on counter)	
1. Lay out a nicely cut piece of parchment paper on a baking sheet. 2. Spread the almonds across the surface. 3. Remove the baking sheet from the scene.	▪ Overhead or a ¾ shot will show the action best; play with the composition of the baking sheet at an angle or slightly off center. ▪ Use hand or large spoon to spread almonds. ▪ Text overlay: oven temperature and time to roast the almonds.
Second scene: mix (overhead on counter)	
1. Return the baking sheet to the scene and place on a trivet or kitchen towel. 2. Bring over a medium glass bowl; start adding each coating ingredient to the bowl: sriracha, soy sauce, oil, and red pepper flakes. Mix together using a rubber spatula or wooden spoon. 3. Add the almonds into sriracha mixture; mix to coat almonds evenly. 4. Spread coated almonds on baking sheet.	▪ Keep the baking sheet peeking into the scene. ▪ Leave time and space between adding each ingredient to list ingredient by name with a text overlay. ▪ Use same rubber spatula or wooden spoon to mix in almonds. ▪ Text overlay: oven temperature and time to roast the almonds for second roasting.
Third scene: serving (overhead on craft paper or any table worksurface)	
1. Show almonds on the pan after second roasting. 2. Capture a serving scene with a napkin or beverage and a bowl of almonds.	▪ Use the swap of finished almonds in a serving dish. Consider adding text—perhaps a link to the recipe.

- "Don't learn in the moment. Test recipes and make sure they work before you start shooting."

- "Buy more food than you think you'll need. For example, if you want to capture that one perfect egg-cracking shot, you might need a dozen eggs or more before getting the shot you like."

- "Try for visual variety when shooting a video. People get bored easily."

- "Be realistic about time commitment needed for food videos: it's not uncommon for a 20-second video to take at least a half day's worth of work or more for shopping, prepping, shooting, and editing."

- "Estimate your time commitment based on the complexity of the final deliverable. You might be able to shoot three recipe-focused videos in a day with the support of a food stylist and an assistant, plus additional time for preproduction preparation and postproduction editing."

—Joanie Simon, food photographer, educator, and author of *Picture-Perfect Food*

"Be prepared and organized when prepping ahead for news station culinary demos. Store prepped ingredients in clear glass bowls, individually cover [them] with plastic wrap (or a compostable cling wrap), and then label each one. This makes ingredients clear if someone is assisting you. Place the bowls on a quarter sheet pan and then 'hotel wrap' the entire sheet pan. Hotel wrapping is a practical technique used to save and transport food by tightly wrapping the entire sheet pan (not just the top) with plastic wrap. If possible, use a restaurant bus tub to transport the sheet tray and other items into the TV studio set. Don't forget to bring the items you assume will be there but might not be, like garbage bags, water, paper towels, extension cords, and disinfecting wipes!" —Sara Haas, RDN, culinary nutrition consultant

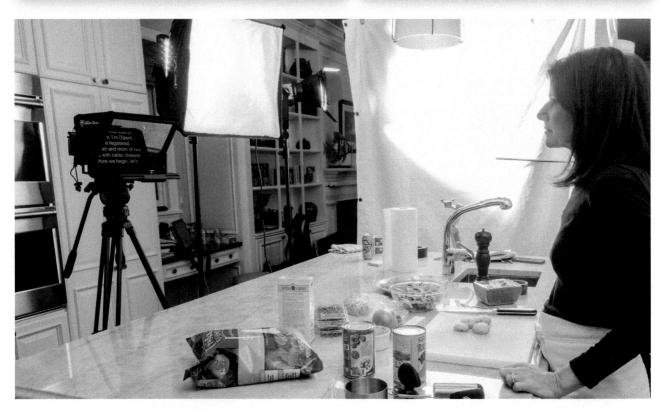

Practicing the script before filming by using an iPad teleprompter mounted over the camera lens.

Production: Shooting the Video

Whether you're shooting your video using a professional camera or a smartphone, certain technical elements always apply, just as with food photography. And while it's true that a video can be successful or go viral without expensive equipment and years of filming experience—especially if the story or host is unique or funny—it's still important to know some basics of lighting and shooting.

Lighting

The goal of the video's lighting scheme is to make the food and talent look their best by eliminating shadows and creating soft, diffused, and flattering light on the food and the talent's face. It's critical to get the lighting right, since it can be difficult—if not impossible—to "fix" a poorly lit scene in postproduction. Use natural light, if possible, or a softened artificial light source (such as a softbox) pointed down at the food if shooting it alone or more to the side or behind the camera if shooting a scene with talent in it. Make sure no windows or lights are set up behind the talent, as they will appear in silhouette.

While natural light is free and is arguably the best choice for quick shoots, it shifts and changes according to the time of day and the weather. Artificial light provides consistency, and it can be used at any time of day or night. The downsides are the additional expense and space needed to store the lights. Consider workarounds, such as renting lighting equipment or creating your own lighting using inexpensive LED light sources.

THREE-POINT LIGHTING FOR VIDEO PRODUCTION

A common setup for video production (and also photography) is known as three-point lighting. This basic lighting technique highlights the subject, allowing it to stand out from the background. In the setup:

The **camera** is at 6:00.

The **key light**, or the brightest light, is set at 4:00. Adjust the angle of the key light to create a shot that has depth.

A **fill light** (a light that's half the intensity of the key light), a white foam board, or another reflective surface is set at 8:00 to bounce light back onto the subject. The fill light helps eliminate the shadows the key light causes.

A **back light** is set between either 10:00 and 11:00 or 1:00 and 2:00. This light separates the subject from the background and helps give the subject more shape and depth.

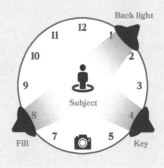

Quick Tip

"When deciding how to light your subject (and food), be aware that lights have color. Pick either daylight (natural light) or artificial light and stay consistent with it during the shoot. Using mixed light sources can create an imbalance [that looks] unnatural. For example, if there is a window in your kitchen, but it's not enough to light your subject, either use the window and supplement with daylight-colored light bulbs (5,600 Kelvin, available at most places that sell lights) or block the window light and use artificial lighting set to look like daylight at 5,600 Kelvin. A useful tool is a light that can be set to either daylight, artificial light, or somewhere in between. These types of lights offer the most flexibility. Some LED ring lights, which many people use for laptop video calls, offer this type of light choice. Keep in mind that you can set your camera settings to capture the type of light you are using, giving you control over the shoot. Most smartphones, however, are automatic, so as the host moves through the frame, exposures and colors can change." —Michael Sutz, professional filmmaker, Twelve Plus Media

Point of View

The compositional tactics used in photography, such as the rule of thirds (objects of interest placed at one of the intersections or along one of the grid lines), leading lines (lines leading the viewer's eyes where you want them to go), and depth of field (deciding what is and isn't going to be in focus) are also used in video. Some additional points to keep in mind when shooting food videos include:

- **Carefully choose what ends up in the video frame.** As a general rule, keep the set uncluttered. Unnecessary items lead to distraction. Only include elements on set that are relevant to and supportive of the video's topic, and carefully think through the color choices for these items and the set lighting, as these help create mood.

- **Shoot in a two-camera setup with different angles** to make the video more interesting. Having two perspectives allows for more choices when editing. The first camera could be used for wide shots and keep focus on the talent, while the second camera could come in for close-ups and focus on the food as it's prepared and cooked. Whether the close-ups are overhead or at a 45-degree angle, they're crucial for highlighting truly mouthwatering shots like bubbling cheese or sizzling steak. If you only have one camera, consider shooting the video twice: once with a wide shot and then again with close-ups.

Quick Tip

"When doing a cooking demo with a host, your focal point is on the host. It's okay to look at the camera—the audience—to address them, but your eyes should always return to the host." —Steve Dolinsky, Food Reporter, NBC 5 Chicago

Quick Tip

"Take videos while on the go and save them in organized video folders by content type. You can easily access and combine any of these videos at a later time." —Rachel Paul, PhD, RDN, The College Nutritionist

- **Capture cooking actions and sounds.** Actions may include a sauce simmering, steam rising from a pot, or a last-minute sprinkle of fresh herbs. Sounds to feature could include stir-frying vegetables, panfrying chicken breasts, or a blender on high speed. All these actions and sounds help tell the story. If a desired sound wasn't captured during filming, remember that sound can be recorded separately and then added to the video during the post-production editing process.

- **Keep the video's shape in mind while shooting.** Technically, this is known as the *aspect ratio* or *width-to-height ratio* of the video. A square video has an aspect ratio of 1:1; a vertical-orientation video has an aspect ratio of 9:16; and a horizontal-orientation video has an aspect ratio of 16:9, the most common size of computer and television monitors. The best idea is to shoot in a way that can be used in all three orientations or to shoot in a horizontal aspect ratio and edit the video in an alternate aspect ratio or resize the aspect ratio in post-production. If the video is shot in the horizontal aspect ratio and the resolution is 4K, more options will be available in post-production, including zooming or resizing to a vertical or square crop. Another option is to shoot in a vertical orientation and then crop the video so it's square.

- **Use a recommended video format (.MP4 or .MOV).** The format you choose will depend on how you plan to share the video. If you are editing for film and television, MOV is best. If you are creating video for websites and social media, MP4 is a good choice, since it produces smaller file sizes. MOV format can be converted to MP4 if needed.

Quick Tip

"Before filming, double check how the video is being used to determine if you need to do it in portrait or landscape mode. I've screwed this up before and had to redo the whole video! Also, do a mini test video to make sure you are looking at the right spot and that you approve of where your eye line is before officially beginning to film." —Dawn Jackson Blatner, RDN, author of *The Flexitarian Diet* and *Superfood Swap*

Equipment

If you are just starting out in creating food videos, use the equipment you already have. Once you gain more experience, add on new items slowly, and consider renting equipment instead of buying it. The type of equipment you will need depends on the type of video you're trying to make, but for all types of video, making sure the lighting and audio are good will mean the difference between a video that looks amateurish and one that's professional looking. Following are descriptions of some common equipment used to shoot videos (see pages 317 to 320 for more on equipment).

Lighting kits Most professionals recommend having two or three softbox lights or LED lights. LEDs are quite versatile, as they can be softened by being bounced onto reflective surfaces, or they can be modified to include soft boxes or other softening devices (e.g., a bed sheet). They may also include an option for adjusting the color temperature (e.g., daylight simulation), and may have the ability to be battery operated. One of the greatest advantages of LED lighting in food photography is that they emit almost no heat. LED ring lights are often used for self-hosted videos shot with a smartphone.

Reflectors Reflective surfaces like white foam board can reflect or bounce light where it's needed—onto the talent or the food—and can fix shadows by filling in the light.

Microphone Most professionals prefer using an external wired microphone (sometimes referred to as a lavalier mic) clipped on the talent's clothing for the best sound. Use a connector to plug it into your smartphone or camera; alternatively, use a wireless Bluetooth connector and microphone for more freedom. Be sure to test the built-in microphones provided with smartphones. You should be able to clearly hear the talent but not the competing sounds in the room.

Headphones A set of headphones allows the videographer or sound technician to monitor the sound quality live during the shoot.

Camera The best options for video capture are either a smartphone or a digital single-lens reflex camera (DSLR). DSLR cameras provide a much wider variety

> *Quick Tip*
>
> **"Don't use the phone holder in a ring light. Instead, use a separate phone stand to hold your phone. Place this stand with your phone attached in front of and at the height of the bottom of your ring light for better, more even lighting."** —Kiano Moju, founder and principal of Jikoni, a food video production company

> *Quick Tip*
>
> **"If it's all voiceover in the video, consider doing that in a closet full of clothes—a homemade sound booth—to help reduce echoes and external noises."** —Dawn Jackson Blatner, RDN, author of *The Flexitarian Diet* and *Superfood Swap*

of prime (fixed focal length) and zoom lenses that can greatly affect the quality of the video. DSLR camera bodies can be upgraded as needed, and the lenses are typically compatible with newer models. Of course, smartphones are easy to upgrade over time, and also work well as secondary cameras. See pages 317 and 318 for more on cameras and lenses.

Tripod Tripods are invaluable for shooting video, as they allow for a steady shot, time after time. Choose a tripod with a lateral arm that adjusts to different heights (clip locks are easier than screw locks; they only need to be tightened when the height is adjusted). You'll need two tripods if you're setting up for overhead (one with an arm) and regular wide shot views. To rotate and tilt the camera or smartphone smoothly, you'll need a tripod mount.

Camera stabilizer Videos require movement, so having a camera stabilizer is always a wise idea. It keeps the camera horizontally balanced as you move. Gimbal stabilizers (motorized steadicams) and sliders help your camera move smoothly, making your videos look more professional.

HD monitor or computer Using a separate monitor is key since you can miss a lot if you can only review the video with a small screen or camera viewfinder. A monitor will allow you to see details more clearly while you shoot.

Wireless video remote and wireless monitoring system You can easily monitor dynamic shots by using a wireless monitoring system that connects your smartphone or camera to a computer monitor through a Wi-Fi, Bluetooth, or other wireless connection. If you're both the talent and the videographer, a wireless video remote will allow you to remotely start and stop recording between takes.

Laptop stand A stand is great for recordings made using Zoom or other live video recording applications.

Teleprompter While many professional-grade teleprompters are available to choose from, you can improvise by downloading a teleprompter (e.g., PromptSmart Pro, Padcaster Parrot) on your laptop, tablet, or smartphone. Position the device just under the camera using either a teleprompter kit that mounts over the camera lens, a stack of books, or a laptop stand so your eyes will line up well with the camera's lens. The further away you stand from the teleprompter, the less noticeable your eye movements will be. The best option is to have a dedicated teleprompter operator on the team.

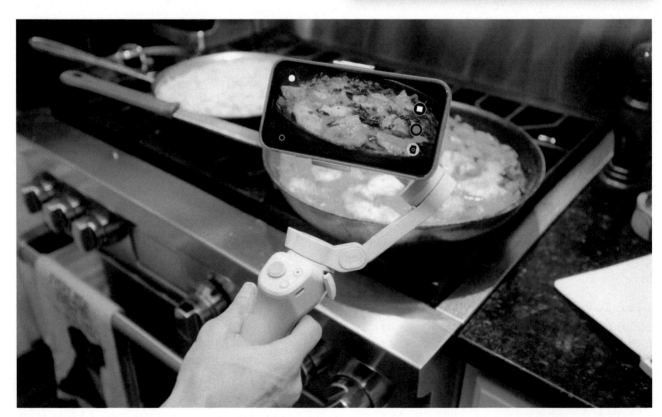

A handheld gimbal stabilizer helps to smooth out footage and prevent shakiness while the smartphone camera is moving.

SHOOTING VIDEO WITH A SMARTPHONE

Whether you're shooting short (15- to 60-second) videos or longer video projects, a smartphone is a convenient way to make engaging quality content. Regardless of the video's type, follow these general tips for planning, shooting, and producing video with a smartphone:

- Make sure your video includes these critical elements:

  - the hook, to grab your audience's attention and make them keep watching

  - an introduction to yourself, your brand, or your company

  - content that is clearly structured and easy to follow

  - a call to action that is clear, compelling, personalized, and obvious.

- Before finalizing the shoot location, decide on the vibe you wish the video to have. Your location should match it.

- Be sure to clean the camera lens, just as you would if you were doing a demo on a laptop.

- Place the smartphone in airplane or do-not-disturb mode so you're not interrupted by notifications, texts, emails, or calls.

- Decide whether to use natural or artificial light, or a mix of both. This may be as simple as choosing one light (e.g., a LED ring light or a large softbox shining in the direction of the talent), two lights (one light shining on the talent and the second light behind the talent to light the background), or a traditional three-point lighting setup (see Three-Point Lighting for Video Production page 337).

- A smartphone microphone is often fine for a quick social media video. But for better sound quality, use an external wired microphone (also known as a lavalier mic) or a wireless microphone. External microphones can reduce unwanted background noise and provide superior sound quality.

- Check your smartphone to make sure it has plenty of space to store the video and is fully charged. Immediately transfer the video to a computer or an external hard drive after shooting to free up space on your smartphone.

- Shoot in 4K: The higher your video's resolution, the better it will appear. You can always convert the file from high resolution to a lower resolution, but it doesn't work the other way around. In the camera settings, choose 4K for the best resolution, and lock the auto exposure and auto focus. To lock the focus, tap the specific point you want to focus on the screen.

- Optimize your video for the platform on which it will be published. Videos with a vertical orientation (aspect ratio) are preferred on many social media platforms, including Snapchat, Instagram, and TikTok, as they usually end up being viewed on smartphones. Never shoot a video that will be posted on a platform that prefers a horizontal aspect ratio in a vertical format, as the black bars that appear on the sides of a vertical video when it's played in a horizontal format are distracting and unappealing.

- Stabilize the smartphone using a tripod mount or stand. The lens should be pointed slightly below eye level. A **gimbal stabilizer** (a handheld mechanical stabilizer) will allow you to stabilize the smartphone even when it's moving.

- Shoot a short test video first and then let it roll!

- Edit your videos directly on your smartphone using a video editing app or download your video to your computer or an external drive and use a desktop version of a video editing software program. Adding music will enhance the viewer's experience.

- Research and learn about the latest in video optimization strategies to increase your videos' rankings in internet searches.

Postproduction: Editing the Video

Most professionals estimate that you'll spend 1 hour of editing time for every minute you shoot of video. A 3-minute video could take 2 to 3 hours of editing time, and a 15-minute video can take anywhere from 10 to 40 hours to edit. The editing time varies greatly depending on the type and complexity of the video.

Keep in mind that SEO [search engine optimization] rules apply to videos as well. So make sure you use relevant titles, captions, descriptions, and tags to give your videos a higher profile.

Editing Software

Many nonlinear editing (NLE) software options for editing video are available. They range from relatively expensive programs (Adobe Premiere Pro) to free (DaVinci Resolve). Either program can achieve the same result: raw footage assembled into a cohesive video in a nondestructive way (meaning that the original footage is not permanently altered). While the work of editing can be extremely time consuming, the creative options editing software provides are endless. It's in the best interest of all creators, regardless of their role in the process, to gain some familiarity with these software packages to get a broader sense of what's possible. Professional editors usually prefer a particular NLE program, and theirs may or may not play well with the software you choose.

If desktop video editing isn't for you, consider using a smartphone video editing app. Many options work well for editing videos destined for Instagram Reels, TikTok, and other social media platforms. Smartphone video editing apps are efficient, as they're designed to quickly edit clips and then upload to the platform of choice, and many are capable of automatically converting videos to the specifications (e.g., the specific aspect ratios) required by each platform.

Editing Tips

While you're editing, refer to the script frequently. Think about the running time, captions, music, visual effects, and instances where it may be worthwhile to include supplemental B-roll footage, such as paid or free stock media (e.g., photos, graphics, videos) to enhance the video's story. Experts suggest keeping

transitions and techniques like fading and zoom to a minimum and to use fast- or slow-motion footage as a way to adjust the video's time without losing the viewer's interest. Since many videos are watched with sound turned off, a catchy title and the use of captions can help grab and hold viewers' attention.

Workflow

Just as with food photography, having a workflow process set up in advance means that you don't have to reinvent the process each time you take on a new video project. Consider keeping all your content in one spot, such as on your local hard drive, an external drive, or a cloud-based folder (e.g., Dropbox) organized in a folder structure. The main folder could have the name of the project and subfolders for main footage, B-roll footage (secondary or supplemental footage), audio, images, graphics, text overlays, and other elements can rest inside.

Background Music

While a well-made video *should* be just as effective with or without sound, choosing background music is still an important editing decision that can enhance the tone and mood of a food video. Many professionals suggest using the same background music in each video in a series for the sake of consistency. Be aware that many video platforms censor videos that use copyrighted music without permission. A quick online search will reveal many resources for free and royalty-free music options. Be sure to read through the licensing information carefully and explicitly follow the guidelines of how and where the music can be used.

VIDEO EDITING TERMINOLOGY FOR SOCIAL MEDIA

Many consider video to be the format of choice for social media. The following terms are helpful to know.

Resolution: The number of pixels (data) in each frame that a monitor can display. A higher number of pixels indicates a higher resolution, and a lower number of pixels indicates a lower resolution (e.g., higher resolution is 4,000 pixels (4K); lower resolution, which is fine for social media posts, is 1,080 pixels.

Aspect ratio: The ratio of an image's width to its height in photography and video. For example, the horizontal or landscape aspect ratio is 16:9, the square aspect ratio is 1:1, and the vertical (full portrait) aspect ratio is 9:16 (2:3 and 4:5 are also vertical aspect ratios). Before creating your video (or digital still), research the current recommendations for aspect ratios for the social media platform you plan to use.

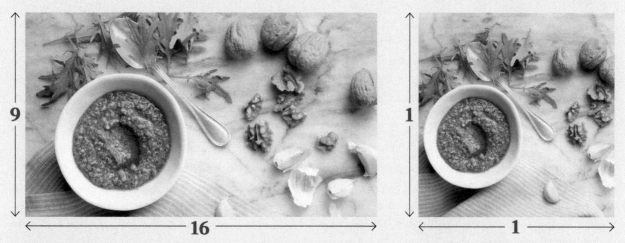

Look at the cropping (16:9 or 1:1) to ensure you have the shots you want for your intended use, e.g., desktop versus mobile.
Photo credit: Renée Comet Photography

File size: The higher the video's resolution is (and the longer the video is), the larger the file size will be. File sizes are dependent on whether the data is compressed and if it's compressed, by how much. A minute of uncompressed video and an hour of compressed low-resolution video could conceivably have the same file size: 1 gigabyte. The software applications that compress video are getting increasingly sophisticated, which means that even smaller or more compressed videos look better than ever. Nonetheless, it's still true that the more compressed a video's data is from its original state, the more degraded it will become.

Bitrate: The rate at which bits are transferred from one location to another. When it comes to video, the bitrate refers to the amount of video data that's transferred either by upload or download over a certain period of time. The video's quality is measured by its bitrate, so if a video is referred to as being "high bitrate," that's just another way of saying that the file will look more like the original footage as it was shot. While high bitrate equals high quality, it also means larger files (e.g., 13 megabits per second [Mbps]).

Creating effective content for social media platforms starts with knowing the goals of the content and creating a content strategy. This strategy helps guide the planning, creating, and distribution of all types of recipe content, including written (e.g., e-newsletter, short tweets, Instagram captions), audio, photography (e.g., process shots, finished dish), video (e.g., live, time lapse, behind the scenes), GIFs (i.e., moving images), and more.

Plan out the process

Use a calendar as big-picture approach to social media content planning. This can help you visualize ideas and organize them in a way that makes the strategy easier to execute. Before creating content, plan a production process that is efficient (and cost effective) by thinking in advance how to turn one piece of content into multiple uses, known as repurposing content. For example, if you plan to develop a YouTube video on making a margherita pizza, you can also use parts of the video on Instagram or TikTok. Since you will have the filming production set up and the recipe's ingredients, take the time to develop a list of content ideas beforehand to ensure you capture any additional short videos or still images needed for future posts (e.g., julienning basil leaves, spinning the dough in the air, cutting the pizza, eating the pizza).

Schedule the content

You can then schedule the different pieces of content across various social media platforms to get the most out of it. When deciding where to post what content, also consider what types of content perform well on that particular platform based on an audit—for example, which three posts had the greatest impact on the social media metric that matters to you (e.g., engagement, audience growth rate, referrals to your website or newsletter).

Leigh Loftus, founder of TheChefShots.com, recommends maximizing the production of content by brainstorming ideas for content you want to capture. Here are a few ideas for creating content for a margherita pizza recipe.

One minute (or less) video ideas:
- How the dough and sauce are made
- How to cut basil
- Which cheese to use and why
- Using a brick oven
- Talking about my specific cooking process

Photo and timelapse opportunities:
- Preparing and kneading the dough
- Spinning the dough in the air
- Saucing and/or topping the dough
- Pizza in the oven
- Cutting the pizza to serve
- Various completed "money shots" including full and taken apart images of the pizza

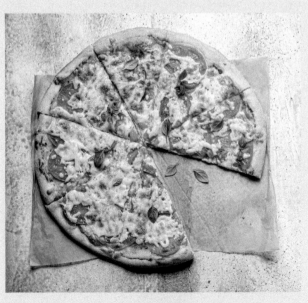

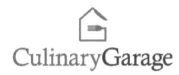

Brand: Ooey Gooey Cheese Co.

Background: What is the brand/product/market situation driving the project?

In 2022, the plant-based cheese category grew by 18%, compared to just 1.4% for conventional dairy-based cheese. Concerns around health, environment, and animal welfare are the key drivers behind consumers' increased interest in plant-based alternatives. Recognizing the increased competition presented by these alternative products, Ooey Gooey Cheese Co. (OGCC) seeks to reinforce its position among current and next-generation consumers as a thoughtful producer of premium, artisan-quality dairy-based cheeses.

Brand/Marketing Objective: What is the overriding brand or marketing objective? To inform or educate consumers about product/brand features? To elevate or evolve the brand's positioning/perceptions?

Reinforce OGCC's authenticity, quality, and deliciousness by showcasing its line of premium artisan cheeses as an everyday indulgence.

Target Audience: What consumer segment is the brand trying to connect with? What are their needs? What's motivating these consumers to be interested in and purchase the brand's product?

We seek to connect with existing and new consumers seeking premium-quality cheese they can feel good about buying and serving to their families.

Project Objective: What is the scope of the assignment/project? What is the deliverable?

Create a series of four 45- to 60-second videos that showcase the quality and deliciousness of OGCC's artisan cheeses in everyday recipes and applications. Videos will be featured on OGCC's website and social media channels.

Featured Products & Messaging: What specific product(s) and/or recipe will be featured in the videos? What are the key messages to be communicated/conveyed?

1. Alpine-Style Cheese | Recipe: Country Ham, Apple, & Swiss Quesadilla

    a) Reflective of cheeses made in the Alps
    b) Semi-firm or hard cheese
    c) Typically sweet and nutty in flavor; sharpness increases with age
    d) Good for melting

2. Double-Cream Brie Cheese | Recipe: Honeyed Apricot & Brie Tartine

    a) Cream is added to lend creaminess and richness
    b) Typical bloomy rind
    c) Great as a centerpiece for cheeseboards and indulgent appetizers and snacks

3. Blue Cheese | Recipe: Blue Cheese, Pear & Walnut Slaw

   a) Blue cheese is OGCC's best seller
   b) Pungent, earthy flavor and blue-green veins derived from the addition of Penicillium fungi
   c) Ranges from creamy to fudgy and crumbly
   d) Varying degrees of sweetness and saltiness

4. Smoked Gouda Cheese | Recipe: OGCC Farmhouse Burger

   a) More buttery and creamy than regular Gouda
   b) Mildly smoky; smoked in brick ovens
   c) Aged 2 to 3 months

Creative Direction: Being mindful of existing brand guidelines and standards, what creative elements should be considered when developing the videos in order to successfully portray the brand and communicate key brand/product messages (e.g., look, feel, tone, personality, etc.)

- Each video should include a 10- to 15-second introduction to the cheese product, leveraging existing farm and creamery footage as needed to illustrate its production to the final packaged product
- Only hands should be featured in the video; there should be no on-camera talent
- Music track should be royalty free
- The voice-over preference is for an articulate, friendly/conversational male
- The overall look and feel of the video and graphics should be sophisticated, yet approachable and must align with brand standards
- The kitchen setting should be appropriate for a middle-income home; modern farmhouse style; stainless steel appliances are okay
- Food/recipe footage should incorporate close-ups to play up the food's deliciousness and crave ability
- The food styling should come across as gourmet and indulgent, but also fresh, natural, and uncomplicated; it should be approachable and not overly styled
- Props should incorporate rustic, natural materials and surfaces (e.g., wooden boards, linen napkins, earthenware, cast iron, etc.)

Technical Details: Final edited videos will be provided in .MOV format

Timeline:

Task	Due Date
Creative brief alignment and approval	
Draft script	
Revised script	
Draft storyboards	
Revised storyboards	
Final storyboard approval	
Preproduction call	
Shoot date(s)	
Editing and graphics	
Final videos delivered	

Used with permission from Culinary Garage/ Susan Parenti & Kathy Takemura

Food Styling, Photography, and Video Resources and Bibliography

Food Styling

The Food Stylist's Handbook: Hundreds of Media Styling Tips, Tricks, and Secrets for Chefs, Artists, Bloggers, and Food Lovers by Denise Vivaldo with Cindie Flannigan. 2017. Skyhorse.

Food Styling: The Art of Preparing Food for the Camera by Delores Custer. 2010. John Wiley & Sons.

Food Photography

Food Photography: From Snapshots to Great Shots, 2nd Edition by Nicole Young. 2015. Peachpit Press.

Food Photography: Pro Secrets for Styling, Lighting, and Shooting by Lara Ferroni. 2012. Union Square & Co.

Food Photography & Lighting: A Commercial Photographer's Guide to Creating Irresistible Images by Teri Campbell. 2012. New Riders.

How to Photograph Food: Compose, Shoot, and Edit Appetizing Images by Beata Lubas. 2020. Running Press Adult.

Picture Perfect Food: Master the Art of Food Photography with 52 Bite-Sized Tutorials by Joanie Simon. 2021. Page Street Publishing.

Plate to Pixel: Digital Food Photography & Styling by Helene Dujardin. 2011. Wiley.

Photography Work Surfaces and Backdrops

Erickson Surfaces:
ericksonsurfaces.com

Capture by Lucy:
capturebylucy.com

Bessie Bakes Backdrops:
bessiebakesbackdrops.com

Ink & Elm:
inkandelm.com

Photo Editing

Smartphone
Adobe Photoshop Express:
adobe.com/products/photophop-express

Adobe Lightroom Photo Editor:
adobe.com/products/photoshop-lightroom/mobile.html

Snapseed:
snapseed.online

VSCO:
vsco.co

Foodie:
foodie.snow.me

LiveCollage:
livecollage.net

PhotoGrid:
photogrid.app/en/

Desktop
Adobe Photoshop:
adobe.com/products/photophop

Adobe Lightroom:
adobe.com/products/photoshop-lightroom.html

Capture One Pro:
captureone.com

Online Resources for Food Styling, Photography, and Videos

Digital Photography School:
digital-photography-school.com

Food Photography Education: The Bite Shot with Joanie Simon:
thebiteshot.com

Foodtography School:
foodtographyschool.com

Food Photography for your Smartphone:
thechefshots.com

Professional Food Styling Videos:
foodstylingvideoclasses.podia.com

Facebook: *The Food Stylist's Handbook* Group

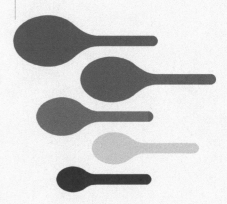

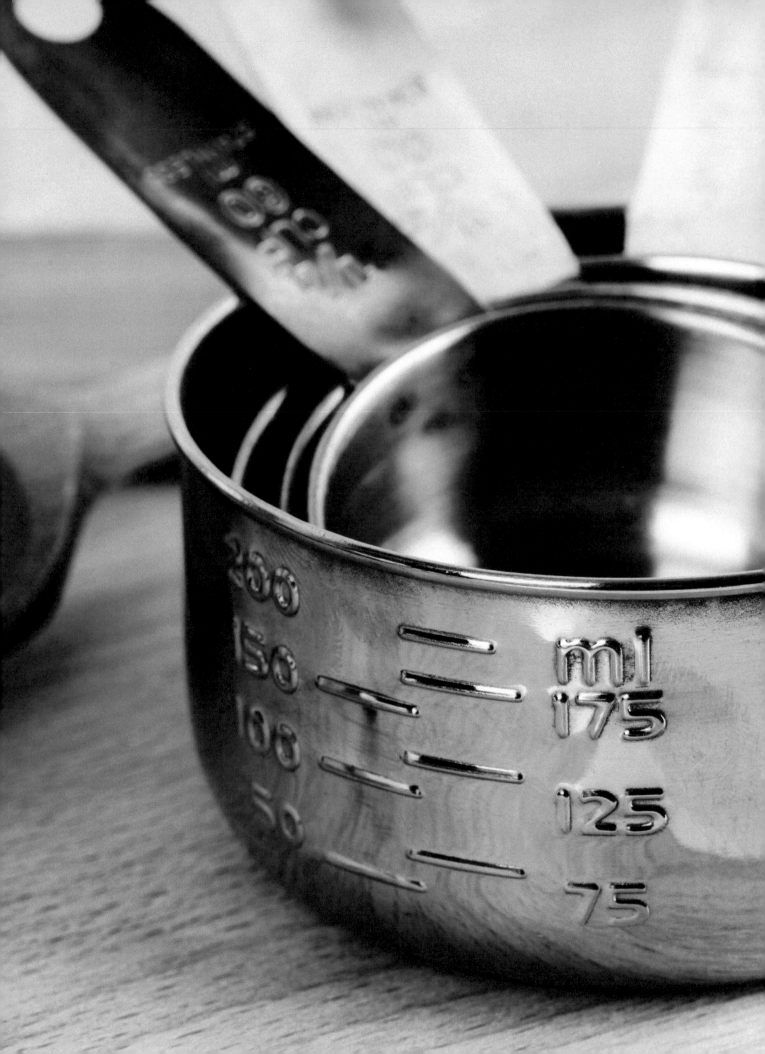

Appendix: Common Ingredient Equivalencies and Conversions

In recipe development, a personal document detailing the volume and weight equivalents of frequently used recipe ingredients can be very helpful when converting volume to weight measurements or adjusting food amounts in recipes and for nutrition analysis. Consider sharing your document with your editor or copy editor to ensure consistency within your recipe project.

This appendix presents general approximate weight and volume equivalencies for many common ingredients. Keep in mind that discrepancies in weight and volume measurements exist, even between the most respected food publications. Factors such as density, moisture, and temperature can influence the volume of ingredients, making weight a more accurate measurement than volume. For example, 1 cup of brown sugar (measured by volume) can change depending on whether it is loosely or tightly packed into the measuring cup. On the other hand, 213 grams of brown sugar will always be 213 grams of brown sugar. Remember that consistency is critical in a multirecipe project, so be sure to use a consistent volume measure or weighed amount of an ingredient across different recipes.

Experienced recipe developers who also specialize in nutrition analysis often create a similar document as a cheat sheet and use it as a reference to ensure consistency when performing nutrient analysis.

Refer to Measurement Conversions, Measurement Equivalencies, and Temperature Conversions on pages 360 and 361 for formulas to easily convert US customary measurements to metric and vice versa.

Types of Ingredient Measurements

There are different ways to describe measured ingredients in a recipe, depending on the type of ingredient and how much accuracy is needed.

Number measurement (i.e., number of items): Use number measurements, such as 3 medium mangoes, when accurate measurement is not critical for the success of the recipe and close-in-size is good enough.

Volume measurement (e.g., teaspoon, tablespoon, cup, etc.): The volume, or the measure of how much space something takes up, is most often used for liquids and dry ingredients in American home cooking recipes.

Weight (ounces or grams): Weight is the most accurate, reliable, and consistent way to measure recipe ingredients and portion sizes—whether liquids, dry ingredients, or solids. When measurement accuracy is critical, in baking for example, provide recipe measurements in weight using a digital scale. Liquids with a high sugar content, such as honey and syrup, ideally should be weighed. In general, small quantities (less than 4 tablespoons), such as 2 tablespoons of olive oil or 1 teaspoon of baking soda, are given in volume, not in weight.

Fruits

Ingredient	Volume/count	US customary weight	Metric weight
Apple	1 medium (1 cup diced/sliced)	5½ ounces	161 grams
Applesauce	1 cup	9 ounces	255 grams
Apricots, dried	½ cup	3 ounces	80 grams
Avocado	1 medium (1 cup cubed)	5¼ ounces	150 grams
Banana	1 medium (about ½ cup mashed)	3½ ounces	100 grams
Bananas, mashed	1 cup	7½ ounces	212 grams
Berries, frozen	1 cup	5 ounces	142 grams
Blueberries	1 cup	5 ounces	148 grams
Cantaloupe	1 medium (4 to 4½ cups cubed) 1 cup cubed	3 pounds AP* –	1,362 grams 125 grams
Cherries, fresh with pits	1 cup (about 21 cherries)	5 ounces	138 grams
Cranberries, fresh	1 cup	3½ ounces	99 grams
Currants	1 cup	5 ounces	142 grams
Dates, dried	½ cup	3 ounces	76 grams
Dried fruits, in general	1 cup	5½ ounces	160 grams
Figs, dried	1 cup	5¼ ounces	150 grams
Grapes	1 cup	5¼ ounces	150 grams
Lemon	1 medium = • 2 to 3 tablespoons juice • 1 tablespoon zest	6¼ ounces – –	180 grams 30 to 45 milliliters 2 grams
Lemon juice, strained	1 cup	8¾ ounces	240 milliliters (244 grams)
Lime	1 medium = • 2 tablespoons juice • ½-1 teaspoon zest	3½ ounces – –	95 grams 30 milliliters 1 gram
Mango	1 medium (1 cup chopped)	5¾ ounces	165 grams
Orange	1 medium = • ¼ cup juice • 1½ tablespoons zest	9½ ounces – –	265 grams 60 milliliters 1.5 grams
Orange juice, strained	1 cup	8½ ounces	240 milliliters (248 grams)
Peaches, peeled and diced	1 cup	6 ounces	170 grams
Pears, peeled and diced	1 cup	5¾ ounces	163 grams
Pineapple	1 medium (about 5 cups cubed) 1 cup chunks	3 pounds AP* 6 ounces	1,362 grams 170 grams
Pineapple chunks, canned	1¼ cups chunks	15.25-ounce can (8.25 ounces drained weight)	234 grams, drained weight
Raisins	1 cup	5¼ ounces	149 grams
Raspberries	1 cup	4¼ ounces	120 grams
Rhubarb, sliced	1 cup	4¼ ounces	120 grams
Strawberries	1 cup sliced	6 ounces	165 grams
Watermelon, cubed	1 cup	5¼ ounces	150 grams

* AP is as purchased, in the raw state before any cutting, processing, or cooking has occurred.

Vegetables

Ingredient	Volume/count	US customary weight	Metric weight
Asparagus	16 to 20 spears	1 pound	454 grams
Beets	1 (2-inch diameter) About 5 medium (2½ cups diced)	3 ounces 1 pound	82 grams 454 grams
Broccoli	1 cup florets 3 cups florets	3 ounces 1 pound (AP)*	85 grams 454 grams (AP)
Cabbage	1½ cups 4½ cups shredded	3 ounces 1 pound (AP)*	85 grams 454 grams
Carrots	1 cup chopped (2 to 2½ medium) 3½ cups sliced or grated	5 ounces 1 pound	142 grams 454 grams
Cauliflower	1 cup florets 1 medium head (about 6 cups florets)	3½ ounces 2 pounds	100 grams 908 grams
Cauliflower, riced	¾ cup	3 ounces	85 grams
Celery	About 1½ large ribs (1 cup chopped) 4 cups chopped	3½ ounces 1 pound	100 grams 454 grams
Collard greens	6 to 7 cups 1½ cups cooked	1 pound 7 ounces	454 grams 195 grams
Corn, canned	1¾ cups	15.25-ounce can (8.25 ounces drained weight)	234 grams, drained weight
Corn kernels	1 medium ear (1 cup)	5 ounces	145 grams
Cucumber	1 medium (about 2 cups sliced)	7 ounces	201 grams
Eggplant	About 6 cups cubed	1 pound (AP)*	454 grams
Garlic	1 clove (1 teaspoon chopped)	0.2 ounce	6 grams
Ginger	1-inch piece (about 1 tablespoon chopped)	0.3 ounces	7 grams
Green beans	About 3 cups, trimmed	1 pound	464 grams
Herbs, leafy, chopped	¼ cup	0.2 ounce	6 grams
Leeks, diced	1 cup	3¼ ounces	92 grams
Lettuce, iceberg	1 medium head (about 9 cups shredded)	1½ pounds	680 grams
Mushrooms, sliced	1 cup	2½ ounces	70 grams
Olives, sliced	1 cup	5 ounces	142 grams
Onion, yellow	1 large (1 cup chopped)	5½ ounces	160 grams
Onions, green	1 cup chopped (about 9)	3½ ounces	100 grams
Peas, frozen	1 cup	5 ounces	134 grams
Peppers, bell	1 medium (about ¾ cup chopped or heaping 1 cup sliced)	3½ ounces	100 grams
Potatoes	2½ cups diced	1 pound	454 grams
Potato flakes, dried	1 cup	2 ounces	54 grams
Potatoes, cooked, mashed	1 cup mashed (1 large potato)	7½ ounces	213 grams
Shallot	1 medium (1 tablespoon minced) 1 cup	0.4 ounce 5½ ounces	10 grams 156 grams
Spinach, baby and other greens	1 cup 10 cups 1 cup cooked	1 ounce 10 ounces 1 pound	30 grams 283 grams 454 grams

Table continues >

Vegetables (continued)

Ingredient	Volume/count	US customary weight	Metric weight
Spinach, chopped, frozen (cooked)	1½ cups	10 ounces	283 grams
Sweet potatoes, cooked, mashed	1 cup mashed (1 large)	8½ ounces	240 grams
Tomato paste	2 tablespoons	1¼ ounces	33 grams
Tomatoes, dried	1 cup	6 ounces	170 grams
Tomatoes, fresh, chopped	1 cup	7 ounces	200 grams
Tomatoes, grape, halved	1 cup	5¼ ounces	150 grams
Zucchini, shredded	1 medium (⅔ cup grated; 1 to 1¼ cups sliced)	4¼ to 5¼ ounces	121 to 150 grams

* AP is as purchased, in the raw state before any cutting, processing, or cooking has occurred.

Nuts and Seeds

Ingredient	Volume/count	US customary weight	Metric weight
Almonds, whole	1 cup	5 ounces	142 grams
Almonds, sliced	1 cup	3 ounces	85 grams
Almonds, slivered	1 cup	4 ounces	110 grams
Almond paste	1 cup	9⅛ ounces	259 grams
Caraway/cumin/fennel seeds	2 tablespoons	½ ounce	18 grams
Cashews, whole	1 cup	4 ounces	113 grams
Chia seeds	2 tablespoons	1 ounce	24 grams
Flaxseeds	¼ cup	1¼ ounces	35 grams
Flaxseed meal	½ cup	1¾ ounces	50 grams
Hazelnuts, whole	1 cup	5 ounces	142 grams
Hazelnut spread	1 cup	11 ounces	320 grams
Macadamia nuts, whole	1 cup	5¼ ounces	145 grams
Peanuts, whole	1 cup	5 ounces	142 grams
Peanuts, chopped	1 cup	5¼ ounces	150 grams
Peanut butter, smooth	2 tablespoons ½ cup	1 ounce 4¾ ounces	32 grams 135 grams
Peanut butter, chunky	2 tablespoons ½ cup	1 ounce 4¾ ounces	32 grams 135 grams
Pecans, halved	¼ cup (about 19 pieces) 1 cup	1 ounce 4 ounces	28 grams 108 grams
Pecans, chopped	1 cup	4 ounces	114 grams
Pepitas (pumpkin seeds)	¼ cup	1 ounce	32 grams
Pine nuts	½ cup	2½ ounces	71 grams
Pistachio nuts, shelled	1 cup	4½ ounces	128 grams
Poppy seeds	2 tablespoons ¼ cup	0.6 ounce 1¼ ounces	18 grams 36 grams
Sesame/sunflower seeds	½ cup	2½ ounces	71 grams
Tahini paste	½ cup	4 ounces	112 grams
Walnuts, halved, pieces	¼ cup (10 to 12 pieces) 1 cup	1 ounce 4 ounces	28 grams 112 grams
Walnuts, coarsely chopped	1 cup	4 ounces	114 grams

Beans, Peas, Lentils, Soy Products

Ingredient	Volume/count	US customary weight	Metric weight
Dried beans, most types (1-pound pkg)	2 cups (uncooked) 6 cups (cooked)	16 ounces 34 ounces	454 grams 960 grams
Beans, cooked, most types	1 cup (⅓ cup cooked)	5½ ounces	160 grams
Beans, canned	1½ cups	15-ounce can, drained	240 grams, drained weight
Lentils, most types (1-pound pkg)	2⅓ cups (uncooked) 6 cups (cooked)	16 ounces 42 ounces	210 grams 1,188 grams
Lentils, cooked	1 cup	7 ounces	198 grams
Miso	¼ cup	2½ ounces	70 grams
Tempeh	1 piece 1 cup	3 ounces –	84 grams 166 grams
Tofu, firm/extra-firm	1 piece 3 cups cubed	3 ounces 14-ounce package	84 grams 397 grams

Breads and Grains*

Ingredient	Volume/count	US customary weight	Metric weight
Barley, cooked	1 cup	6½ ounces	157 grams
Barley, pearled, uncooked	1 cup	7½ ounces	216 grams
Breadcrumbs, dried	1 cup (about 4 slices of bread)	4 ounces	112 grams
Breadcrumbs, fresh	1 cup (about 3 slices of bread)	3 ounces	85 grams
Breadcrumbs, Japanese panko	1 cup	2 ounces	60 grams
Bulgur (cracked wheat), uncooked	1 cup	6¾ ounces	190 grams
Cornmeal (medium grind), uncooked	1 cup	5½ ounces	156 grams
Couscous (fine), uncooked	1 cup	6 ounces	173 grams
Couscous (pearl/Israeli), uncooked	1 cup	5 ounces	150 grams
Crackers, Ritz	24 crackers (1 cup fine crumbs)	2½ ounces	72 grams
Millet, whole, uncooked	1 cup	7½ ounces	204 grams
Millet, whole, cooked	1 cup	6 ounces	174 grams
Spaghetti (1-pound package)	8¾ cups (cooked)	16 ounces	454 grams
Penne (1-pound package)	8 cups (cooked)	16 ounces	454 grams
Polenta (coarsely ground), uncooked	1 cup	5¾ ounces	163 grams
Popcorn, popped	1 cup	½ ounce	11 grams
Quinoa, uncooked	1 cup	6 ounces	170 grams
Rice (basmati, long-grain), uncooked	1 cup	7 ounces	195 grams
Rice (basmati, long-grain), cooked	1 cup	5½ ounces	158 grams
Tapioca, quick-cooking	2 tablespoons	¾ ounce	21 grams
Wheat berries, uncooked	1 cup	6½ ounces	184 grams
Wheat germ	1 cup	4 ounces	113 grams

* Also refer to quick-cooking and long-cooking grains yields (in cups) on pages 78 and 79.

Meat, Poultry, Seafood, and Eggs

Ingredient	Volume/count	US customary weight	Metric weight
Bacon, raw	16 to 24 slices (varies by how sliced)	1 pound	453 grams
Beef, ground, raw (1 pound)	1¾ cups cooked	12 ounces cooked	340 grams cooked
Chicken, boneless breast, raw (7 ounces)	about 1 cup cooked, diced/shredded	5 ounces cooked	140 grams cooked
Chicken, whole rotisserie, cooked (Costco, about 3 pounds)	6 cups shredded meat (4 cups breast meat; 2 cups dark meat)	1¾ pounds	840 grams
Chicken, whole rotisserie, cooked (average 2 pounds)	3 cups (about 2 cups shredded white meat; 1 cup dark meat)	1 pound	420 grams
Egg, large	1 egg 1 yolk 1 white	1¾ ounces 0.65 ounce 1.05 ounces	49 grams 18.6 grams 30 grams
Salmon, canned	½ cup	5-ounce can (4 ounces drained weight)	102 grams drained weight
Scallops, sea	20 to 30 scallops	1 pound	454 grams
Scallops, bay	70 to 120 scallops	1 pound	454 grams
Shrimp, in shell	small (51 to 60 count) medium (41 to 50 count) large (31 to 35 count) extra-large (26 to 30 count) jumbo (21 to 25 count) colossal (10 to 15 count)	1 pound	454 grams
Tuna, canned	½ cup	5-ounce can (4 ounces drained weight)	113 grams drained weight
	about 1 cup	12-ounce can (9 ounces drained weight)	255 grams drained weight

Dairy and Plant-Based Milks

Ingredient	Volume/count	US customary weight	Metric volume/weight
Butter	1 tablespoon ½ cup (1 stick) 1 cup 2 cups	½ ounce 4 ounces 8 ounces 16 ounces (1 pound)	14 grams 113 grams 227 grams 454 grams
Butter, clarified	1 cup	6.8 ounces	195 grams
Buttermilk	1 cup	8½ ounces	240 milliliters (242 grams)
Cheese, aged (such as Parmesan), finely grated	½ cup	2 ounces	50 grams
Cheese, hard (such as cheddar, mozzarella), shredded	1 cup	4 ounces	112 grams
Cheese, soft (such as blue cheese, feta), crumbled	¼ cup	1 ounce	28 grams
Cheese, cream	1 cup	8 ounces	227 grams
Cheese, mascarpone	1 cup	8 ounces	227 grams
Cheese, ricotta	1 cup 1¾ cups	8 ounces 15-ounce container	228 grams 425 grams

Table continues >

Ingredient	Volume/count	US customary weight	Metric volume/weight
Cream, heavy/half-and-half	1 tablespoon 1 cup	– 8¼ ounces	15 milliliters 240 milliliters (235 grams)
Crème fraîche	1 cup	8 ounces	226 grams
Malted milk powder	¼ cup	1¼ ounces	35 grams
Milk	1 cup	8½ ounces	240 milliliters (246 grams)
Milk, coconut, canned	1 cup 1⅔ cups	8½ ounces 13.5-ounce can	240 milliliters (241 grams) 400 milliliters (383 grams)
Milk, evaporated	1 cup 1½ cups	8 ounces 12-ounce can	240 milliliters (226 grams) 354 milliliters (339 grams)
Milk, sweetened condensed	1 cup 1 cup plus 2 tablespoons	11 ounces 14-ounce can	240 milliliters (312 grams) 397 grams
Milk powder, dried nonfat	¼ cup	1 ounce	28 grams
Sour cream	2 tablespoons 1 cup 2 cups	– 8½ ounces 16-ounce container	30 grams 242 grams 454 grams
Soy milk	1 cup	8½ ounces	244 grams
Yogurt, Greek	1 cup About ⅔ cup (1 single serving container)	8 ounces 5.3-ounce container	227 grams 150 grams

Flours and Starches

There is no universally accepted weight measurement for 1 cup of flour. Flour can differ wildly in terms of weight, depending on the type of flour, if the flour is sifted, stirred, or fluffed before measuring, and then if it is spooned or scooped into the measuring cup. A recipe developer can write and test recipes using the gram weight measurements in this chart, create their own custom conversion chart for flour weights, or use a publisher's weight for 1 cup of flour. The most important factor is that the recipe is tested and works as written with the volume and weight measurements provided in the recipe.

Ingredient[a]	Volume/count	US customary weight[b]	Metric weight
Almond flour	1 cup	3½ ounces	96 grams
All-purpose flour (dip and sweep)	1 cup	5 ounces	140 grams
All-purpose flour (light spoon and sweep)	1 cup	4¼ ounces	120 grams
All-purpose flour (sifted)	1 cup	4 ounces	114 grams
Amaranth flour	1 cup	3½ ounces	103 grams
Arrowroot starch	2 tablespoons	½ ounce	18 grams
Barley flour	1 cup	4 ounces	120 grams
Bread flour (dip and sweep)	1 cup	5.2 ounces	157 grams
Bread flour (light spoon and sweep)	1 cup	4½ ounces	130 grams
Bread flour (sifted)	1 cup	4¼ ounces	121 grams
Buckwheat flour (light spoon and sweep)	1 cup	4 ounces	115 grams
Buckwheat flour (dip and sweep)	1 cup	4½ ounces	125 grams
Cake flour (sifted)	1 cup	3½ ounces	100 grams
Cake flour (light spoon and sweep)	1 cup	4 ounces	114 grams
Cake flour (dip and sweep)	1 cup	4½ ounces	130 grams
Cassava flour	1 cup	5 ounces	140 grams
Chestnut flour (sifted)	1 cup	3.8 ounces	109 grams
Chickpea flour	1 cup	3 ounces	85 grams

Table continues >

Flours and Starches (continued)

Ingredient[a]	Volume/count	US customary weight[b]	Metric weight
Coconut flour	1 cup	4½ ounces	128 grams
Cornstarch	2 tablespoons	½ ounce	16 grams
Double Zero (00) flour	1 cup	4 ounces	116 grams
Durum flour (high-protein flour)	1 cup	4½ ounces	124 grams
Gluten-free all-purpose baking mix (King Arthur)	1 cup	4¼ ounces	120 grams
Gluten-free all-purpose flour (King Arthur)	1 cup	5½ ounces	156 grams
Gluten-free measure-for-measure flour (King Arthur)	1 cup	4¼ ounces	120 grams
High-gluten flour	1 cup	4¼ ounces	120 grams
Oat flour	1 cup	4 ounces	120 grams
Pastry flour	1 cup	3¾ ounces	106 grams
Potato flour	1 cup	6½ ounces	180 grams
Potato starch	2 tablespoons	1 ounce	24 grams
Pumpernickel flour	1 cup	3¾ ounces	106 grams
Quinoa flour	1 cup	4 ounces	115 grams
Rice flour, brown	1 cup	4½ ounces	130 grams
Rice flour, white	1 cup	5 ounces	142 grams
Self-rising flour	1 cup	4 ounces	113 grams
Semolina flour	1 cup	5¾ ounces	163 grams
Sorghum flour	1 cup	4.9 ounces	138 grams
Soy flour	1 cup	5 ounces	140 grams
Spelt flour	1 cup	3½ ounces	99 grams
Sprouted wheat flour	1 cup	4 ounces	113 grams
Tapioca flour	1 cup	4 ounces	120 grams
Teff flour	1 cup	4¾ ounces	135 grams
Tapioca starch (instant)	2 tablespoons	½ ounce	12 grams
White Lily flour	1 cup	4½ ounces	130 grams
Whole wheat flour	1 cup	5 ounces	143 grams
Whole wheat flour (sifted)	1 cup	4½ ounces	125 grams
Whole wheat pastry flour	1 cup	3.4 ounces	96 grams

[a] Measured by spoon-and-sweep method, except as noted

[b] Ounce measurements are rounded

Chocolate

Ingredient	Volume/count	US customary weight	Metric weight
Cacao nibs	1 cup	4¼ ounces	120 grams
Chocolate chips and chunks	1 cup	6 ounces	170 grams
Chocolate chips, mini	1 cup	6¼ ounces	177 grams
Cocoa powder, Dutch-processed (dip and sweep)	1 cup	3.3 ounces	95 grams
Cocoa powder, Dutch-processed (lightly spooned)	1 cup	3¼ ounces	92 grams
Cocoa powder, Dutch-processed (sifted)	1 cup	2.6 ounces	75 grams
Cocoa powder, nonalkalized, unsweetened (lightly spooned)	1 cup	3 ounces	84 grams

Sweeteners

Ingredient	Volume/count	US customary weight	Metric weight
Agave syrup	1 tablespoon ½ cup	– 6 ounces	21 grams 168 grams
Corn syrup	1 cup	11½ ounces	328 grams
Glucose, liquid	1 cup	11¾ ounces	336 grams
Honey	1 tablespoon 1 cup	¾ ounce 11¾ ounces	21 grams 336 grams
Jam or preserves	¼ cup	3 ounces	85 grams
Maple syrup	½ cup	5½ ounces	156 grams
Molasses	¼ cup 1 cup	3 ounces 11¼ ounces	85 grams 322 grams
Refiner's syrup	1 cup	12 ounces	340 grams
Sugar substitute (Splenda)	1 cup	Almost 1 ounce	25 grams
Sugar, coconut	1 cup	7 ounces	180 grams
Sugar, dark brown, packed	1 cup	8.4 ounces	239 grams
Sugar, demerara	1 cup	7¾ ounces	220 grams
Sugar, granulated	1 cup	7 ounces	200 grams
Sugar, light brown, packed	1 cup, packed	7½ ounces	217 grams
Sugar, powdered, sifted	1 cup	4 ounces	115 grams
Sugar, sparkling	¼ cup	2 ounces	57 grams
Sugar, turbinado	1 cup	6½ ounces	180 grams

Fats

Ingredient	Volume/count	US customary weight	Metric weight
Butter	1 tablespoon ½ cup (1 stick) 1 cup 2 cups	½ ounce 4 ounces 8 ounces 16 ounces (1 pound)	14 grams 113 grams 227 grams 454 grams
Butter, clarified	1 cup	6.8 ounces	195 grams
Lard	½ cup	4 ounces	113 grams
Oil, coconut	1 tablespoon 1 cup	½ ounce 8 fluid ounces	14 grams (15 milliliters) 224 grams
Oil, olive	1 tablespoon 1 cup	½ ounce 8 fluid ounces	14 grams (15 milliliters) 224 grams (236 milliliters)
Oil, vegetable (canola, sunflower, avocado)	1 tablespoon 1 cup	½ ounce 8 fluid ounces	14 grams (15 milliliters) 218 grams
Oil, walnut	1 cup	8 fluid ounces	224 grams
Shortening	1 tablespoon 1 cup	– 6¾ ounces	12 grams 191 grams

Miscellaneous Baking

Ingredient	Volume/count	US customary weight	Metric weight
Baking powder	1 teaspoon	0.14 ounce	4 grams
Baking soda	1 teaspoon	0.18 ounce	5 grams
Citrus peel, candied	½ cup	3 ounces	85 grams
Coconut, dried (sweetened or unsweetened)	1 cup	3 ounces	85 grams
Coconut, dried, flakes	1 cup	2.1 ounces	60 grams
Cookie crumbs	1 cup	3 ounces	85 grams
Cream of tartar	1 teaspoon	0.11 ounce	3.1 grams
Espresso powder	1 tablespoon	¼ ounce	7 grams
Extract, vanilla or almond	1 tablespoon 1 teaspoon	½ ounce –	12 grams 4 grams
Gelatin	1 teaspoon	0.11 ounce	3.1 grams
Ginger, crystallized	½ cup	3¼ ounces	92 grams
Graham cracker crumbs, boxed	1 cup	3½ ounces	99 grams
Heath or toffee bar, chopped	1 cup	5½ ounces	156 grams
Marshmallow creme	About 1½ cups	7-ounce jar	198 grams
Marshmallow Fluff	About 1½ cups	7½-ounce jar	213 grams
Marshmallows, mini	8½ cups 1 cup	16-ounce bag	464 grams 50 grams
Marshmallows, regular	64 marshmallows (8 = 1 cup)	16-ounce bag	464 grams
Meringue powder	¼ cup	1½ ounces	43 grams
Pumpkin puree	1 cup 1¾ cups	8 ounces 15-ounce can	227 grams 425 grams
Yeast, active dry	2¼ teaspoons	¼ ounce	7 grams

Salt

Ingredient	Volume/count	US customary weight	Metric weight
Salt, kosher (Diamond Crystal)	1 teaspoon	0.123 ounce	3.5 grams
Salt, kosher (Morton)	1 teaspoon	0.175 ounce	5 grams
Salt, sea, flakes (Maldon)	1 teaspoon	0.211 ounce	6 grams
Salt, table	1 teaspoon	0.25 ounce	6.5 grams

Condiments

Ingredient	Volume/count	US customary weight	Metric weight
Gochujang	1 tablespoon	¾ ounce	21 grams
Harissa	1 tablespoon	½ ounce	15 grams
Hoisin sauce	1 tablespoon	0.7 ounce	20 grams
Hot sauce (sriracha)	1 tablespoon	¾ ounce	20 grams
Jam or preserves	2 tablespoons	1½ ounces	40 grams
Ketchup	1 tablespoon ½ cup	0.6 ounce 4.5 ounces	17 grams 130 grams
Mayonnaise	1 tablespoon ½ cup	– 4 ounces	13 grams 113 grams
Mustard, Dijon	1 tablespoon	½ ounce	15 grams
Mustard, stone ground	1 tablespoon	½ ounce	15 grams
Mustard, yellow	1 tablespoon	½ ounce	15 grams
Pesto, basil	2 tablespoons	1 ounce	28 grams
Pizza sauce	¼ cup	2 ounces	57 grams
Soy sauce	1 tablespoon	–	15 milliliters

Alcohol

Ingredient	Volume/count	US customary weight	Metric weight
Gin, vodka, rum, whiskey, 100 proof	1 cup	8 ounces	222 grams
Wine, white or red	1 cup	8 ounces	235 grams

Bibliography

Barns W. Bob's Red Mill flour weight chart. Accessed January 3, 2022. bobsredmill.com/blog/featured-articles/bobs-red-mill-flour-weight-chart

Boeckmann C. Measuring vegetables for recipes: pounds to cups. Accessed January 3, 2022. Almanac website. almanac.com/content/measuring-vegetables-recipes-pounds-cups

Dusoulier C. Ingredient conversions. Chocolate and Zucchini food website. Accessed January 3, 2022. cnz.to/conversions

Herbst R, Tyler Herbst S. *The New Food Lover's Companion*. 5th ed. Sourcebooks; 2013.

King Arthur Baking Company. Ingredient weight chart. King Arther Baking Company website. Accessed January 3, 2022. kingarthurflour.com/learn/ingredient-weight-chart.html

Lopez-Alt KJ. *The Food Lab: Better Home Cooking Through Science*. W.W. Norton and Company; 2015.

Lynch FT. *The Book of Yields: Accuracy in Food Costing and Purchasing*. 8thed. John Wiley & Sons; 2011.

Sarazen R. Personal equivalency chart.

Rattray D. A to Z Food and cooking equivalents and yields. The Spruce Eats website. Accessed January 3, 2022. thespruceeats.com/food-and-cooking-equivalents-and-yields-3054044

Rodgers R. Personal equivalency chart.

US Department of Agriculture. FoodData Central. FoodData Central website. Accessed January 3, 2022. fdc.nal.usda.gov

MEASUREMENT CONVERSIONS

Converting US customary measurement to metric

Ounces (weight) to grams	Multiply ounces by 28.35
Pounds to grams	Multiply pounds by 453.5
Cups to liters	Multiply cups by 0.24
Ounces (fluid) to milliliters	Multiply ounces by 29.57

Converting metric measurements to US customary

Grams to ounces (weight)	Multiply grams by 0.0352
Grams to pounds	Multiply grams by 0.0022
Liters to cups	Multiply liters by 4.226
Milliliters to ounces (fluid)	Multiply milliliters by 0.0338

MEASUREMENT EQUIVALENCIES

Liquid volume equivalencies

US customary volume measurement	Alternate measurement(s)	Metric measurement
1 teaspoon	–	5 milliliters
1 tablespoon	3 teaspoons; ½ (fluid) ounce	15 milliliters
2 tablespoons	1 (fluid) ounce	30 milliliters
¼ cup	4 tablespoons; 2 (fluid) ounces	60 milliliters
⅓ cup	5 tablespoons plus 1 teaspoon; about 3 (fluid) ounces	80 milliliters
½ cup	8 tablespoons; 4 (fluid) ounces	120 milliliters
1 cup	16 tablespoons; 8 (fluid) ounces	240 milliliters
2 cups	1 pint; 16 (fluid) ounces	480 milliliters
4 cups	1 quart; 2 pints; 32 (fluid) ounces	946 milliliters (about 1 liters)
1 gallon	4 quarts; 128 (fluid) ounces	3,785 milliliters (about 4 liters)

Weight equivalencies

US customary weight measurement	Alternate measurement(s)	Metric measurement
1 ounce	–	28.35 grams
1 pound	16 ounces	453.5 grams
2 pounds	32 ounces	907 grams
2.2 pounds	35.2 ounces	1 kilogram

TEMPERATURE CONVERSIONS

Use this conversion table to convert oven temperatures from Fahrenheit to Celsius (and vice versa).

Fahrenheit to Celsius

$(°F - 32) \times 0.555 = °C$

Example: $(350° F - 32) \times 0.555 = 177° C$

Celsius to Fahrenheit

$(°C \times 1.8) + 32 = °F$

Example: $(200° C \times 1.8) + 32 = 392° F$

Oven temperatures in Fahrenheit and Celsius

140° F	60° C		275° F	140° C		400° F	200° C
150° F	70° C		300° F	150° C		425° F	220° C
170° F	80° C		325° F	160° C		450° F	230° C
200° F	100° C		350° F	180° C		475° F	240° C
250° F	120° C		375° F	190° C		500° F	260° C

Appendix: Recipe Writing Style Guides

Recipe style guides, also referred to as style sheets, provide the recipe writer guidance on how a recipe should be written and ensures consistent language throughout product lines, publications, recipe-related projects, or across different publishing platforms. Recipe style guides are *usually* provided to recipe writers, and if not, a writer should create their own. Style guides are also used by the editor, copy editor, and proofreader.

A recipe style guide can range from a simple, one-page guide ("cheat sheet") to a long and detailed document, depending on the publication or project. There is no single authority or reference on recipe style. The two examples that follow—a style guide for a cookbook and a style guide for a food company—can be used as a starting point and modified to meet your needs. And always treat a style guide as a working document, regularly adding updates based on new or commonly used culinary words, terminology, and phrases.

Recipe Style Guide for a Cookbook

A cookbook style guide is used by cookbook authors, editors, copy editors, and proofreaders. While every publisher has their own style rules, a style guide is meant to keep editorial decisions organized and help ensure that the language and recipe style choices are consistent within the project and that the recipes are accurate, clear, and concise. This example of a cookbook style guide (pages 363 through 370) can be used as a reference when creating your own recipe style guide.

Recipe Style Guide for a Food Company

Food companies, and often each brand within a food company, have their own style rules. The example of a food company style guide on pages 372 through 376 can be used as a starting point for anyone involved in producing and marketing recipe content for a food company.

EXAMPLE: (XYZ PUBLISHER) COOKBOOK STYLE GUIDE

Formatting

- *All* copy should be flush left, including ingredient lists; 12-point Helvetica font.
- Don't try to make text look like a finished book page. Don't add extra line spaces (except where noted below), don't center, don't use tabs. The designer will take care of all these things.
- Skip a line between paragraphs or numbered steps. Don't indent.
- Insert a page break between recipes.
- **Do not** use boldface or underlining. First letter capitalized. Never use all capitals.

General Writing Style

- Most important: Be consistent throughout your manuscript.
- Different recipe writing style preferences are fine; however, please send us three separate recipe samples in your preferred style for approval before your project begins.
- Use this style guide first for spelling, hyphenation, capitalization, and italicization. If not found in this style guide, use *The Chicago Manual of Style* as a general reference. (Or, if preferred, the *Associated Press Stylebook*). If your questions are not answered, use these other resources: Merriam-Webster dictionary and *The New Food Lover's Companion*, by Sharon Tyler Herbst and Ron Herbst.
- Use the serial comma ("flour, baking soda, and baking powder").

Front Matter

Include any ingredient or equipment information that will help readers prepare the recipes in your book.

Recipe Organization Within Chapters

Within each chapter, put the recipes in a logical order. Three examples:
- Main ingredient: all beef together, all pork, all chicken, all fish and shellfish, all vegetables, all grains, etc.
- Type of recipe: all pies together, all cakes, all cookies
- Order of courses: beverages, appetizers, soups, salads, side dishes, entrées, desserts

Within those sections of the chapters, also follow some logical order. A few examples:
- Cut of poultry (skinless boneless breasts, chicken thighs, etc.); fish and seafood by species (bass, snapper, shrimp, trout, etc.), or grouped alphabetically by fish (bass to trout), followed by shellfish (clams to shrimp)
- Grains by type (pasta, corn, quinoa, rice, etc.)
- Similar fruits or veggies (apples and pears; peaches, plums, and apricots; potatoes and sweet potatoes)
- Similar cooking style (bake, roast, stovetop)
- Lightest to heaviest (broths, soups, chowders, stews, chilis)
- Flavor profile (winter herbs, summer herbs; or vanilla, chocolate, caramel, coconut)
- Cuisine (Italian, Mediterranean, etc.)

Recipe Elements

Place the elements in the following order with a single space between each element:
- Title
- Headnote
- Preparation Time
- Cooking Time
- Yield
- Ingredient List
- Directions
- Tips
- Make Ahead (if applicable)
- Nutrition Analysis (if agreed upon or if recipes make a health or nutrition claim)

Example continues>

Title
Should be clear.

Headnote
Limit to 75 words.

Preparation Time
Give time in increments of 5 minutes: Prep time: 15 minutes

Cooking Time
Give cooking time in a range (if needed) and in minute increments: Cook time: 10 to 12 minutes

Yield
Decide on the format(s) and be consistent. Examples of how the different kinds of yields (servings, size of pie, number of cookies) could be styled:

- 12 servings, 1 muffin per serving
- 6 servings, 1 cup (200 grams)
- 10 servings, 1¼ cups per serving (320 milliliters)

- Makes two 9-inch (23-cm) pie crusts
- Makes about 40 cookies, 1 per serving

Ingredient List

Organization
- List the ingredients in the order they are used and largest to smallest when ingredients are added at the same time.
- Arrange subrecipe ingredients in the logical order of preparation. For example, subrecipes that take longer or are needed ahead of time should be listed first: pesto (first), pasta (second); and sauce (first), meat (second).
- List dry ingredients before wet in baking.

Amounts and Measures
- For an international audience or if recipes include a nutrient analysis, provide US customary measures *and* metric measures. In ingredient text, place metric measures in parentheses after the US customary measures: 2 cups (500 milliliters). If the text is already in parentheses, use a slash instead: chopped fresh oregano leaves (¼ cup/13 grams).
- Obtain approval from editor if only providing US customary measurements.
- Spell out all US customary measurements (e.g., ounce, pound, teaspoon, tablespoon, cup) and metric measurements (milliliter, liter, gram, kilograms). If there are space constraints, abbreviate metric measurements with a space after the numeral (25 mL, 1 L, 25 g, 1 kg).
- Do not use decimals to indicate US customary measurements. Instead, use fractions: 1½ ounces (45 grams) dark chocolate, *not* 1.5 ounces.
- When two numbers follow one another, spell out one of them, most often the one that's more easily spelled out: one 3-inch cinnamon stick; or Yield: 22 three-inch cookies.
- Market measure: Provide information as close as possible to how you purchase it at a grocery store. That is: a count, plus a weight measurement if it is crucial to the recipe: 1 medium onion, chopped (about 1 cup/200 grams); 2 eggplants (about 2 pounds each/1 kilogram); 4 boneless, skinless chicken breasts (about 2 pounds/1 kilogram)
- Cans and packages: Use commonly purchased can/package sizes whenever possible. When calling for a whole can, package, or bottle, the exact size, including both US customary and metric, must be specified: 2 cans water-packed tuna, (6 ounces/170 grams each); 1 package pasta (8 ounces/250 grams).
- Do not call for a portion (such as half) of a can or package. Instead, provide a volume/weight amount: 1 cup (250 grams) drained canned pineapple chunks.
- Ingredients typically purchased by weight/ounces (e.g., cheese, dried mushrooms): Give in ounces, metric, and US customary measure: 4 ounces (120 grams) shiitake mushrooms (about 1 cup)
- Shrimp: Specify size (small, medium, large, extra large) and specify "peeled and deveined" if necessary.
- Liquids: Give liquids in cups/milliliters unless amount equals 4 quarts or more (exception: ice cream); For liquid amounts less than 1 cup, give in fluid ounces/milliliters.
- Weight: If weight is less than 1 pound, give in ounces/grams.
- Divided use: When the amount is divided into tablespoons in the directions, list it as tablespoons in the ingredient list. For example, 4 tablespoons (60 milliliters/40 grams), divided use; not ¼ cup (60 milliliters/40 grams), divided use. For awkward amounts, do not try to calculate it in tablespoons or in cups only, but rather use "plus": 1 cup plus 2 tablespoons (270 milliliters), *not* 18 tablespoons (270 milliliters).

Style Guidelines

- Be consistent with how an ingredient is specified throughout the cookbook. For example, do not call for green onions in one recipe and scallions in another.
- Each ingredient should be listed on its own line. Do not combine ingredients even if they are used in the same quantity.
- For measurement ranges, use "to," not a dash: 3 to 4 ounces, *not* 3–4 ounces.
- Use an initial capital for ingredients without an amount: Freshly ground pepper.
- When ingredient amount is not given, specify the use: Flour for dredging; Powdered sugar for dusting.
- Ingredient suggestions and preferences: When including a suggestion for a specific ingredient or a preference, put in parentheses: 6 ounces (170 grams) mixed wild mushrooms (such as cremini, chanterelle, and porcini), chopped (about 1½ cups); ½ cup (75 grams) yellow cornmeal (preferably stone-ground)
- Stock/broth: If a recipe calls for homemade chicken broth or stock and a recipe is included in the book, refer to it after ingredient: Chicken Stock (page 000). Or specify canned chicken broth. If reduced-sodium is preferred: "reduced-sodium canned chicken broth."
- Salt: In baking recipes specify amount of table salt. In savory recipes specify amount and type of kosher salt (Morton or Diamond Crystal). Do not say "Salt, to taste" in the ingredient list. Instead, list salt without a measurement in the ingredient list, and in the directions say, "season with salt to taste." If there is *additional* salt to taste, keep measurement in ingredient list (1 teaspoon kosher salt) and indicate to taste in directions: season with additional salt to taste.
- Pepper: in ingredient list, use "fresh ground pepper"; in directions, use "pepper."
- Herbs and spices: Indicate whole or ground, fresh or dried. Ideally, give an option for either fresh or dried with the different amounts.
- Garlic: X garlic cloves, *not* X cloves garlic.
- Butter: When needed, specify at room temperature, not softened.
- Flour: Specify all types of flour except all-purpose (then, use just "flour"). Exception: Specify all-purpose *if* there are other types of flour in the recipe.
- Sugar: Do not specify granulated sugar unless there are other sugars in the recipe. Specify packed brown sugar.
- Optional ingredients: Use "(optional)" after the ingredient: 2 green onions, chopped (optional). In the direction, use "if using" or similar: Sprinkle with the green onions if using.
- When an ingredient list includes another recipe in the book, the name of the recipe should appear in title case followed by the page reference: Basil Pesto (page 000). (Note: in cookbook manuscripts, page numbers are represented by "000" as the actual page numbers are unknown until the proofs are typeset.)

Ingredient Preparation

- Give simple preparation instructions in ingredient list:1 bunch kale, stems removed.
- Give more complicated instructions in the recipe directions, such as peeling and seeding tomatoes. If it doesn't fit in directions, write a note, then cross-reference in the ingredient list: 5 pounds tomatoes (see Note).
- Whenever possible, begin with a whole piece of food and give instructions for cutting it up: 3 apples (about 1½ pounds/680 grams), cored and chopped.
- Be aware of the difference of the prep listed before and after the ingredient. If an ingredient is prepped before it is measured, the preparation directions should directly follow the measurement: 1 cup chopped walnuts. This yields a different amount than if it is measured and then prepped: 1 cup walnuts, chopped.
- It is not necessary to specify peeling for onions, garlic, and shallots.
- Preparation of ingredients is usually assumed. For example, 1 red pepper, chopped: There is no need to say "seeded and ribs removed"). **Exceptions:** Specify prep for ingredients that may or may not be peeled, such as apples, potatoes, carrots, ginger, etc.: e.g., 1-inch piece ginger, peeled and minced.
    - Use "dice" when you want uniform-sized cubes: ¼, ½, or ¾ inch.
    - Use "cut into," *not* "sliced into": 1 stalk celery, cut into 2½- to 3-inch pieces; 1 onion, cut into 3-inch-thick slices.
    - Use "slice" when uniform slices are needed: 1 carrot, thinly sliced lengthwise into ⅛-inch-thick slices.
    - Specify "crosswise" and "lengthwise" slices if needed for clarity: 1 (6-inch) baguette, halved lengthwise
- Hyphenate measurements or amounts used as adjectives that precede the noun: 1 loaf bread, cut into 1-inch-thick slices.
- For canned goods, always specify whether the packing liquid is to be included in the recipe or drained. For example, if drained: 1 can (6 ounces) water-packed tuna, drained. If the liquid is to be included, use "with juice" or "with liquid" (whichever is applicable), *not* "undrained." If the liquid is being used, repeat the information in the directions: e.g., Add the celery, tomatoes with juice, beans, and oregano.

Example continues>

Directions

General Style

- Write directions in a numbered or paragraph style. If a step is getting too lengthy, divide into two steps at a logical point.
- Use only one space after all punctuation, including periods.
- Use "*the*" before ingredients. "Combine *the* flour, baking powder, and salt," not "Combine flour, baking powder, and salt."
- Use "*a*" or "*an*" before a container or tool: "In *a* small bowl"; "In *a* Dutch oven."
- Use serial commas (comma before the word "and" in a series of three or more items): onions, garlic, and mushrooms.
- When a number begins a sentence, spell it out or recast the sentence.
- General fractional amounts are written out in the directions: Fill each muffin cup about two-thirds full; add one-third of the flour.
- Use "place" for precise placement, "put" for casual placement: Place the fillets on warm serving plates; Put the mussels in a large pot.
- Use "drain" when you want to save the solids only and "strain" when you want to save the liquid (and perhaps the solids as well). If unclear, note whether the strained liquid or drained solids should be reserved for later use or discarded.
- When giving subrecipe instructions in the directions, orient the reader with phrases such as "To make the tomato sauce, . . . "

Equipment

- Either begin or end all cooking steps with the vessel used: In a large bowl, beat the egg whites until stiff peaks form. Or: Beat the egg whites to stiff peaks in a large bowl. Decide and be consistent.
- Always specify the size of the bowl or pan (small, medium, or large) and kind of pan (skillet, saucepan, pot, Dutch oven, etc.).
- Hyphenate compound measurements that act as an adjective preceding a noun: 9-by-13-inch dish.
- Specify utensils when necessary: Whisk the sauce. With a slotted spoon, transfer the potatoes to a paper towel–lined plate to drain.
- When possible, give an alternate technique for recipes using equipment that people may not have, such as food mill, food processor, or heavy-duty mixer. For example, give instructions for making dough both with a food processor and by hand.
- Use "cookie sheet" instead of "baking sheet;" use "sheet pan" instead of "jelly roll pan."
- Use "slow cooker" instead of Crock-Pot, which is a brand name.

Referring to Ingredients in the Directions

- All ingredients in the ingredient list must be used in the directions, in the order they appear in the ingredient list.
- Refer to each ingredient in as succinct a way as possible without sacrificing clarity. For example, if the ingredient list includes sherry wine vinegar and extra-virgin olive oil, use "Add the vinegar and oil" in the directions. Exception: Use modifiers if more than one type of an ingredient is in the recipe: Add the canola oil . . . add the olive oil.
- When two amounts of the same ingredient are used at different times in the directions, combine them in the ingredient list and indicate in the directions when the ingredient is first used. For example, in the ingredient list: 1¼ cup sugar, divided use; in the directions: Add 1 cup of the sugar . . . add the remaining ¼ cup sugar.
- When an alternate ingredient is listed in the ingredient list, do not refer to it in the directions unless there is an alternate preparation: 4 tablespoons butter or plant-based butter. Directions: Melt the butter.

Cooking and Adding Ingredients

- Use the same (or very similar) succinct but detailed phrases throughout for cooking steps such as melting chocolate, sautéing, beating egg whites, kneading dough. Use the same wording for the same tasks throughout the project or manuscript.
- Provide a suggested cooking time as well as a visual indicator of doneness: Add the onions and garlic and cook, stirring occasionally, until very tender and deeply golden brown, about 30 minutes.
- Be descriptive. Don't use terms such as deglaze, but instead explain the action: "Add the wine and stir to scrape up the browned bits from the bottom of the pan." Instead of reduce: "Cook over medium heat to reduce by one half."
- Use succinct phrases, such as "let cool," "remove from heat," "let sit for 30 minutes."
- Give stovetop heat: low, medium, medium-high, or high.
- Use "heat to a boil" and "simmer."
- Say "cook *for* 3 minutes," not "cook 3 minutes."
- For heating the oven: "Heat the oven to 350° F," *not* preheat. Provide oven heating instructions in the logical place—at the beginning of the directions or about 20 minutes before oven is needed. For long-term recipes like bread or marinated meats: Heat the oven about 20 minutes before baking.
- For chilling: "Cover and refrigerate," *not* Chill.

Make Ahead

When applicable, include information to successfully make the recipe ahead: how to store it safely, assemble before serving, and cooking or reheating instructions if necessary.

Nutrition Analysis

Books with a health focus should include the following nutrients in the order shown, with the amounts rounded according to the US Food and Drug Administration rounding rules. Recipes should be analyzed by a registered dietitian or professional nutrient analyst.

Nutrients per serving
Calories
Fat: (grams)
Saturated fat: (grams)
Sodium: (milligrams)
Total carbohydrate: (grams)
Fiber: (grams)
Total sugars: (grams)
Added sugars: (grams)
Protein: (grams)
Calcium: (milligrams)
Vitamin D: (micrograms)
Iron: (milligrams)
Potassium (milligrams)

Food Safety

Eggs

If a recipe contains raw eggs, include a note with a caution or an alternative ingredient. For example:

This recipe contains raw eggs. If you are concerned about the food safety of raw eggs, substitute pasteurized eggs in the shell or ¼ cup (60 milliliters) pasteurized liquid whole eggs.

Meat and Poultry

When giving instructions for cooking meat and poultry, include the following information:
- Do not rinse chicken.
- Do not reuse marinade as a sauce (unless instructions are given to boil marinade before reusing).
- Proper internal cooking temperatures for doneness.

Example continues>

Common Spelling

A

about, *not* approximately

agave nectar

aïoli

airtight

al dente

alcohol: capitalize if brand name or name is derived from proper noun, (e.g., Champagne, chardonnay)

allspice: specify ground allspice *or* whole allspice

aluminum foil (first mention; just "foil" thereafter)

ancho chile powder

anise seeds, *not* aniseed

apples: most varieties are capitalized, including Cortland, Golden Delicious, Granny Smith, Honeycrisp, and McIntosh

Arborio rice

Asian chile-garlic sauce

Asian markets and Asian food, *not* Oriental

avocado, avocados (no "e" in plural)

B

baba ghanouj

bacon: call for slices (not strips)

barbecue

barley: specify pearl barley, whole (hulled) barley, *or* pot barley

béarnaise

béchamel sauce

Belgian waffle

bite-sized

BLT

bran: specify natural bran, bran flakes cereal, *or* bran cereal (such as xyz); these are generally *not* interchangeable

bread crumbs (two words): specify dry *or* fresh

Brussels sprouts

buttercream

C

cannellini beans: specify cannellini (white kidney) beans

cardamom, *not* cardamon

cast-iron (adj), cast iron (noun): a cast-iron pot; pan is made from cast iron

celery: call for stalks, *not* ribs

cheese (capitalization and spelling): Asiago, bocconcini, Boursin, brick, Brie, Camembert, cheddar, chèvre, Colby, Edam, Emmental, feta, fontina, Gorgonzola, Gouda, Gruyère, haloumi, Havarti, Jarlsberg, manchego, mascarpone, Monterey jack, mozzarella, Munster, Oka, paneer, Parmesan (or Parmigiano-Reggiano), pecorino, pepper jack, Port Salut, provolone, quark, queso blanco, queso fresco, ricotta, Romano, Roquefort, Stilton, Swiss

cheese: softer cheeses are shredded; hard cheeses are grated; feta and blue are crumbled. Give measurements in cups and weight: ¼ cup (1 ounce) grated Parmesan cheese

chicken breasts: boneless skinless chicken breasts (not breast halves), *or* bone-in skin-on chicken breasts

chickpeas (one word), *not* garbanzo beans

chili (for the dish)

chili powder (except when made from a single type of chile pepper: e.g., ancho chile powder *or* chipotle chile powder)

chili sauce

Chinese five-spice powder

chocolate: specify milk chocolate, semisweet chocolate (not semi-sweet), *or* bittersweet (dark) chocolate; give a cacao percentage when it's crucial to the success of the recipe (70% bittersweet (dark) chocolate); in general, it is best to call for a weight than a volume amount.

cider vinegar, *not* apple cider vinegar

cilantro: specify fresh cilantro

citrus juice: specify fresh lemon juice unless bottled is preferred

citrus zest: call for grated lemon zest; always list zest before juice in ingredient list regardless of order used in directions (why: it's hard to zest a juiced lemon)

Cobb salad

cocoa: specify unsweetened cocoa powder in ingredients list, just "cocoa" in method

coconut: specify sweetened *or* unsweetened, and "flaked, shredded, *or* desiccated; e.g.: sweetened flaked coconut

coleslaw (one word)

confectioners' sugar, *not* confectioner's

coriander: use fresh cilantro when referring to fresh leaves; ground coriander for the spice

cornmeal (one word)

cornstarch

crabmeat: specify backfin (lump) crabmeat

cream: specify heavy cream, whipping cream, *or* half-and-half

crème caramel

crème fraîche

cremini mushrooms, *not* crimini

puffed rice cereal, *not* Rice Krispies

D

dal, *not* dhal

deep-fry

Dijon mustard, *not* just Dijon

doughnut, *not* donut

Dutch oven

E

English muffin

entrée

F

farm-to-table

farmers market

fillet (for fish); filet mignon

fish sauce: specify fish sauce (nam pla)

flat iron steak

flaxseed *or* ground flaxseed, *not* flaxseed

flour: specify kind (cake flour, whole wheat, all-purpose;
    unbleached all-purpose preferred for baking)
French bread, French dressing, French toast
french fries (no cap because refers to cut, *not* the country)

G
ginger: specify fresh *or* ground
gluten-free: hyphenate when used as an adjective or noun
Greek salad
green onions: specify white part only *or* both white and
    green parts

H
half-and-half
hard-boil (v); hard-boiled (adj)
heatproof (adj)
herbes de Provence
homemade
horseradish: specify prepared horseradish
hot pepper sauce (*not* Tabasco): if a specific variety is
    essential, use hot pepper sauce (such as [Brand] sauce)

I
Italian seasoning: specify dried Italian seasoning

J
Jell-O

K
ketchup, *not* catsup
Key lime
kosher food; kosher salt

L
lasagna ("lasagne" is plural)
leeks: specify white part only *or* both white and green parts
low-fat: with hyphen if it's an adjective preceding the noun;
    otherwise low fat
lemongrass (one word); specify white part only
lychee, *not* litchee *or* litchi

M
M&M's
mandarin orange
mango, mangos (no "e" in plural)
Marsala
meatloaf, *not* meat loaf
medium heat, *not* moderate
medium pan, etc., *not* medium-sized
medium-rare
milk shake
milk: only specify fat content (e.g., whole milk *or* 2% milk)
    when crucial to success of the recipe
multigrain bread

N
napa cabbage
niçoise olive
niçoise salad, *or* salade niçoise
nonfat
non-GMO
nonstick
nonstick cooking spray

O
ovenproof
oil: specify kind (extra-virgin olive oil, use vegetable oil,
    unless canola is essential)

P
paleo
panfry
papaya (sing. and pl.)
parchment paper (give an alternative, such as nonstick
    aluminum foil, *or* greasing pan
Parmesan cheese: specify freshly grated Parmesan cheese
Parmigiano-Reggiano (always made in Italy)
parsley: if using curly, just say parsley; for flat-leaf, specify
    flat-leaf (Italian) parsley
pâté
pâte à choux
pecorino romano cheese
pepitas: specify raw green pumpkin seeds (pepitas)
pepper: black pepper (not just "pepper");
    assumed black: freshly ground pepper; specify if white
        peppercorns;
    cayenne: specify cayenne pepper in ingredients list; just
        "cayenne" in method;
    chipotle peppers: specify drained canned chipotle
        peppers *or* canned chipotle peppers with adobo
        sauce; if dried, specify dried chipotle peppers
    crushed red pepper flakes
phyllo pastry, *not* filo
pierogi
pimientos
poppyseed (one word)
powdered sugar: use confectioners' sugar (not
    confectioner's sugar)

R
ragout
rib-eye steak
rice: specify white *or* brown, and long-grain *or* short-grain
    (or other specific variety)
rice vinegar, *not* rice wine vinegar
romaine lettuce
Russian dressing

S
sauté pan *or* skillet, *not* frying pan
sauté, sautéed, sautéing

Example continues>

sesame oil: specify Asian if this is the kind wanted

shiitake mushrooms

soufflé

spareribs (one word)

Sriracha sauce

stir-fry, stir-frys (n.)

stockpot

sugar, brown sugar: specify packed *or* lightly packed, even
for small volumes; specify light *or* dark; in directions,
use brown sugar (rather than just "sugar")

sun-dried tomatoes

sweet-and-sour

Swiss chard, *not* just "chard"

Szechuan

T

Tabasco, a trademark for a brand of hot sauce

taste buds

Thousand Island dressing

turmeric

U

umami

upside down (adv.)

upside-down cake

W

wheat germ

wheatgrass

whole grain bread, whole grain mustard

whole wheat bread, whole wheat flour

Worcestershire sauce

Z

zip-close plastic bags, *not* Ziploc

Sample Recipe

Green Beans with Roasted Fennel and Shallots

This recipe, given to me by Evie Lieb who adapted it from *Bon Appétit*, affords lots of flexibility for holiday preparation. You can make the entire dish at one time. Or, to cut down on holiday stress, make it ahead of time by cooking the beans and roasting the fennel and shallots a day or two beforehand. Refrigerate until you need them, then reheat before serving and enjoy!

Preparation time: 20 minutes
Cooking time: 35 minutes
Yield: 6 servings (about 1 cup per serving)

2 large fennel bulbs
¾ pound shallots, halved (quartered if large)
1 tablespoon fresh thyme leaves (optional)
5 tablespoons olive oil, divided use
Kosher salt
Freshly ground pepper
1 pound haricots verts or slender green beans, ends trimmed

1. Heat the oven to 450° F. Spray a sheet pan with nonstick cooking spray or line it with nonstick aluminum foil or parchment paper.

2. Cut the fennel bulbs in half lengthwise; then, leaving some of the core still attached, cut into ½-inch wedges. Place the fennel, shallots, and thyme, if using, in a large bowl; toss with 3 tablespoons of the oil to coat evenly. Spread the fennel and shallots in a single layer on the prepared sheet. Sprinkle generously with salt and pepper. Roast, tossing every 10 minutes, until the vegetables are tender and starting to brown, 30 to 35 minutes. If making ahead, cool the vegetables and store in a covered container in the refrigerator for up to 2 days.

3. Bring a large saucepan of water to a boil and add about 1 tablespoon salt. Add the haricots verts and cook until crisp tender, about 3 minutes. Drain and rinse with cold water or plunge into a bowl filled with ice water. Drain the beans again and spread on a paper towel. If making ahead, gently roll up the towel with the beans inside and place in a zippered plastic bag. Store in the refrigerator for up to 2 days.

4. About 1 hour before serving, spread the fennel, shallots, and beans on a sheet pan coated with nonstick cooking spray or lined with nonstick aluminum foil or parchment paper. Toss with the remaining 2 tablespoons oil. Reheat in a 400° F oven until hot, about 10 minutes. Transfer to a serving bowl.

Recipe style guide example adapted from: Chronicle Books cookbook style sheet | Robert Rose cookbook style guide | *The Recipe Writer's Handbook* by Barbara Gibbs Ostmann and Jane L. Baker. 2001. Harvest. | *Recipes Into Type* by Joan Whitman and Dolores Simon. 1993. HarperCollins | Mark Graham, New Food Studios | Raeanne Sarazen, Culinary and Nutrition Consulting

EXAMPLE: FOOD COMPANY STYLE GUIDE

Brand Vision: Products that improve the lives of people we touch every day.

Audience: From Generation Z to retirees, our customers span a range of ages, professions, income, and interests. Keep brand messaging as inclusive as possible, and when needed, segment recipes to appeal to a specific demographic. Focus on what unites customers: a need for convenience and a love for delicious foods.

Brand Voice: Knowledgeable and instructive in content; warm and enthusiastic in tone.

General Copy Standards

- For spelling and grammar, use this style guide first, then consult the *AP Stylebook*, *Webster's New World College Dictionary*, and *The New Food Lover's Companion* by Sharon Tyler Herbst and Ron Herbst.
- Use contractions (we've, you're, etc.) to convey friendliness.
- Always capitalize the name of brand product when written out in full: BRAND NAME Red Chile Slow Cook Sauce); do not capitalize categories of products, such as "sauces" or "salsas."
- Capitalize cheeses if based on a proper noun: Monterey Jack, Parmigiano Reggiano
- For hyphens, the general rule of thumb is use them in adjectives before a noun but not after: "easy-to-use recipe" and "the recipe is easy to use"). Exceptions: Don't hyphenate "all natural" or "gluten free."
- Use accents on words such as jalapeño.
- Do not use ampersands (&) in text, title, or directions.

Recipe section	Style guidelines for print (space constraints) and digital	Variations for digital
Headnote	Should be brief, explanatory, and aspirational.	No more than 75 words.
Yield	List number of servings per recipe and amount per serving: • Yield: 6 (½-cup) servings • 1 (9-inch) pie, 8 servings	
Preparation and Cooking Time	Give prep time in increments of 5 minutes: • Prep Time: 15 min. Give cook time in minute increments: • Cook Time: 10–12 min. Use an en dash for a range of numbers, with no spaces.	Use "to" for a range of numbers.

Measurement Abbreviations	Use abbreviations:
	 • tablespoon: Tbsp
	 • teaspoon: tsp
	 • cup: cup/cups
	 • quart: qt
	 • gallon: gal
	 • package: pkg
	 • ounce: oz or fl oz
	    • If there is space, spell out ounces: 1 (15-ounce) can
	    • For weight, list oz up to 1 lb
	 • pound: lb
	 • gram: g
	 • milliliter: mL
	 • inch: in
	 • minute: min
		Do not abbreviate; spell out all measurement units.

Recipe section	Style guidelines for print (space constraints) and digital	Variations for digital
Ingredient Amounts	Use 1½ tsp, *not* ½ Tbsp Use Tbsp when less than ¼ cup: 2 Tbsp Use ¼ cup, *not* 4 Tbsp, unless amount is divided. Use qts when whole, otherwise use cups: 2 qts (*not* 8 cups) or 6 cups (not 1½ qts). Do not use hyphen between whole number and fractions: 1½	Same instructions, with units spelled out: • Use 1½ teaspoons, not ½ tablespoon. • Use tablespoon when less than ¼ cup: 2 tablespoons. • Use ¼ cup, not 4 tablespoons, unless amount is divided. • Use quarts when whole, otherwise use cups: 2 quarts (not 8 cups) or 6 cups (not 1½ quarts).
Ingredient List	List ingredients in the order they are used in the directions, and from largest to smallest amount when added at the same time. Combine ingredients if it's the same amount and order used in the ingredient list, bold **each**: • 1 teaspoon **each:** oregano, salt, pepper (no ands) If one ingredient is used twice, say "divided" and clarify amounts in recipe directions: • *in ingredient list:* ¾ cup shredded mozzarella cheese, divided • *in directions:* Add ¼ cup of the mozzarella. . . . . add the remaining ½ cup mozzarella. Miscellaneous: • butter: 1 stick (½ cup) unsalted butter. Specify if unsalted; otherwise salted is assumed in all recipes. • oil: use "oil" or "olive oil"; no need to specify vegetable oil or canola oil • eggs: not necessary to specify egg size, as large is standard • milk: assume whole milk unless specified nonfat, 1%, or 2% • spices: list all spices as ground, dried, whole, or fresh • garlic: 2 cloves garlic, *not* 2 garlic cloves • vanilla extract (in the ingredient list); vanilla (in the directions) • sugar: packed brown sugar; granulated sugar • nuts: ½ cup (00 ounce.) chopped walnuts • salt and pepper: provide specific amount of salt and pepper; only use "to taste" in directions, not in the ingredient list. Never say season to taste if food can't be tasted. For example, raw meatloaf mixture cannot be seasoned to taste • List optional ingredients as "(optional)" Provide subheads in ingredient list and directions if there are multiple recipe components and there is a logical separation, e.g.: Dressing, Filling, Topping	Each ingredient should be listed on a new line. Do not combine ingredients even if they are used in the same quantity.
Ingredient List: Packaged Ingredients	Put brand names in all caps. Make brand name and specific name of product in bold or different color: • ¾ cup **BRAND NAME' Shredded Mild Cheddar Cheese** Specify jar, can, or package size: • 1 can (15 ounces) diced tomatoes • 1 pkg (8 ounces) **BRAND NAME Cream Cheese** Specify if ingredient is purchased prepared: • 1 cup jarred roasted bell peppers Do not use trademark ingredient in recipe if not our Brand product, instead use a generic description: • puff pastry sheet, *not* Pepperidge Farm Puff Pastry Sheet	

Example continues>

Recipe section	Style guidelines for print (space constraints) and digital	Variations for digital
Ingredient List: Preparation of Ingredients	Separate ingredient prep with comma: • 2 eggs, beaten • 1 pkg (10 ounces) spinach, thawed and drained List prep technique before measured ingredient: • ¼ cup grated onion (*not* ¼ cup onion, grated) Give equivalents when helpful: • 1 small zucchini, grated (about 1 cup) • ½ pound mushrooms, sliced (about 2 cups)	

Directions	Use paragraph style. No more than four paragraphs, preferably three. First word is an action verb—in bold:
	• **Stir** milk into beans . . .
	
	For product package preparation directions:
	• Initial action verb **bold CAPS:**
	  • **HEAT** water, milk . . . .
	  • **ADD** next 5 ingredients. Stir.
	
	When an ingredient list includes "XYZ product, prepared according to package directions," the ingredients used to prepare this product should not be listed in the ingredient list. However, include a step within the recipe directions for the product preparation.
		Keep numbered steps to no more than five steps, preferably three.
		Do *not* say "add next 5 ingredients or "add all remaining ingredients." List each ingredient separately:
		• **Combine** ground beef, breadcrumbs, onion, salt, and pepper in a large bowl.

Directions: Oven and Stove	**Oven:** Use degree symbol: 350° F. Heat oven, *not* preheat oven. Where the position of oven rack is important, include it in the heating instructions: • Heat oven to 400° F, with rack positioned in top third. • Place a rack in the middle of the oven and heat it to 375° F. **Stove:** Cook over medium-high heat, *not* moderately high heat	**Oven:** Spell out degrees: 350 degrees.
Directions: Articles	Do not use articles with ingredients: • Stir onions, potatoes . . . [no *the* before onions or potatoes]; add cheese . . . [no *the* before cheese] Use articles with equipment: • Whisk together honey, oil, . . . in *a* small bowl. • Place potatoes in *an* ungreased casserole dish.	
Directions: Commas	Use after second to last ingredient in list: • potatoes, *onions,* and cheese.	
Directions: Numerals	Spell out numbers zero through nine. Use digits for numbers 10 and above. **Exception:** Use digits for numbers and fractions that refer to specific measurements in the recipe directions: • 1 teaspoon of the . . . ; ½ cup of the . . . .; set aside 2 dozen.	
Directions: Miscellaneous Language	Always include a direction, visual cue, plus amount of time: • Bake for about 20 minutes, until the tops of the muffins have a pale golden-brown color and a toothpick inserted in the center comes out clean. Avoid the word sauté, instead use "cook and stir" or similar: • Cook and stir until boiling, about 2 minutes. • Cook over high heat until browned, about 4 minutes. Avoid the word braise, instead use "cover and simmer" or "simmer, covered." Examples of other preferred directions: • Lightly spray 12 muffin cups with the nonstick cooking spray. • Toast nuts on a cookie sheet in a 350° F oven until lightly browned, about 10 minutes. Cool and chop.	

Recipe section	Style guidelines for print (space constraints) and digital	Variations for digital
Directions: Equipment	Specify the size of skillets, pots, pans, and bowls based on the following: Common pans: • small skillet/saucepan (8 inches) • medium skillet/saucepan (10 inches) • large skillet/saucepan (12 inches) • small pot (1.5 to 2 quarts) • medium pot (3 to 4 quarts) • large pot (big enough to boil a pound of pasta) • loaf pan (9x5-inch) • square baking pan (9-inch square) • baking *dish* (usually glass or ceramic; 13x9-inch) • baking *pan* (usually metal; 13x9-inch) • cookie sheet (flat) • sheet pan (1-inch rim)	
Kitchen Tips and Notes (two tips are mandatory for each recipe, even if the editor chooses not to use them)	**Substitutions:** Place an asterisk in ingredient list after brand product name, then list the recommended brand product substitute at the bottom of the recipe: • 1 pkg (8 ounces) **BRAND NAME Cream Cheese*** • *You can substitute 1 pkg (8 ounces) **BRAND NAME Neufchatel Cheese** for the cream cheese. **Serving suggestion:** Focus on recommending other brand products, how to round out meal, or provide aspirational ideas: • Serve with large thin wheat or rice crackers or **BRAND NAME Pita Chips.**	
	How-to note: Include detailed instructions in a note at end of recipe: • Use a chef's knife to cut the tough ribs and stems from the kale leaves before using as directed.	**How-to note:** Include detailed instructions in recipe ingredient list **or** directions. In ingredient list: • 1 bunch kale, ribs and stems removed, leaves torn into pieces In directions: • Using a chef's knife, remove the tough ribs and stems from the kale leaves. Tear leaves into pieces and add to the bowl.
	Do-ahead tip: **Make ahead:** Prepare quesadillas as directed; wrap in foil, refrigerate. When ready to eat, remove from fridge. Heat oven to 350° F. Reheat until warm, about 25 min.	**Do-ahead tip:** **Make ahead:** Prepare quesadillas as directed; wrap in foil, refrigerate. When ready to eat, remove from fridge. Heat oven to 350° F. Reheat until warm, about 25 minutes.
Nutrition Information	List nutrition facts as follows: **Nutrition Information per serving:** TK* calories, TK grams fat, TK grams saturated fat, TK milligrams cholesterol, TK milligrams sodium, TK grams carbohydrate, TK grams dietary fiber, TK grams total sugars, TK grams protein * TK= to come	

Example continues>

Style Guidelines for Food Terms

Add terms based on project/brand needs

A	B	C
accent marks: use accent marks on all words with a foreign origin	**barbecue:** *never* BBQ, barbeque, or bar-b-cue **Belgian waffle** **blue cheese:** *never* bleu cheese **breadcrumbs:** one word, *not* bread crumbs **Bundt:** always capitalize	**Caesar salad** **cardamom,** *not* cardamon **chile,** when referring to the peppers **chili,** when referring to the spice or prepared dish **chili powder,** *except* when made from a single type of chile pepper: "ancho chile powder" or "chipotle chile powder" **confectioners sugar** (no apostrophe) **heavy cream** *not* whipping cream
D **Dijon mustard** **doughnut,** *not* donut	**E** edamame	**F** **fajita** **farmers' market,** *not* farmer's market **all-purpose flour** *not* white flour
G **garlic:** 1 clove garlic, *not* 1 garlic clove **ginger:** fresh ginger, *not* gingerroot **GMO:** non-GMO	**H** **half-and-half** **homemade** (one word)	**I**
J **Jell-O** **jellyroll**	**K** **ketchup,** *not* catsup **Kool-Aid** **kosher salt**	**L** **low-fat**
M **M&M's** **Marshmallow Fluff** **meatloaf** **medium-rare**	**N** **nonstick** **nonstick cooking spray,** *not* nonstick vegetable spray **Neufchâtel cheese**	**O** **Oreo** **ovenproof**
P **panfry** **Parmesan** **potpie**	**Q**	**R** **ranch dressing** **refried beans** **Rice Krispies**
S **sauté pan** **scallions** **sloppy Joes** **stir-fry**	**T** **Toll-House cookie**	**U** **upside-down cake**
V	**W** **wheatgerm** **whole-grain** (adj.): whole-grain mustard **whole wheat** (noun) **whole-wheat** (adj.): whole-wheat bread **Worcestershire sauce**	**X**
Y	**Z** **zest:** grated zest, *not* rind or peel **zip-close bag,** *not* Ziploc	

Sample Recipe

Example of digital recipe with no space constraints

Chicken and Bacon Potpie

Chicken potpie is a favorite comfort meal for the entire family. The addition of bacon and mushrooms adds a delicious savory depth to the filling.

Preparation Time: 35 minutes
Refrigerator Time: 1 hour
Cook Time: 1 hour
Yield: one 9-inch potpie, 8 servings

Pie Crust
1 cup all-purpose flour
4 ounces (½ of 8-ounce package) **BRAND NAME Cream Cheese**, softened
½ cup butter, softened

Filling
6 slices **BRAND NAME Bacon**, cut into ½-inch pieces
½ pound mushrooms, sliced
1 large baking potato, peeled and cut into ½-inch pieces
1 large onion, chopped
1 carrot, peeled and chopped
2 cloves garlic, minced
3 tablespoons all-purpose flour
3 cups reduced-sodium chicken broth
4 ounces (½ of 8-ounce package) **BRAND NAME Cream Cheese,** cubed
3 cups cubed cooked chicken

1. For pie crust, place flour in a large bowl. Cut in cream cheese and butter with pastry blender or 2 knives until the mixture resembles coarse crumbs. Shape dough into a ball; flatten into a disk. Wrap tightly with plastic wrap. Refrigerate 1 hour.

2. Meanwhile, for filling, cook bacon over medium heat in a large deep skillet or Dutch oven until crisp, about 5 minutes. Remove bacon from pan using a slotted spoon; drain on a paper towel–lined plate; set aside. Discard all but 2 tablespoons of pan drippings.

3. Add mushrooms, potatoes, onion, carrot, and garlic to pan; cook 5 minutes, stirring occasionally. Add flour; cook and stir 1 minute. Gradually stir in broth and heat to a boil. Add cream cheese; cook and stir until cream cheese is melted and mixture is well blended, about 1 minute. Remove from the heat; stir in chicken and bacon. Spoon mixture into a 9-inch deep-dish pie plate sprayed with nonstick cooking spray.

4. Heat oven to 400° F. Roll out pie crust dough into a 10-inch round between 2 sheets of waxed paper; place over chicken mixture. Flute edge, sealing crust to edge of pie plate. Cut several slits in crust to allow steam to escape. Place on cookie sheet.

5. Bake until top is golden brown, about 40 minutes. Cover edge of crust with foil the last 10 minutes to prevent overbrowning.

Tips:

Serving suggestion: Serve this potpie with a seasonal green salad or fruit salad for a delightful brunch.

Make-ahead: Wrap unbaked pie in foil, then freeze up to 3 months. When ready to serve, unwrap and cover edge of crust with foil strips. Bake frozen pie in 425° F oven until crust is golden brown and filling is heated through, about 1 hour 10 minutes.

Nutrition Information

Per serving: 460 calories, 29 grams fat, 16 grams saturated fat, 120 milligrams cholesterol, 510 milligrams sodium, 24 grams carbohydrate, 2 grams dietary fiber, 3 grams total sugars, 24 grams protein

Example continues>

Sample Recipe

Example of a print recipe with space constraints

For back of package recipes, small recipe cards, and any other publishing platform with limited space. Group or number individual action tasks and combine/group action tasks where appropriate. For example:

Cheddar Cheese Muffins

Prep time: 10 minutes
Bake time: 20–25 minutes
Makes: 12 servings

2 cups all-purpose flour
1 package (8 ounce) **BRAND NAME Shredded Cheddar Cheese**
1 tablespoon **each**: baking powder, sugar
½ teaspoon kosher salt
1 cup milk
1 egg
1 stick (½ cup) butter, melted

1. Heat oven to 400° F. Lightly spray 12 muffin cups with nonstick cooking spray.

2. Combine flour, cheese, baking powder, sugar, and salt in a large bowl.

3. Whisk together milk, egg, and butter in another bowl. Pour over dry ingredients and stir until combined.

4. Bake and Serve: Spoon the muffin mixture into the prepared muffin cups. Bake until golden brown, 20 to 25 minutes. Serve warm.

Food company style guidelines included in this example adapted from: Stonewall Kitchen Style Guide | selected food company style guides | Mark Graham, New Food Studios | Raeanne Sarazen, Culinary and Nutrition Consulting

Appendix: Food Safety Instructions in Recipes

Research shows that including food safety instructions in recipes improves consumer food safety behaviors. Four basic food safety practices—clean, separate, cook, and chill—can help ensure that prepared recipes are safe to eat. The Partnership for Food Safety Education developed a Safe Recipe Style Guide that addresses the four most common food safety problem areas in home kitchens. This style guide provides easy edits to any recipe to improve food safety practices. Adapt these and other food safety instructions, when appropriate, into the recipe headnote or instructions. See Foodsafety.gov for additional tips and guidance on food safety.

SAFE RECIPE STYLE GUIDE

The Partnership for Food Safety Education developed this abbreviated *Safe Recipe Style Guide* that addresses the four most common food safety problem areas in home kitchens. The recipe instructions provided here are meant to be adapted to recipes, as appropriate and needed.

🌡️	**Temperature**	Cook until the internal temperature reaches [*insert correct temperature*] on a food thermometer.
🧼	**Handwashing**	Wash hands with soap and water. [*Include this at the beginning of the recipe and after each time the cook must touch raw meats, poultry, seafood, or eggs.*]
⇄	**Cross-contamination**	Wash the [*insert cutting board, counter, utensil, or serving plate*] with hot, soapy water after it touches raw meats, poultry, seafood, or eggs. Do not reuse marinades used on raw foods. Do not rinse raw poultry or meat.
🚰	**Produce**	Gently rub produce under cold running water. Scrub firm produce with a clean vegetable brush under running water.

GENERAL FOOD SAFETY TIPS AND EXAMPLES OF RECIPE INSTRUCTIONS

CLEAN: wash hands and surfaces

- Wash hands with warm water and soap for at least 20 seconds before and after handling food.
- Wash cutting boards, dishes, utensils, and counters with hot, soapy water after preparing each food item and before continuing to the next step.
- Rinse or scrub fresh fruits and vegetables under cool running tap water, even if they are to be peeled.

Examples of recipe food safety instructions:

- Wash your hands well, then chop the herbs.
- Wash the cutting board and your hands after skewering the chicken pieces onto the bamboo sticks.
- To clean lettuce, fill a large bowl or a clean sink with cool water. Add the lettuce pieces and swish them around to loosen and remove the dirt. Wait about 10 minutes. The dirt will settle to the bottom of the bowl or sink. Remove the lettuce from the water and gently dry using paper towels.
- Scrub potatoes, using a vegetable brush, under running water to remove any dirt.

SEPARATE: don't cross-contaminate

- Keep raw meat, poultry, seafood, and eggs separate from other ready-to-eat foods in the refrigerator.
- Use one cutting board for fresh produce and a separate one for raw meat, poultry, and seafood.
- Do not rinse raw meat or poultry, since washing can spread germs as juices may splash onto sink or counter.
- Never place cooked food on a plate that previously held raw meat, poultry, seafood, or eggs.

Examples of recipe food safety instructions:

- Add chicken to marinade. (Raw chicken should not be rinsed, as doing so can spread bacteria in the sink and surrounding surfaces.)
- Transfer the grilled chicken to a clean plate. (Remember, a plate that once held raw meat may contain bacteria and can spread to cooked meat.)
- Remove the meat from the bag and discard the marinade. (If using the marinade for basting or as a sauce, either reserve half of it before pouring it over the raw meat or make extra by doubling the recipe.)

COOK to a safe internal temperature

- Cook beef roasts and steaks to a minimum internal temperature of 145° F.* All poultry should reach a minimum internal temperature of 165° F measured with a food thermometer.
- When meat is ground up, bacteria can spread. Cook ground meats to at least 160° F, and remember, color is not a reliable indicator of doneness. Use a food thermometer to check the internal temperature of burgers.
- Cook fish to a minimum internal temperature of 145° F or until the flesh is opaque and separates easily with a fork.

Examples of recipe food safety instructions:

- Roast turkey until thermometer inserted in the meaty part of the thigh reads 165° F, about 3 hours.
- Grill burgers until the internal temperature is at least 160° F. Checking the color of the juices or the interior is not a reliable way to determine doneness.

CHILL: refrigerate promptly

- Use the 2-hour rule: Refrigerate or freeze perishable foods within 2 hours after cooking or buying them from the store. (When the temperature exceeds 90° F, the window of safety shrinks to 1 hour.)
- There are only three safe ways to defrost frozen food: in the refrigerator, in cold water, or in the microwave. Food thawed in cold water or in the microwave should be cooked immediately.
- Always store foods that are marinating in the refrigerator.
- If there are large amounts of leftovers, divide them among a series of shallow containers for quicker cooling in the refrigerator.

Examples of recipe food safety instructions:

- Defrost frozen chicken pieces in refrigerator overnight.
- Place the meat and marinade in an airtight container and store in the refrigerator for 4 to 6 hours, until ready to grill.
- To cool the soup down faster, divide it among several clean, shallow containers and stir occasionally. Once it has fully cooled, cover and refrigerate for up to 4 days.

Tips adapted from Foodsafety.gov.

* Note that professional chefs often use different internal temperatures for cooking beef and lamb (roasts, steaks, chops); see page 215.

Appendix: Understanding Meat Cuts for Recipe Development

The availability of many different cuts of meat can be confusing for the home cook, not to mention for recipe developers. To ensure that recipes with meat are written with clarity, recipe developers should be familiar with the parts of an animal and the terms used to describe retail cuts. When an animal is butchered, it is broken down into large sections called "primal cuts" (e.g., loin). These sections are broken down into smaller "subprimal cuts" (e.g., whole beef tenderloin). The subprimal cuts are then cut into individual steaks, roasts, chops, and other retail cuts (e.g., tenderloin steak). However, this isn't always straightforward when looking at the retail cut name on a package of meat. For example, the shoulder area primal cut of beef (chuck) has a subprimal cut (blade) that is further cut into retail cuts that may be labeled as flat iron, top blade, top blade filet, or shoulder top blade steak.

When using a specific cut of meat in a recipe, it's important to understand the characteristics of the primal (or section of the animal) where a cut comes from so the correct cooking method can be used. Retail cuts from the same primal cut generally share similar traits so the recommended cooking methods will often be the same. For example, a porterhouse or New York strip steak from the loin can be cooked with direct dry heat such as pan searing, roasting, broiling, and grilling. Being familiar with the general parts and cuts for one animal also makes it easier to apply that knowledge to other animals, such as lamb or bison.

BEEF RETAIL CUTS

Chuck
Beef stew
Top blade/flat iron steak
Chuck roast/chuck eye/pot roast
Blade roast
Arm roast
Denver steak
Short ribs
Ground chuck

Rib
Short rib
Prime rib (bone-in)
Rib roast (boneless)
Ribeye/Delmonico/cowboy steak
Beef back rib (not much meat)

Short loin
Top loin steak, boneless
Porterhouse steak
T-bone steak
New York strip steak
Beef tenderloin: tenderloin roast/Chateaubriand
Beef tenderloin: filet mignon steaks/tournedos
Club steak/wing steak

Sirloin
Top sirloin steak
London broil
Ground sirloin

Bottom sirloin
Tri tip roast/
    triangle roast
Bavette steak

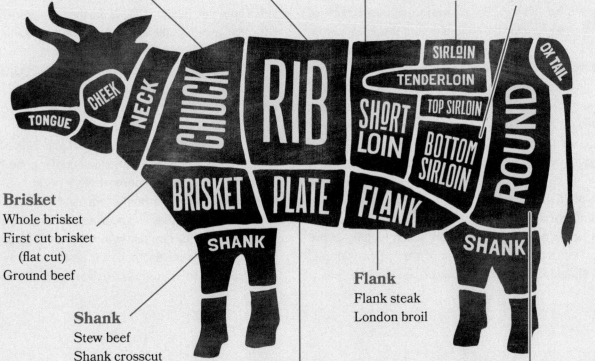

Brisket
Whole brisket
First cut brisket
    (flat cut)
Ground beef

Shank
Stew beef
Shank crosscut

Plate
Skirt steak/fajita meat
Hanger steak
Ground beef

Flank
Flank steak
London broil

Round
Round steak
Top round roast
Bottom round/
    boneless rump roast
London broil
Eye of round
Ground round

COOKING METHODS FOR BEEF CUTS

Primal	Subprimal	Common retail cut names *(meat may be labeled differently based on geographic region)*	Cooking method *Moist heat: braising, stewing* *Dry heat: roasting, broiling, grilling*
Chuck	Neck Blade Shoulder clod Chuck roll	Beef stew Top blade/flat iron steak Chuck roast/chuck eye roast/pot roast Blade bone pot roast (7 bone) Arm roast Denver steak Country style ribs Short ribs[a] Ground chuck	Moist heat Dry heat: • Flat iron steak (collagen removed from top blade muscles and portioned into steaks) • Ground chuck used to make burgers
Rib	Short rib Seven-bone rib	Short rib[a] Prime rib Ribeye steak/Delmonico steak/cowboy steak Beef back ribs (not a lot of meat)	Moist heat Dry heat
Loin[b]	Short loin	Porterhouse steak T-bone steak New York strip steak/strip steak, bone-in or boneless Filet/filet mignon steak/Chateaubriand Club steak/wing steak	Dry heat
Sirloin[b]	Sirloin butt Top sirloin Bottom sirloin	Top sirloin steak Tri tip roast Bavette steak London broil[c] Ground sirloin	Dry heat
Round[b]	Inside round Outside round	Round steak (tenderize first) Top round roast Bottom round/rump roast (for roast beef) London broil[c] Eye of round (least tender; best for jerky) Ground round	Dry heat
Shank (foreshank, hind shank)	No further breakdown	Stew beef Crosscut beef shank (common cut for osso buco)[d]	Moist heat
Brisket	Brisket point Brisket plate	Whole brisket (to make corned beef) First cut brisket (flat cut) Ground beef (can be mixed in with other ground beef cuts, such as chuck and short rib)	Moist heat Dry heat for ground beef for burgers
Plate		Skirt steak/fajita meat Hanger steak Ground beef	Dry heat
Flank[b]		Flank steak London broil	Moist or dry heat

[a] Short ribs can come from either the chuck, the rib, or the plate; the best comes from the rib.

[b] Leaner cuts typically come from these primal cuts.

[c] London broil is a thick, lean piece of meat, rather than a specific cut. Most often it's from the bottom or top round, the cap of the top of the sirloin, or the tri tip; sometimes it comes from the flank.

[d] Osso buco traditionally uses a shank of veal (baby calf).

Loin

Pork tenderloin
Center cut pork loin roast or chop
Porterhouse pork chop
Pork rib roast or chop
Pork sirloin roast or chop
Boneless pork loin
Butterfly pork chops/America's chop
Schnitzel
Country-style ribs
Baby back ribs
Pork back ribs
Canadian bacon
Leaf lard (around kidneys)

Leg

Ham steak
Fresh ham
Ham (cured and smoked)
Prosciutto (Italian)
Serrano or Ibérico ham (Spanish)
Hock/shank

Fatback

Key ingredient in sausages,
    pâté, salami, and mortadella
Salt pork, salted and cured

FATBACK

SHOULDER: BLADE

LOIN

NECK

HEAD

SHOULDER: ARM

SIDE (BELLY)

LEG (HAM)

HOCK

HOCK

Blade

Pork shoulder blade steak
Pork shoulder blade roast
Pork butt, Boston butt,
    Boston shoulder
Pork blade chops

Arm

Picnic roast or picnic shoulder
Picnic ham
Shoulder arm steak/arm roast
Sausage and deli meats
Ground pork

Side

Spareribs
St Louis ribs
Bacon, cured
Pancetta
Pork belly, fresh
Lard

COOKING METHODS FOR PORK CUTS

Primal	Subprimal	Common retail cut names *(fresh, cured, or smoked)*	Cooking methods *Moist heat: braising, stewing* *Dry heat: roasting, broiling, grilling*
Shoulder	Shoulder blade (butt)	Pork shoulder blade steak Pork shoulder blade roast, boneless or bone-in Pork butt, Boston butt, pork shoulder (e.g., for pulled pork or carnitas) Pork blade chops	Dry heat or moist heat
	Shoulder arm (picnic)	Picnic roast or picnic shoulder Picnic ham Shoulder arm steak/arm roast Sausage and deli meats (such as capocollo) Ground pork	
Loin		Pork tenderloin Center cut pork loin roast or chop Porterhouse pork chop Pork rib roast or chop Pork sirloin roast or chop Boneless pork loin Butterfly pork chops/America's chop Pork cutlets Schnitzel[a] (pork chops or steaks pounded thin) Country-style ribs Baby back ribs Pork back ribs Canadian bacon (cured boneless pork loin) Leaf lard	Dry heat

Leg		Fresh ham
		Hock/shank (cured and smoked)
		Ham steak (cooked and smoked)
		Ham (cured and smoked)
		Prosciutto (Italian) and Serrano and
		   Ibérico (Spanish) ham: uncooked, salt-cured,
		   and aged
			Dry heat

Fatback		Key ingredient in sausages, pâté, salami, and mortadella Salt pork, salted and cured	
Side (belly)		Spareribs St Louis ribs Pork belly, fresh Bacon, smoke-cured pork belly Pancetta, seasoned, salt-cured (not smoked) pork belly Lard	Dry heat

[a] Veal cutlets are often used to make schnitzel.

Acknowledgments

I could not have written this book without the wisdom, experience, and support of other professionals, all of whom I want to acknowledge. Your contributions, generosity of time, and help in making me feel not so alone in what can be the isolating task of writing is greatly appreciated. And to all of the chapter reviewers who provided constructive criticism, added suggestions for improvements on content, and helped ensure that each chapter includes professional best practices, you have my sincere thanks. Each of you (listed on pages 388 and 389) are true subject matter experts: clinical dietitians, private practice dietitians, food service chefs, test kitchen directors, recipe developers, recipe testers, culinary school chef instructors, food writers, cookbook authors, food editors, food stylists, food photographers, and videographers. I appreciate your wisdom and suggestions to make this book even better. My gratitude and a heartfelt thank-you go to these reviewers particularly, for going over and above:

Rick Rodgers, Michael Sutz, Lisa Cherkasky, Renée Comet, Wendy Hess, Mark Boughton, Mary Valentin, and Cindie Flannigan

To the professionals who contributed recipes, your recipes are not only well-written but also, they work! Thank you for allowing me to feature them.

To those whom I interviewed for this book, I appreciate you answering my endless and nuanced questions. Your Quick Tips are insightful and practical. It was a pleasure to geek out on the seemingly simple but quite complex and, at times, controversial topic of recipes. I already knew this, but writing this book officially confirmed that food professionals carry around a lot of expertise in their heads. This book includes the wisdom and expertise from so many of you who shared your expertise and real-life experiences as a chef, food photographer, food stylist, food editor, food writer, cookbook author, or marketing professional:

Ken Albala, Robin Asbell, Mary Ashkar, Andrew Batten, Bonnie Benwick, Rose Levy Beranbaum, Sarah Billingsley, Lynn Blanchard, Rob Bleifer, Linda Brewer, JeanMarie Brownson, Frances Bucien, Joy Butler, Lisa Cherkasky, Renée Comet, Kathryn Conrad, Richard Coppedge, Steve Dolinsky, Andrew Dornenburg, Chris Eakin, Kara Elder, Shelley Feist, Cynthia S. Ferron, Cindie Flannigan, Suzanne Florek, Huge Galdones, Christine Gallary, Darra Goldstein, Michael Grady, Mark Graham, Lisa Gross, Jill Haas, Carol Haddix, Mary-Frances Heck, Laura Heineman, Denise Herrera, Sandra Holl, Catherine Huchting, Dianne Jacob, Jauveneeka Jacobs, Chris Koetke, Dean J. Lavornia, Evie Lieb, Cindie Little, Leigh Loftus, Nancy Macklin, Rosemary Mark, Jeff Martin, Don McCormick, Alice Medrich, Jill Melton, Kiano Moju, Joan Nathan, Kara Neilson, Susan Parenti, Kathryn Pauline, Victor Penev, Todd Pierson, Ann Taylor Pittman, Donna Pierce, Jonathan Poyourow, Chandra Ram, Deri Reed, Peter Reinhart, Rick Rodgers, Dan Sachs, Adam Salomone, Leda Scheintaub, Joanie Simon, Mary Margaret Sinnema, Diane Sokolofski, Zach Steen, Allison Stout,

Michael Sutz, Kathy Takemura, Mary Valentin, Denise Vivaldo, Hava Volterra, Stephanie A. Wilkins, Dédé Wilson, Allan Windhausen, and Daniel Zadoff

And special thanks to the many nutrition professionals who shared their knowledge of food and health with me throughout the writing process:

Laura Ali, Diane Abrams, Jane Andrews, Catherine Barry, Dawn Jackson Blatner, Kirby Branciforte, Andrea Canada, Maria Caranfa, Jo Ann Carson, Patsy Catsos, Amy Cifelli, Erin Coffield, Patty Coleman, Natalie Cooke, Andrea Custer, Sanna Delmonico, Cheryl Dolven, Meghan Donnelly, Karen Drummond, Karen Duester, Roberta Duyff, David Grotto, Sara Haas, Sovanny Hartnett, Janet Helm, Sarah Hendren, Mindy Hermann, Mary Abbott Hess, Wendy Hess, Rachel Huber, Amy Keller, Breana Killeen, Marlene Koch, Jaclyn Konich, Ellie Krieger, Joanne Larsen, Emily Latchtrupp, Stephanie Lichtman, Nancy Macklin, Marlee Marrotta, Ashley Martinez, Marisa Moore, Jane Muir, Marion Nestle, Lydia Nader, Kerry Neville, Jackie Newgent, Nikki Nies, Jill Nussinow, Carolyn O'Neil, Sharon Palmer, Rachel Paul, Cathy Powers, Jessie Price, Krishnendu Ray, Michele Redmond, Krystal Register, Shemera Robinson, Kate Scarlata, Dianne Sutherland, Pat Tanumihadja, Bonnie Taub-Dix, Marissa Thiry, Tricia Thompson, Kelly Toups, Alissa Triplett, Kelly Vaccaro, Alisa Via-Reque, Hope Warshaw, Ali Webster, Jill Weisenberger, Margie Woch, and Lindsey Yeakle

To my editor at the Academy of Nutrition and Dietetics, Betsy Hornick, I give a special thank you. You worked tirelessly with me at every stage of the book process, from development to publication. At times the book topics seemed unwieldy, especially with my tendency to go down a rabbit hole on the smallest but always interesting detail. You were right there, pulling me out and keeping me on track. You gave me the freedom to focus on the nitty gritty while offering a firm and knowledgeable hand in moving the book forward.

Many thanks to Morgan Krehbiel and Erin Fagan Faley, for your editorial and design guidance; Perrin Akins Davis, for your copyediting; Deri Reed, for recipe editing; and Susan Roberts McWilliams for proofreading. And thank you to my two sisters, Frances Sutz, a gifted writer and incredible cook who gave invaluable chapter feedback and edits on my introduction; and Debra Baker, nurse extraordinaire, who asked me daily, "So how's your book going?" and never tired of hearing about it.

Lastly, thank you to my husband, Rob, and three kids, Aidan, Michael, and Elaine, for your love and support, without whom I would never have learned the real-life skills of cooking. A special recognition to Michael and Elaine, who were diagnosed with celiac disease in their teens. Their condition enabled me to deepen my empathy for individuals forced to make permanent changes to their diets and the grief and difficulty that can follow. While pasta and all-purpose flour were once staples in my kitchen, I took on how to use gluten-free substitutes and gluten-free flours in cooking and baking. The discoveries were endless. And that really sums up what I love about food, nutrition, and cooking: there is always more to learn, and share. Thank you to everyone who shared so much with me.

Reviewers

Laura M. Ali, MS, RDN, LDN
Nutrition Consultant and Freelance Writer
Pittsburgh, PA

Julie Andrews, MS, RDN, CD, FAND
Cookbook Author, Chef, Food Photographer
The Gourmet RD, LLC
Grand Rapids, MI

Jennifer Armentrout
Former Editor-at-Large
Fine Cooking Magazine
Newtown, CT

Bonnie Benwick
Former Deputy Food Editor
The Washington Post
Washington, DC

Garrett Berdan, RDN
Culinary Nutrition Consultant and Educator
Portland, OR

Mark Boughton
Professional Photographer
Mark Boughton Photography
Nashville, TN

Andrea Custer, MS, RDN
Mérieux NutriSciences
Chicago, IL

Dawn Jackson Blatner, RDN
Nutrition Consultant and Communications Expert
Chicago, IL

Maria Caranfa, RDN, LDN
Global Food and Nutrition Strategist
Chicago, IL

Patsy Catsos, MS, RDN
Medical Nutrition Therapist and FODMAP expert
Patsy Catsos Advanced Nutrition, LLC
New London, NH

Lisa Cherkasky
Professional Food Stylist and Writer
Arlington, VA

Renée Comet
Professional Food Photographer
Renée Comet Photography
Washington, DC

Kristy Del Coro, MS, RDN
Culinary Nutritionist and Co-Founder of the
Culinary Nutrition Collaborative
North Yarmouth, ME

Sanna Delmonico, MS, RDN
Associate Professor
Culinary Institute of America
Saint Helena, CA

Cheryl Dolven, MS, RDN
Corporate Dietitian
Orlando, FL

Meghan Donnelly, MS, RDN, CDN
Senior Manager of Nutrition Services
Dr. Schär
New York, NY

Cindie Flannigan
Professional Food Stylist, Recipe Developer
C.L. Flannigan, Inc.
Venice, CA

Huge Galdones
Professional Food Photographer
Galdones Photography, LLC
Chicago, IL

Carol Mighton Haddix
Former Food Editor
Chicago Tribune
Chicago, IL

Sarah Hendren, MS, RDN, LD, CD
Regulatory Affairs Scientist
Frito Lay North America
Irving, TX

Wendy Hess, MS, RD
Owner, Consulting in Nutrition Analysis
Burlington, VT

Ellie Krieger, MS, RDN
Food Network and PBS Host, Author, Columnist
New York, NY

Trinh Le, MPH, RD
Food Writer
Berkeley, CA

Nancy Macklin, MS, RDN
Food, Nutrition, and Test Kitchen Professional
Dallas County, IA

Rosemary Mark
Culinary Consultant, Recipe Developer, Test Kitchen Professional
Walnut Creek, CA

Jeff Martin
Professional Food Stylist, Founder of Food Photo Affair,
Food Photographer and Stylist Conference
Covington, KY

Marisa Moore, MBA, RDN, LD
Registered Dietitian Nutritionist
Marisa Moore Nutrition, LLC
Atlanta, GA

Jackie Newgent, RDN, CDN
Plant-Based Culinary Nutritionist, Recipe Developer, Food Writer
Brooklyn, NY

Nikki Nies, MS, RD
Nutrition Associate Manager
Aramark
Dallas, TX

Sharon Palmer, MSFS, RDN
Writer, Editor, Blogger, Plant-Based Food and Nutrition Expert
Ojai, CA

Todd Pierson
Professional Photographer and Video Producer
Pierson Studios
Oswego, IL

Catharine Powers, MS, RDN, LD
Partner, Culinary Nutrition Publishing LLC
Akron, OH

Michele Redmond, MS, RDN, FAND
Dietitian Chef and Food Enjoyment Activist
The Taste Workshop
Scottsdale, AZ

Rick Rodgers
Cookbook Author, Recipe Developer
West Orange, NJ

Michael Sutz
Filmmaker and Video Producer
Twelve Plus Media
Saint Paul, MN

Marissa Thiry, MS, RD
Senior Associate Manager, Global Nutrition and Sustainability
Taco Bell Corp
Irvine, CA

Tricia Thompson, MS, RD
Founder, Gluten Free Watchdog, LLC
Manchester, MA

Mary Valentin
Professional Food Stylist and Educator
Mary Valentin Food Stylist, LTD
Chicago, IL

Alisa Via-Reque, MS, RD, LD
Registered Dietitian, Eat Fit Dallas
Coppell, TX

Denise Vivaldo
Professional Food Stylist
President, Denise Vivaldo Group
Oxnard, CA

Dédé Wilson
Co-author of *The Low-FODMAP Diet Step by Step*
Former *Bon Appétit* contributing editor
Co-Founder and Editor-in-Chief of FODMAP Everyday
Amherst, MA

Taylor Wolfram, MS, RDN, LDN
Owner of Taylor Wolfram LLC
Chicago, IL

About the Author

Raeanne Sarazen is a registered dietitian and chef who specializes in food writing and recipe development. She is known for translating complex nutrition recommendations into recipes for people with diet-related health conditions and simplifying the complicated recipes of professional chefs for the home cook. Her philosophy is that food is more than just sustenance—it is a source of healing and joy.

Raeanne has more than two decades of food industry experience. She has worked in hospitals as a clinical dietitian, at the *Chicago Tribune* as test kitchen director and assistant food editor, and in restaurant kitchens, including Charlie Trotter's. Raeanne has written articles, developed recipes, and produced videos for the *Chicago Tribune*, *The Wall Street Journal*, *Cooking Light*, *Better Homes and Gardens*, and national food companies.

Raeanne completed her professional cooking studies at Le Cordon Bleu. She received her Bachelor of Science in Nutrition and Medical Dietetics from the University of Illinois, and a Master of Arts in New Media Studies from DePaul University. She is a Distinguished Fellow of the Academy of Nutrition and Dietetics and a founding member of the Academy of Nutrition and Dietetics Food and Culinary Professionals dietetic practice group.

A mother of three, Raeanne lives in Chicago with her husband Rob. Her greatest joys are hiking and traveling the world with her family and learning about local foods and culture.

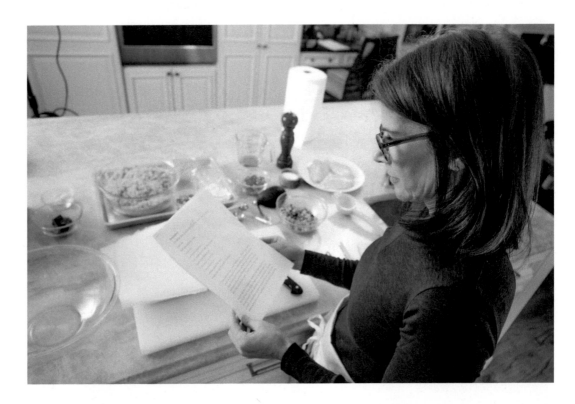

Continuing Professional Education

This edition of *The Complete Recipe Writer's Guide* offers readers 7 hours of Continuing Professional Education (CPE) credit expiring December 31, 2025. Readers may earn credit by completing the interactive online quiz at:

https://publications.webauthor.com/complete_recipe_writing_guide

Index

sugar(s): added, data, 269*b*; alternatives to granulated, in recipes, 114–116; culinary functions of, 113*b*; functional role of, 46; healthy-sounding, 115*b*; high FODMAP ingredient substitutions, 177*b*; nutritional comparison of added, 116*b*; reducing, in recipes, 111–116; reducing added, in traditional holiday dish, 118*b*; tips for reducing, in baking, 113; tips for reducing, in savory recipes, 111; types of carbohydrates in food, 112*b*

sugar alcohols, 120*b*

sugar substitute(s), 122–123*b*; recipe development with, 119; reducing carbohydrates and added sugars, 121*b*; tips for using, in recipes, 120

sulfite sensitivity, 148; developing recipes for people with, 148

superfoods, term, 37

sustainability: resources related to, 39; term, 38

sustainable, term, 43

Sutz, Michael, 320, 337

sweeteners: high FODMAP ingredient substitutions, 177*b*; volumes and weights, 357*t*

T

Takemura, Kathy, 304

target audience: demographics, 8; lifestyle and behavioral characteristics, 8; recipe, 7–8; recipe considerations, 9*b*

taste, 5*b*; aroma, 4; developing your palate, 3–5; experience, 5; mouthfeel, 4; recipe testing, 234; sensations, 4*b*

Taub-Dix, Bonnie, 340

teff, 75*b*, 78*b*

teleprompter, videos, 340

tempeh, plant-based meat substitute, 71

Tempeh Mock Chicken Salad (recipe), 72*b*

testing. *See* recipe testing

tethering tools, photography, 318–319

thermometers, recipe testing, 229*b*

Thiry, Marissa, 289

Thomas, Ashley, 104

Thompson, Tricia, 155

3-R's, sustainability, 38

TikTok, 334, 341*b*, 342, 344*b*

timing, recipe testing, 233–234

title(s): categories and examples, 185*b*; grammar, 185*b*; recipe writing and editing, 184–185

tofu: plant-based meat substitute, 71–72; substitution for heavy cream, 145*b*

tolerance testing, recipe testing, 236

trans fats, 94*b*

tree nut allergy, 130; developing recipes for people with, 130; substitutions, 130*b*

turbinado sugar, alternative to granulated sugar, 116

U

umami ingredients, 108*b*

undercooked food, 213

University of the Pacific, 15

U.S. Copyright Act, 327*b*

US Copyright Office, 20

US Department of Agriculture (USDA), 31, 128*b*; Certified Organic, 148; Food and Nutrient Database for Dietary Studies (FNDDS), 284; FoodData Central, 174, 251, 280, 286; Global Branded Food Products Database, 284; MyPlate, 29; National Nutrient Database for Standard Reference Legacy Release (SR Legacy), 284; resources, 294

US Food and Drug Administration (FDA), 189*b*, 246; food allergen labeling laws, 127, 128*b*; labeling compliance standards (80–20 rule), 289–290; natural sugars, 115*b*; Nutrition Labeling and Education Act (NLEA), 291*b*; reporting nutrition information, 289–290

US Food Safety and Inspection Service (FSIS), 214

V

Valentin, Mary, 299, 300, 310

vegetable oils, 94*b*

vegetables: carbohydrates in food, 112*b*; in common plant-based foods, 87*t*; descriptions of ingredient amounts, 194; dietary fiber in common plant-based foods, 87*t*; high FODMAP ingredient substitutions, 176*b*; modifying the amount or type of fat in recipes, 95*b*; as plant-based alternative to meat, 80*b*; recipe testing, 232; styling tips, 312; tips for, in recipe development, 63–64; triggering foods,

148*b*; volumes and weights, 351–352*t*

vegetarian diets, types of, 63

vegetarian/vegan, resources, 23

vertical farm, term, 43

vertical images, 325*b*

Via-Reque, Alisa, 269, 281

vine- or tree-ripened, term, 43

visual, recipe testing, 235

visual experience, 5

Vivaldo, Denise, 304, 305

volume, measurement, 197

W

Warshaw, Hope, 120

website plug-ins, recipe, 220*b*, 249

weight, measurement, 197

Welstead, Lori, 159

wheat: gluten, 153*b*; whole options, 75*b*

wheat allergy, 134–135; developing recipes for people with, 135; substitutions, 135*b*

wheat berries, 79*b*

wheat flour: functional role of, 46; types of and uses for, 81*b*

whole food, term, 43

whole grain food, identifying, 76

whole grains: baking with, 81–82; longer-cooking, 79*b*; options for recipe development, 75*b*; quick-cooking, 78*b*; in recipe development, 75–76; storing flours of, 80*b*; tips for use in baking, 82; tips for using in savory recipes, 77

Whole Grains Council, 75–76

wild rice, 75*b*

Wilson, Dédé, 175, 179*b*

wireless monitoring system, 340

wireless video remote, 340

Wolfert, Paula, 5

WordPress, 220; recipe website plug-ins for, 288*b*

workflow, editing video, 342

working recipe, testing, 226

worksheet, taste panel, 235*b*

writing recipes. *See* recipe writing and editing

X

xanthan gum, gluten-free baking, 167*b*

Y

yeast ingredients, gluten in, 157*b*

yield: evaluating recipe, 264; percentage, 259; recipe testing, 234; recipe writing, 188–189

Z

zoom feature, 325